CONCEPTUAL MODELS
FOR NURSING PRACTICE

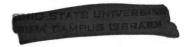

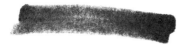

CONCEPTUAL MODELS FOR NURSING PRACTICE
SECOND EDITION

Joan P. Riehl, R.N., M.S., Ph.D

Adjunct Professor, School of Nursing
University of California at Los Angeles
Los Angeles, California

Sister Callista Roy, R.N., M.S., Ph.D

Chairperson, School of Nursing
Mount St. Mary's College
Los Angeles, California

APPLETON-CENTURY-CROFTS/New York

80 81 82 83 84 / 10 9 8 7 6 5 4 3 2 1

Prentice-Hall International, Inc., London
Prentice-Hall of Australia, Pty. Ltd., Sydney
Prentice-Hall of India Private Limited, New Delhi
Prentice-Hall of Japan, Inc., Tokyo
Prentice-Hall of Southeast Asia (Pte.) Ltd., Singapore
Whitehall Books Ltd., Wellington, New Zealand

Library of Congress Cataloging in Publication Data

Riehl, Joan P.
    Conceptual models for nursing practice.

    Includes bibliographies and index.
    1. Nursing—Philosophy. I. Riehl, Joan P.
II. Roy, Callista. III. Title.
RT84.5.R53   1980   610.73'01   79-28305
ISBN 0-8385-1200-3

Text design: Deborah Payne
Cover design: Susan Rich

To our contributors,
whose willingness to share their lives with others
has helped to make this work possible

*Experience without theory is blind
but theory without experience is mere intellectual play*

KANT

Contents

Contributors

Donna Aamodt, R.N., M.S.
Assistant Professor, Department of Nursing, Union College, Denver, Colorado

June Abbey, R.N., Ph.D., FAAN
Professor and Director, Physiological Nursing Program, College of Nursing, University of Utah, Salt Lake City, Utah

Brenda Beitler, R.N., M.S.
Instructor, Department of Nursing, Union College, Lincoln, Nebraska

Mary C. Blake, R.N., B.S.
Instructor, Nursing, Portland Community College, Portland, Oregon

Pamela J. Brink, R.N., Ph.D., FAAN
Associate Professor of Nursing and Anthropology, School of Nursing, University of California, Los Angeles, California

Joan M. Caley, R.N., B.S.N.
Nursing Supervisor, Veterans Administration Medical Center, Vancouver, Washington

Robert Chin, Ph.D.
Professor of Psychology, Boston University, Boston, Massachusetts

Marilyn K. Chrisman, R.N., M.N.
Coordinator of Staff Development, Kaweah Delta District Hospital, Visalia, California
Respiratory Clinical Nurse Specialist in private practice and consultant in respiratory care

Leatrice J. Coleman, R.N., M.S.N.
Director of Nursing, Augustana Hospital and Health Care Center, Chicago, Illinois

Ruth B. Craddock, R.N., MSNE
Assistant Professor, School of Nursing, University of Louisville, Louisville, Kentucky
Doctoral Student, School of Nursing, University of Alabama, Birmingham, Alabama

Karla Damus R.N., Ph.D.
Epidmiological Consultant, National Institute for Child Health and Human Development, Bethesda, Maryland

Lucille Davis, R.N., Ph.D.
Director, School of Nursing, Saint Xavier College, Chicago, Illinois

Marilyn J. Dirksen, R.N., B.S.
Supervisor, Community Health Nursing, Multnomah County Division of Direct Health Services, Portland, Oregon

Maryln Engalla, R.N., B.S.N.
Staff Nurse, Providence Medical Center, Portland, Oregon

Marsha D. Fowler, R.N. M.S.
Kennedy Fellow in Medical Ethics, Harvard University, Cambridge, Massachusetts
Respiratory Clinical Nurse Specialist and consultant in respiratory care

Claire G. Glennin, R.N., M.N.
Assistant Chief of Nursing Services, Veterans Administration Medical Center, San Francisco, California

Judy Grubbs, R.N., M.S.N.
President, Ellison, Grubbs and Ellison, Hospital Counseling and Architectural Planning, Los Angeles, California

Mary L. Hennrich, R.N., B.S.
Child/Young Adult Program Manager, Multnomah County Division of Direct Health Services, Portland, Oregon

Bonnie Holaday, R.N., M.N., D.N.Sc.
Associate Professor, School of Nursing, Emory University, Atlanta, Georgia
Clinical Specialist, Emory Perinatal Center, Atlanta, Georgia

Mary Lebold, R.N., M.S.
Associate Professor, School of Nursing, Saint Xavier College, Chicago, Illinois

Betty Neuman, R.N., M.S.
Curriculum Consultant, School of Nursing, and Director of Nursing and Allied Health, Continuing Education, Ohio University, Athens, Ohio

Dorothy Ann Nordal, R.N., B.S.
ADN Nursing Instructor, Chemeketa Community College, Salem, Oregon

Josephine M. Preisner, R.N., M.N.
Mental Health Consultant, Baltimore, Maryland

Martha E. Rogers, Sc.D., FAAN
Professor, Division of Nursing, New York University, New York, New York

Arnold M. Rose (deceased)
Department of Sociology, University of Minnesota, Minneapolis, Minnesota

Alyce Sato, R.N., M.Ed.
Instructor, Department of Nursing, Idaho State University, Pocatello, Idaho

Mary Schmitz, R.N., M.S.
Instructor, Mount St. Mary's College, Los Angeles, California

Beverley M. Small, R.N., M.S.
Instructor, College of Nursing, Texas Woman's University, Dallas, Texas

Marsha K. Stanhope, R.N., M.N.
Doctoral Student, School of Nursing, University of Alabama, Birmingham, Alabama

Suzan L. Starr, R.N., B.S.N.
Staff Nurse, Oncology, Los Angeles New Hospital, Los Angeles, California

Barbara Tkachuck, R.N., M.S.
Instructor, Department of Nursing, Union College, Lincoln, Nebraska

Janet F. Venable, R.N., M.N.
Lecturer, California State University, Los Angeles, California

Marilynn J. Wood R.N., Ph.D.
Chairperson, Division of Nursing, Azusa Pacific College, Azusa, California

Margaret Wyatt, B.S.N., M.A., Ph.D.
Director, School of Nursing, Ohio University, Athens, Ohio

Preface

Since the appearance of the first edition of this book in 1974, nursing has continued to grow as a field of scientific inquiry and in this growth has continued to analyze and utilize conceptual models for practice. This growth, reflected in the survey reported in Chapter 32, is contributing to nursing's evolution into a scientific discipline. The revision of this text attempts to bring up to date in one book much of the current work being done in the development of nursing models. The models presented herein represent a broader philosophical and geographical perspective than did those in the earlier edition. Furthermore, the opening considerations of the meanings of models and theories as well as the concluding remarks about a unified model have resulted from both authors' recent educational and professional experiences.

As in the first edition, the conceptual frameworks in this text are organized into three major types: developmental, system, and interaction. In Part I we discuss theory and models and briefly review the history of nursing models in education, research, and service.

In Part II, Conceptual Frameworks, we again include the basic theory of system, developmental, and interaction models from which most of our nursing models are derived. In Part III, our contributors present the theory of developmental models and illustrate their use in clinical practice. Systems models and interaction models for nursing practice are similarly discussed in Parts IV and V.

Part VI constitutes our final unit. In this section, we present one patient and do a case analysis, utilizing representative models from each of the three major types reviewed in this text. We also present a survey of current models that are taught and implemented in schools of nursing across our nation. Our last chapter is devoted to the discussion of a unified model of nursing.

As in our first edition, we believe this book may be employed in diverse ways by numerous health personnel.

Educators of undergraduate and graduate students in nursing may use the book as a text and as a reference. Similarly, students will utilize the book in courses on the conceptual basis for nursing. Nurse administrators who are interested in improving the quality of patient care will find this text valuable in attaining that goal and in helping them and their staffs to understand and implement models of nursing. Some examples of this appear in Chapters 23 and 27 of this book. To medical and paramedical personnel this text will serve as a communication aid in assisting these health team members to comprehend part of the scope of nursing.

Personally, we found our first edition useful in our work with students as we assisted them to realize the value of models, to grasp nursing's theoretical concepts, and to implement the concepts in clinical nursing practice. This text, which is broader in scope, should prove even more valuable to us, to our students, and to others who have an interest in this field.

We again express our gratitude to our contributors who have submitted papers for this edition and to the publishers who granted permission for the reprinted selections.

J.P.R.
Sr. C.R.

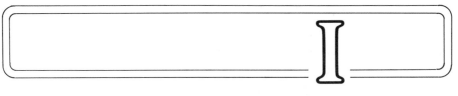

The Nature of
Nursing Models

Nursing is establishing itself as a scientific discipline. Its thrust toward scientifically sound social usefulness includes the development of conceptual models. The nursing model provides the basis for selecting knowledge to be transmitted in nursing education, the framework for nursing practice, and the impetus and direction for nursing research. This text presents some developing nursing models and illustrates their use in nursing practice.

Chapter 1 describes the nature of models and theory and the relationship between the two. Chapter 2 reviews the history of nursing models in education, research, and service. The pursuit of all three of these components of nursing is due, in part, to a statement made at the Nursing Development Conference Group in 1973 which pointed out that the strength of nursing rests in the ability of nurses to tolerate the strain of initiating and keeping preferred nursing systems operational in multiple environments, at the same time deriving satisfaction from their effective actions. Such nursing systems and resulting satisfactions have been developed through research, operationalized in practice, and transmitted through nursing education.

Joan P. Riehl
Sister Callista Roy

1

Theory and Models

Theory development is important to the growth of any discipline; models are constructs related to theory. An understanding of models can be had by comparison of a model with theory. In this chapter we will define and describe the terms *theory* and *model,* and then attempt to relate them.

THEORY

A theory may be defined as a scientifically acceptable general principle which governs practice or is proposed to explain observed facts. Another definition of theory is that it is a logically interconnected set of propositions used to describe, explain, and predict a part of the empirical world. Theories can be constructed in two ways, either deductively or inductively.

In deduction theory construction the method proceeds from a generalization to specific deductions. This type of theory begins with a set of concepts. The purpose of a concept is to point out the phenomenon under consideration. Labels like nurse, patient, and anxiety are concepts or intellectual pointers to the phenomena under consideration. Hage (1972) distinguishes two kinds of theoretical concepts: (1) those that label categories or classes of phenomena, like nurse and patient; and (2) those that label dimensions of phenomena, like degree of anxiety and level of mobility. Hage calls the latter general variables and sees them as more significant for theory development. In speaking of general variables, Stinchcombe (1968) points out that these concepts can have various values and are defined in such a way that one can tell by means of observation which value one has in a particular occurrence.

Deductive theories are not merely conceptual schemes, but rather the concepts, or variables, must be interrelated in the theoretical statements.

Reynolds (1971) describes five different types of theoretical statements: laws, axioms, propositions, hypotheses, and empirical generalizations. Laws are statements of relationships which have enough support to be generally accepted as true. An example would be the second law of thermodynamics. Axioms and propositions are generally used in deductive theories. Axioms are statements which are independent of other statements in the theory and from which all other statements of the theory may be logically derived. The statements that are derived from axioms are called propositions. A hypothesis is a proposition stated in terms that can be measured directly. An empirical generalization is an hypothesis that has been validated. Deductive theories develop concepts by a logical process, relate these in statements, and then deduce other statements from the original statement.

The inductive process of theory construction works from the specifics of empirical situations to generalizations about the data. This approach is perhaps best exemplified in the grounded theory of Glaser and Strauss (1967). These authors prescribe that the researcher immerse himself or herself in the data of the research project and attempt to generate new theoretical insights.

The steps in this inductive process are not unlike the elements of deductive theory. For Glaser and Strauss, the elements of theory are first the conceptual categories and their conceptual properties, then the hypotheses, or generalized relations among the categories, and their properties. The difference is in the process used to derive these elements. In developing grounded theory, initially the researcher enters the field with only a general perspective and a general subject or problem area, not with a preconceived theoretical framework. For example, one might begin with the general notion of a nurse's care of the dying patient. The conceptual categories and their conceptual properties are then indicated by the data. For example, Glaser and Strauss found that two categories of nursing care are the nurse's "professional composure" and the "perceptions of social loss" of a dying patient. One property of the category of social loss is "loss rationales"—that is, the rationales nurses use to justify to themselves their perceptions of social loss.

Once categories and their properties emerge the researcher's observations also lead to the generation of relations among categories, or the steps of hypothesis-making. In the clinical situation these may be a suggestion of a relationship between categories or properties. The accumulating interrelations form an integrated central theoretical framework. For example, two relationships that Glaser and Strauss hypothesize are that the higher the social loss of the dying patient, the greater the tendency of nurses to develop loss rationales to explain away the death and the better the care. This can be generalized to the proposition that the higher the social value of a person, the less delay they experience in receiving services from experts. Thus inductive theory also is a system of concepts and relationships in the form of propositions.

NURSING THEORY

Nursing theory specifically can be defined as a conceptual structure of knowledge useful and necessary to attain the goals established by nurses (Berthold, 1968).

Some nursing theoreticians follow the deductive method and select relevant concepts from other bodies of knowledge such as sociology, psychology, physiology, and business management. They begin with general concepts and use these as parameters for looking at specific nursing situations. Murphy (1971) summarizes the view of deductive theoreticians by stating that "in essence, proponents of this approach suggest that theorizing in nursing is the result of modification, reconceptualization, and synthesis of concepts from other fields of knowledge as they describe and predict nursing practices." Other theoreticians clearly present the inductive approach to theory building in nursing. For example, Wald and Leonard (1964) suggest that the theorists begin with practical nursing experience and develop concepts from their inductive analysis of this experience rather than borrowing concepts that they feel will fit.

The relationship of both inductive and deductive theory to practice is well discussed by Dickoff and James (1968). Their treatment of the topic will be the basis for the following discussion of levels of theory. These authors clearly point out that a theory is neither idle speculation nor a picture-image of reality. Rather, theory is an invention of interrelated concepts, and this invention is to some purpose. As such, the various kinds of theory are grouped into four levels: factor-isolating theories, factor-relating theories (situation-depicting theories), situation-relating theories (predictive theories and promoting or inhibiting theories), and situation-producing theories (prescriptive theories). In this scheme, each higher level of theory presupposes the existence of theories at the lower levels. A situation is depicted in terms of factors already isolated; predictive or promoting theories conceive relationships between depictable situations; and situation-producing theories prescribe in terms of available predictive and promoting theories, and use depicting theories in the characterization of goal content.

First of all, in regard to factor-isolating theories, it should be remembered that all scientific theory begins with the naming of factors. Dickoff and James consider that lack of attention to this level of theory building is detrimental, especially when theory is being self-consciously developed for the first time, as it is in nursing.

Second, after factors are identified, they should be seen in relationships. The first order of relationship is correlation; that is, the joint presence or absence of two factors. Two factors are related by their proximity in the given situation. This relation does not imply causation and does not take into account time sequence—the two factors merely coexist. This level of theory is called situation-depicting in that it does more than give names to isolated factors.

Third, factors must be related in such a way that predictions can be made. Predictions are based upon causal relationships between factors in a situation. Causal relationships must show the dynamic qualities of priority and direction among the factors or variables. Thus, to say that A causes B one must be able to show that A exists before B, and that when A increases, B increases, and when A decreases, B also decreases. Situations may thus be connected causally.

Finally, after a predictive theory is identified, it is possible to move to the highest level of theory building, called situation-producing theory. This level surpasses predictive theory by stating that, not only if A happens then B occurs, but also that A is an appropriate cause of B, and that certain methods will bring about B, or will facilitate A's causation of B.

Dickoff and James suggest that nursing theory should be largely situation-producing theory. The day-to-day practice of nursing is made up of prescriptive elements. Given any one of the hundreds of situations that the nurse faces daily, she must have a prescription for action. This prescription comes from situation-producing theory.

MODEL

A model can be defined as a symbolic depiction in logical terms of an idealized, relatively simple situation showing the structure of the original system (Hazzard and Kergin, 1971). A model, then, is a conceptual representation of reality. It is clearly not the reality itself, but an abstracted and reconstructed form of reality. This can be simply illustrated by examining a toy model of, say, a car. Such a model is not actually a car, but its pieces represent the features of the actual car or even of cars in general. These models are abstractions in that they display the outline or architectural sketch of the genuine article. It is similarly possible for a model to show the features of a discipline and give direction to the cluster of laws that are selected to form a theoretical system.

NURSING MODEL

A conceptual model for nursing practice is a systematically constructed, scientifically based, and logically related set of concepts which identify the essential components of nursing practice together with the theoretical bases for these concepts and the values required in their use by the practitioner (Johnson, 1975). It is a mental image of the realm of nursing—how it is put together and how it works. A nursing model is made up of general ideas and concepts. The parts are related to each other through a cohesive and systematic approach to the patient.

In her discussion of the requirements of an effective conceptual model for nursing, Johnson (1975) states that the assumptions and values upon which the major units of the model are based must be clearly stated. Furthermore, the concepts which are expressed in the major units of the model must be clearly defined and the terms used reducible to observable indices in the general and in the concrete case. There must also be internal consistency between units. Johnson lists the essential units as:

1. A goal of action: the mission or ideal goal of the profession expressed as the end product desired (a state, condition, situation).
2. A descriptive term for patiency: that concept which best isolates who or what is acted upon to achieve the goal of action, i.e., those aspects of the person (as patient) or the organization of his functioning toward which attention is to be directed; the target of action.
3. The actor's role: a descriptive label which indicates the nature of the nurse's (as the actor) actions on patiency.
4. Source of difficulty: the originating point of deviations from the desired state or condition.
5. Intervention focus: the kind of problems found when deviations from the desired state occur; the kinds of disturbances in the patiency which are to be prevented or treated. Mode is the major means of preventing or treating such problems; the kinds of levers which can be used to change the course of events toward the desired end.
6. Consequences intended: the outcomes of action desired stated in more abstract or broader terms than the mission and/or including significant corollaries of the intended outcomes. Unintended outcomes are those which are not intended but which might follow, and which may or may not be desirable.

Those who develop models in nursing will therefore be concerned with the following viewpoints: assumptions, values, goal, patiency, actor's role, source of difficulty, intervention focus and mode, and intended and unintended consequences.

RELATIONSHIP OF MODELS TO THEORY

The term *model* is broader than the term *theory* when applied to nursing. That is, the model is the image of the entire field and includes concepts of all its major units—the goal, patiency, and so forth. On the other hand, theory refers to the lawlike propositions of given phenomena within the model. Thus there may be a theory of the patiency of the model, such as a theory of the person as a behavioral system or an adaptive system. Theories from the pure sciences provide the theoretical basis for the model's view of the patiency. Similarly, there may be theories of nursing practice consisting of the sets of propositions about the problems or interventions which arise out of the intervention focus in relation to the sources of difficulty specified by the model. This relationship can be illustrated by the drawing based on Johnson (1975) shown below.

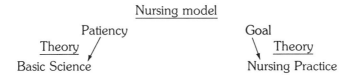

The theory, then, in a sense provides the working insides of the model. The development of models can lead to indications as to where theory is needed. Likewise, the development of theory, for example, a unified theory of the human person, may inspire new models. Both theory and model provide separate conceptions of reality for their own purposes—the theory emphasizing, explaining, and predicting a certain empirical reality, and the model showing the parts of nursing and how they are related so that the nurse can have a cohesive and systematic approach to the patient.

In inquiring into the science of nursing, a number of models of the reality of nursing have been created. Some of these are presented in Parts 3, 4 and 5. The authors of these models, and other interested nurses, continue to examine models to further identify related theory and the working structure of laws which lie behind the model. In service-oriented disciplines the findings of the search become a part of practice. The profession of nursing is a practice-oriented discipline and, as such, its models have been developing over time.

REFERENCES

Berthold JS: Symposium on theory development in nursing. Nurs Res 17:3:196, 1968

Dickoff J, James P: A theory of theories: a position paper. Nurs Res 17:3:197, 1968

Dickoff J, James P, Wiedenbach E: Theory in a practice discipline. Nurs Res 17:5:415, 1968

Glaser B, Strauss A: The Discovery of Grounded Theory. Chicago, Aldine, 1967

Hage J: Techniques and Problems in Theory Construction in Sociology. New York, Wiley, 1972

Hazzard ME, Kergin DJ: An overview of system theory. Nurs Clin North Am 6:3, 1971

Johnson D: Unpublished lecture notes and class handouts: University of California at Los Angeles, Fall, 1975

Murphy J: Theoretical Issues in Professional Nursing. New York, Wiley, 1971

Peplau HE: Interpersonal Relations in Nursing. New York, Putnam's, 1952

Reynolds P. A Primer in Theory Construction. Indianapolis, Bobbs-Merrill, 1971

Rogers ME: An Introduction to the Theoretical Basis of Nursing. Philadelphia, F. A. Davis, 1970

Stinchcombe A: Constructing Social Theories. New York, Harcourt, Brace, 1968

Wald FS, Leonard RC: Towards development of nursing practice theory. Nurs Res 13:4, 1964

Joan P. Riehl
Sister Callista Roy

Nursing Models in Education, Research, and Service

As one reviews the literature, it becomes apparent that conceptual model of nursing have developed over time. The essential elements gaining clarity in these models are (1) the goal of nursing, (2) a concept of the patient, and (3) the mode of nursing intervention. In addition, there is increasing evidence that these models are providing the organized conceptual frameworks that guide nursing education, some nursing research, and nursing service. This chapter provides a brief nursing model history and examines how models influence nursing education, research and service.

NURSING EDUCATION

Nursing curriculums historically evolved from a general notion of nursing in the Nightingale era, through a period of medical model influence, and finally to an era of general use of one of several nursing models which are used to develop curriculums. Only a brief historical review of the events that occurred in the last several decades that seemingly had a direct connection to the evolution of nursing models will be included here.

In the 1940s, nurses' concern for the whole person resulted in the adding of psychosocial studies to the curriculum. This supplemented knowledge of the biologic systems which had previously dominated nursing education. With this change, an emphasis on the interpersonal process in nursing intervention soon emerged. The focus in the 1940s led to the holistic approach in the 1950s in which the patient emerged as a logical focal point of the content presented in nursing schools. This person-centered approach conceptualized the patient as having common human needs, and the goal of nursing was to meet these needs.

By the 1960s, several nursing approaches appeared. In one, the content was organized around the goal of nursing which related to the person. For example, in some schools it was taught that it was the nurse's role to promote the behavioral stability of the patient (Johnson, 1961). In a second approach, nursing was what nurses did. The process of nursing became the content of the curriculum. The student was taught to be a decision maker and analyst (McDonald and Harms, 1966). A third emerging conceptual approach focused on the human developmental process as applied not only to the growing youngster but also to three adult age groups—young adult, middle life, and later years (Smith and Gibbs, 1963). Finally, a patient-oriented concept based upon human needs was also delineated (Abdellah, et al., 1960).

The preceding historical events naturally led to the development of several well delineated nursing models in the 1970s. Smith, Germaine, and Gibbs (1971), for example, identified some specific nursing goals, namely, (1) preventing, modifying, and reducing or removing stressors, (2) supporting adaptive processes utilized by the patient in his attempt to establish a new state of equilibrium, and (3) recognizing that applying stressors is a necessary part of the treatment process and that, in moderation, stress is necessary for life. The models that were developed became widely used in nursing curriculums because the National League for Nursing adopted, in the spring of 1974, accreditation criteria requiring that nursing programs be based upon a conceptual framework.

Certain patterns regarding nursing education have emerged during the mid and late 1970s. Nurse educators have continued with the task of imparting to their students the knowledge and skills necessary to practice nursing. They have fulfilled this charge through the development and implementation of the nursing curriculum. Teaching students about nursing models is an essential part of this. In general, four major aspects of the curriculum are influenced by the model taught in any given school.

Prenursing courses represent one aspect of the planned curriculum. These courses are derived from the nursing model and focus on the model's view of the patiency as their core of knowledge. For example, using Martha Rogers' model (Rogers, 1970) with its emphasis on man/environment/energy interactions, the prenursing courses would have a heavy emphasis on physics. Similarly, using Peplau's developmental nursing model (Peplau, 1952), the prenursing courses focus primarily on personality development and interpersonal relations.

The second major aspect of the curriculum incorporates the objectives of the program, i.e., the behaviors expected of the graduates. For example, Hodgman (1973) described a preventive intervention model and listed the following as a program objective: The student will be able to distinguish between primary, secondary, and tertiary prevention and will specify the terminus of nursing activity for each phase. And, according to Redman's

(1974) article on an adaptation model, an objective is that the student be able to assess the adequacy of the patient's adaptive responses or process in terms of adaptive potential and desirable adaptation.

The third aspect of the curriculum that has been influenced by the selected nursing model is the curriculum design. According to Chater (1975), "A curriculum design must be constructed in order to implement the objectives. Curriculum design is first of all the overall plan or structure of the curriculum, showing the arrangement of the courses and the organization for its operations. Second, curriculum design includes methods and procedures to be used to achieve the objectives." Hodgman (1973) demonstrated this by describing the courses and procedures involved in a curriculum based on a preventive intervention model. The first course focused on primary preventive intervention, and the procedure used was primarily communication techniques, such as role playing. The second course was concerned with secondary prevention and focused on procedures used in the hospital, for example, demonstration and return demonstration. The third course related to tertiary prevention, and the procedure used was to build on the skills of the other two levels and to add the skills of rehabilitation. The fourth and final course emphasized the student's choice. To support these courses, the student concurrently took courses in systems of health care, strategies for change, and introduction to nursing research.

The last phase of curriculum development is the evaluation of the curriculum. The selected conceptual model could also provide guidance for this task. The objective here is to determine if the student is the kind of nurse implied in the nursing model. This could be ascertained by evaluating the performance of the graduate against the terminal objectives, and, of course, the performance of the student at any given level within the educational program.

On another level of academic endeavor, several important meetings on nursing theory were held nationally in the late 1960s. The third of a series of symposiums on nursing theory development was held at the Frances Payne Bolton School of Nursing of Case Western Reserve University in the fall of 1967. The papers presented contributed to a clarification of the current status of theory development in nursing. "A Theory of Theories: A Position Paper" by Dickoff and James (1968) has been used widely as a basis for analysis and development of theoretical models. Two other major nursing theory conferences were held at the University of Kansas in 1969 (Norris, 1969). Current issues concerning the development of nursing were delineated, several models were discussed, and general systems theory was explored. Finally, the Third National Conference on Nursing Diagnoses, held in St. Louis in the spring of 1977 included a work group of nursing theorists who struggled with the problem of establishing a nursing model framework for the development of a taxonomy of nursing diagnoses.

NURSING RESEARCH

The development of nursing models in the history of nursing research involves a much shorter time span than it did in nursing education. It began with the founding of the *Nursing Research* journal in 1952. The categories of research and concerns reported in this journal over a twenty-year period were reviewed by Newman (1972). She noted that studies from 1952 until 1968 relating to the nursing process and human behavior (the patiency of a model) accounted for only about 12 percent of the entries. However, since 1968 the number of such articles had risen to approximately 36 percent. Also in the 1960s, nursing models began to be included in graduate nursing curriculums, where much nursing research was being done. As a result, master's theses and doctoral dissertations began to include nursing models in their theoretical frameworks. Furthermore, in the 1960s and 1970s specific nursing models began to be tested in research designed to validate them. See, for example, Orlando (1961), King (1971), Earle (1969), and Roy (1967, 1977).

According to Murphy (1971) and King (1971) the rapid growth of nursing models in the late 1960s and in the 1970s was based upon a number of factors. Murphy lists the proliferation of new knowledge as a prime motivating force in the search for models and theories to unify existing information. King calls this the vast accumulation of knowledge from research. Murphy lists three influencing factors: recognition of the interrelatedness of knowledge from various disciplines, dissatisfaction with compartmentalized knowledge, and finally, expanding roles, which created the need for new insights. Along the same line, King noted the need to differentiate between professional, technical, and vocational practice by making explicit the scientific foundations. She has offered two other influencing factors: the number of nurses with advanced degrees who ask questions about nursing as a discipline, and the fact that disciplines in higher education are expected to have a theoretical body of knowledge that can be taught.

The research trend is important and will undoubtedly continue for—as Berthold (1968) points out—the ultimate criteria of a theory's usefulness, and hence a model's, are whether it stimulates new observations and insights, and generates predictions of relevant events that are subsequently confirmed.

The research process consists of observing reality according to rules of the scientific method. Four steps are usually involved. In nursing research, the nursing model provides the basis for selecting the aspect of reality to be observed which constitutes the first step in the research process. The model provides the assumptions and values about nursing, the goal of nursing action, and also the focus and means of intervention. Each of these elements, then, can be the subject of scientific exploration. Once the subject is identified and defined, the second step in research is to refine the reality to be observed by the selection of variables. The nursing model conceptualizes the variables that are most important, the mode of intervention, and the consequences of nursing action. As the model points to these variables and their relationships, it becomes a form of what Dickoff and James (1968) refer to as the highest level of theory—situation-producing theory. That is, it is a "conceptualization of the prescription under which an agent or practitioner must act in order to bring about situations of the kind conceived as desirable in the conception of the goal." After the relationship between the variables is specified, the third step in the research process emerges, which is the formulation of the hypothesis. Hypotheses may reflect basic science relationships drawn from the patiency of the nursing model or nursing practice relationships stemming from the goal of nursing.

The final research step consists of testing the hypotheses for validity. In the literature, more and more testable hypotheses are being derived from nursing models. For example, Redman (1974) provides the following two basic science hypotheses based on an adaptation model: (1) The probability of maladaptive processes occurring among subsystems of a living system decreases as the number of parallel modes of functioning or parallel information channels serving it increases; (2) the greater a threat to a living system, the more components of the system are involved in adapting to it. Likewise, Roy (1967) tested a specific nursing practice hypothesis also based on an adaptation model, that is, that the nurse's introduction of role cues to the mother of the hospitalized child will increase the role adequacy of the mother in dealing with her child.

Throughout the total research process, from definition of the problem through confirmation or negation of the hypothesis, the nursing model provides guidance. Selection of subjects is frequently aided by the model's description of the patiency, or recipient of nursing care, and the actor's role in nursing care. After variables are selected, data collection methods are chosen, and these may be further determined by the values implied in the nursing model. For example, methods must not violate the principles of patient welfare or independence that are dictated by the model. Finally, the data that are collected and analyzed either support or refute the hypothesis. Regardless of the outcome, the research invariably identifies other areas that need investigation. In this way, systematic model building in nursing occurs.

NURSING SERVICE

The history of nursing service parallels the growth of nursing models already described in nursing education and research. As in the latter two, there was an early dependence on medicine followed by increasing awareness and explicit development of models for nursing practice.

In the 1950s team nursing was introduced into nursing service. This was an attempt to be patient-centered, not procedure- or task-centered. The holistic view of the patient that had emerged in nursing education in the 1940s was beginning to have its influence on nursing practice. The decade of the 1960s saw the advent of federal legislation, with its emphasis on accountability, which affected nursing service. In response to this demand for accountability, nursing service personnel developed philosophies of patient care and objectives. In these, both the views of the person receiving nursing care and the goal of nursing began to be spelled out. Furthermore, as accreditation standards required the use of nursing care plans, the process of providing care became documented. Inservice education focused on the effective use of these care plans. Also, during the 1960s there was a more widespread use of progressive patient care concepts. Patients were placed into critical, intermediate, and self-care units. As the specific objectives for each type of care were developed, the implicit models of nursing being utilized became more explicit.

With nursing education of the late 1960s and 1970s more firmly rooted in nursing models, the nursing service of the 1970s began to be more consciously influenced by nursing models. This was illustrated by Bowar-Ferres (1975) who described the nursing model in use at the Loeb Center for Nursing Rehabilitation. And others, such as Laros (1977) have also reported on the use of models in practice.

In nursing service there is some evidence of the presence of models in such various aspects as the written philosophy of care, departmental and unit objectives, continuing education activities, and in the standards of practice as a framework for designing outcome criteria. Glennin's article in this text illustrates how the Johnson model, for example, is used in developing standards of practice. It is based upon an assumption about behavioral system balance. One of the data-gathering standards of practice is stated thus: Observes and notes if patients' behavior seems purposeful, orderly, and predictable. In another situation, Laros (1977) showed how the Roy model was used to develop outcome criteria for patients with chronic obstructive pulmonary disease.

When a model is used by an individual, such as a clinical nurse specialist or staff nurse, its most significant function is to provide a diagnostic and treatment orientation for the specific practice of nursing. The model's view of the patiency prescribes what data base is gathered in the patient assessment and the intervention focus dictates what type of patient problems stem from the assessment. Thus, according to the Johnson model, the nurse gathers data about the drive or goal, set, choice, and action for each of the seven behavioral subsystems. The problems identified are insufficiency or discrepancy within a subsystem or incompatibility or dominance involving more than one subsystem. Based on her nursing model, the nurse knows what she is to assess and what specific problems she is capable of diagnosing.

The planning and implementing of care are similarly prescribed by the intervention mode of the model. The intervention mode of the Johnson model is to restrict, defend, inhibit, or facilitate. The nurse then plans and implements care utilizing these modalities.

Lastly, the evaluation phase of the nursing process would be a reassessment of the patient's condition following the nursing intervention. Evaluation would be stated in terms taken from the model's approach to assessment. This methodological approach provides a continuous process that incorporates all elements of the selected model, and it facilitates the nurse's practice.

The use of nursing models in practice can be viewed in broader terms. Models are relevant in examining a number of variables in health care, namely, the setting, the care given, the health-care provider, and the consumer of health-care services. The pertinent factors of each of these is reviewed below.

The Setting

Theoretically, a general, or universal, model can be employed with any group of patients in any setting. A specific framework is used with a particular type of patient and in a given setting. At this point, invariably, a frame of reference vis-à-vis the nurse's model is utilized. In addition to focusing on patients and families, models have also been developed for distributing nursing responsibility and linking nursing care functions between the clinical nurse specialist, the head nurse, and the staff nurse. All of these types of models are discussed and illustrated by the Nursing Development Conference Group (1973). Although the models in this book are oriented toward the specific patient, they are universal enough in concept to be general models. They can thus be used in any setting and by several different levels of personnel.

The Care Given

A special committee appointed by the Secretary of HEW not only identified the setting in which nurses function but also classified their activities. These constituted three groups—primary care, acute care, and long-term care (JAMA, 1972). As nurses assume more responsibility in each of these areas, the scope of their practice will broaden. As this occurs, the problem of role modification becomes prominent and must be resolved. One group has found that such resolution is easier when the patient remains the central focus in the practitioner-patient relationship (Nursing Development Conference Group, 1973). To assure this, it is imperative that nurses use a model to guide them through the nursing process and to direct the channeling of care.

The Health-Care Provider

For effective patient care, several areas of self-knowledge are required. The nurse must know her capabilities and be self-directed; she must identify her own philosophy of nursing; she must have a commitment to the profession; she must select a functional area (education, research, or practice) as well as the type of care that she wants to provide (primary, acute, or long-term). These categories are not inflexible. The nurse may modify them, move from one area to another, and assume more than one role during a given period. For example, a nurse working with a medical group may take histories and conduct physical examinations as a primary care agent, yet perform long-term care functions with medically noncomplex patients as a clinical nurse specialist. In both roles she is viewed in the broad sense as a nurse practitioner—one who provides direct patient care, at least at times. If from practice she moves to teaching or to research, the nurse should persist in using the model she has selected.

The Consumer of Health Care Services

The rights and demands of the health-care consumer must always be considered. In response to consumer need, such new roles as the PNP (pediatric nurse practitioner) and the family nurse practitioner, as well as others, have recently emerged. If this trend continues, services will be expanded to include treatment, rehabilitation, health education, health maintenance, prevention, and early case finding. Nurses who are interested in providing quality and quantity of care in each of these areas are beginning to realize the value and necessity of models. As their responsibility grows and they become more independent, they increasingly require an overall framework as a guideline for health-care decisions.

The nursing model, then, provides the unifying framework for an organized way of looking at nursing. The remainder of this text explores nursing models and their use in nursing practice.

REFERENCES

Abdellah F, Martin A, Beland I, Matheny R: Patient-Centered Approaches to Nursing. New York, Macmillan, 1960

Berthold JS. Symposium on theory development in nursing. Nurs Res 17:3:196, 1968

Bowar-Ferres S: Loeb Center and its philosophy of nursing. Am J Nurs 75:5:810, 1975

Chater S: A conceptual framework for curriculum development. Nurs Outlook 23:428–433, 1975

Dickoff J, James P: A theory of theories; a position paper. Nurs Res 17:3:197, 1968

Earle A: The effect of supplementary post-natal kinesthetic stimulation on the developmental behavior of the normal female newborn. Unpublished doctoral dissertation, New York, University of Nurse Education, 1969

Hodgman E: A conceptual framework to guide nursing curriculum. Nurs Forum 13:2:110–131, 1973

Johnson D: The significance of nursing care. Am J Nurs 61:11, 1961

King I: Toward a Theory for Nursing. New York, Wiley, 1971

Laros J: Deriving outcome criteria from a conceptual model. Nurs Outlook 25:5:33, 1977

McDonald FJ, Harms MT: A theoretical model for an experimental curriculum. Nurs Outlook 14:8:48, 1966

Murphy J: Theoretical Issues in Professional Nursing. New York, Wiley, 1971

Newman M: Nursing's theoretical evolution. Nurs Outlook 20:7:449, 1972

Norris CM: (ed.) Nursing theory conference, 1st Proceedings, Kansas Medical Center, Department of Nursing Education, 1969

Nursing Development Conference Group: Concept Formalization in Nursing. Boston, Little, Brown, 1973

Orlando I: The Dynamics of Nurse-Patient Relationship. New York, Putnam's, 1961

Redman BK: Why develop a conceptual framework? J Nurs Educ 13:240, 1974

Roy C: Role cues and mothers of hospitalized children. Nurs Res 16:2:179–182, 1967

Smith DW, Gibbs CD: Care of the Adult Patient. Philadelphia, Lippincott, 1963

Smith DW, Germaine CPH, Gibbs CD: Care of the Adult Patient, 3rd ed. Philadelphia, Lippincott, 1971

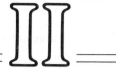

Conceptual Frameworks

Most nursing models are based upon three general types of frameworks: systems, developmental, and interaction. The theoretical concepts for these models are presented in this section in two rather succinct articles, one by Chin and one by Rose. Much has been written on these topics, but these articles were chosen especially for their informative conciseness.

The systems and developmental frameworks are discussed in the article by Chin (1969). He differentiates between analytic and concrete models, defines the key terms and illustrates their relationships, then points out each model's advantages and limitations to the practitioner. In addition, Chin introduces the intersystem model—a concept that has many similarities to interaction theory—and urges its adaptation. Another type of model which Chin proposes characterizes "changing," and incorporates ideas from the systems and developmental models. In comparing these three models, Chin lists the assumptions and approaches to use in regard to content, causation, goal, intervention, and change.

Systems theory has been discussed by many authors. One investigator, Howland (1963), states that there has been an interest in man-machine systems since the beginning of the industrial revolution. In summarizing this development, he reviews the contributions to systems analysis from such broad fields as scientific management, early industrial engineering, operations research, and human engineering. Among the first to write extensively on systems theory was Bertalanffy (1968). His book, *General System Theory*, defines and compares such key terms as the following—equilibrium, homeostasis, steady state, adaptation, adjustment, regulating and control mechanisms, the phenomena of change, differentiation, evolution, entropy and negentropy, models and reality, open and closed systems, the processes of growth, development, creation, and cybernetics. For a comprehensive study of systems theory, Bertalanffy's book is highly recommended. Two other excellent sources are the September, 1971, issue of *Nursing Clinics* and two books by Grinker (1956, 1967). In *Nursing Clinics* systems theory is operationalized in nursing practice, while Grinker and his group met on several occasions to identify what they believed to be a unified theory of human behavior, and discussed systems theory at length. The terms commonly used with this theory were defined in accordance with the group's own professional perspective.

In his summary of interaction theory, Rose (1962) first reviews his major concepts in analytic terms and then in genetic terms— that is, in terms of the socialization process of the child. He limits his comments to the assumptions, definitions, and general propositions that help to make these concepts more understandable. Based on the theory, he derives several assumptions. Then, from these, he deduces a general proposition that applies to human characteristics. In his proposition, Rose attempts to describe and predict human behavior. As nurses proceed in determining the body of knowledge to be included in their profession, they might consider the approach offered by Rose. A model developed by Riehl, in Chapter 28 of this text, is a step in this direction.

In the following sections, the articles selected for inclusion in this edition are representative of the work being done in this field and illustrate how the developmental, system, and interaction models are implemented in nursing practice.

The Utility of System Models and Developmental Models for Practitioners

All practitioners have ways of thinking about and figuring out situations of change. These ways are embodied in the concepts with which they apprehend the dynamics of the client system they are working with, their relationship to it, and their processes of helping with its change. For example, the change agent encounters resistance, defense mechanisms, readiness to change, adaptation, adjustment, maladjustment, integration, disintegration, growth, development, and maturation as well as deterioration. He uses concepts such as these to sort out the processes and mechanisms at work. And necessarily so. No practitioner can carry on thought processes without such concepts; indeed, no observations or diagnoses are ever made on "raw facts," because facts are really observations made within a set of concepts. But lurking behind concepts such as the ones stated above are assumptions about how the parts of the client system fit together and how they change. For instance, "Let things alone, and natural laws (of economics, politics, personality, etc.) will work things out in the long run." "It is only human nature to resist change." "Every organization is always trying to improve its ways of working." Or, in more technical forms, we have assumptions such as: "The adjustment of the personality to its inner forces as well as adaptation to its environment is the sign of a healthy personality." "The coordination and integration of the departments of an organization is the task of the executive." "Conflict is an index of malintegration, or of change." "Inhibiting forces against growth must be removed."

It is clear that each of the above concepts conceals a different assump-

From *The Planning of Change:* Readings in the Applied Behavioral Sciences, edited by Warren G. Bennis, Kenneth D. Benne, and Robert Chin. Copyright © 1961 by Holt, Rinehart and Winston, Inc. Reprinted by permission of Holt, Rinehart and Winston, Inc.

tion about how events achieve stability and change, and how anyone can or cannot help change along. Can we make these assumptions explicit? Yes, we can and we must. The behavioral scientist does exactly this by constructing a simplified *model* of human events and of his tool concepts. By simplifying he can analyze his thoughts and concepts, and see in turn where the congruities and discrepancies occur between these and actual events. He becomes at once the observer, analyzer, and modifier of the system* of concepts he is using.

The purpose of this paper is to present concepts relevant to, and the benefits to be gained from using, a "system" model and a "developmental" model in thinking about human events. These models provide "mind-holds" to the practitioner in his diagnosis. They are, therefore, of practical significance to him. This suggests one essential meaning of the oft-quoted and rarely explained phrase that "nothing is so practical as a good theory." We will try to show how the systems and developmental approaches provide key tools for a diagnosis of persons, groups, organizations, and communities for purposes of change. In doing so, we shall state succinctly the central notions of each model, probably sacrificing some technical elegance and exactness in the process. We shall not overburden the reader with citations of the voluminous set of articles from which this paper is drawn.

We postulate that the same models can be used in diagnosing different sizes of the units of human interactions—the person, the group, the organization, and the community.

One further prefatory word. We need to keep in mind the difference between an analytic model and a model of concrete events or cases. For our purposes, *an analytic model* is a constructed simplification of some part of reality that retains only those features regarded as essential for relating similar processes whenever and wherever they occur. *A concrete model* is based on an analytic model, but uses more of the content of actual cases, though it is still a simplification designed to reveal the essential features of some range of cases. As Hagen† puts it: "An explicitly defined analytic model helps the theorist to recognize what factors are being taken into account and *what relationships among them are assumed* and hence to know the basis of his conclusions. The advantages are ones of both exclusion and inclusion. A model lessens the danger of overlooking the indirect effects of a change of a relationship" (our italics). We mention this distinction since we find a dual usage that has plagued behavioral scientists, for they themselves keep getting their feet entangled. They get mixed up in analyzing "the small group as a system" (analytic) and a school committee as a small group (concrete), or a

---

*"System" used here is any organized and coherent body of knowledge. Later we shall give the term a more specific meaning.

† E. Hagen, chapter on "Theory of Social Change," unpublished manuscript.

national social system (analytic) and the American social system (concrete), or an organizational system (analytic) and the organization of a glue factory (concrete). In this paper, we will move back and forth between the analytic usage of "model" and the "model" of the concrete case, hopefully with awareness of when we are involved in a semantic shift.

THE SYSTEM MODEL

Psychologists, sociologists, and anthropologists, economists, and political scientists have been "discovering" and using the system model. In so doing, they find intimations of an exhilarating "unity" of science because the system models used by biological and physical scientists seem to be exactly similar. Thus, the system model is regarded by some system theorists as universally applicable to physical and social events, and to human relationships in small or large units.

The terms or concepts that are a part of the system model are *boundary, stress* or *tension, equilibrium,* and *feedback.* All these terms are related to open system, closed system, and intersystem models. We shall first define these concepts, illustrate their meaning, and then point out how they can be used by the change agent as aids in observing, analyzing, or diagnosing—and perhaps intervening in—concrete situations.

The Major Terms

System

Laymen sometimes say, "You can't beat the system" (economic or political), or "He is a product of the system" (juvenile delinquent or Soviet citizen). But readers of social science writings will find the term used in a rather more specific way. It is used as an abbreviated term for a longer phrase that the reader is asked to supply. The "economic system" might be read as: "We treat price indices, employment figures, etc., as if they were closely interdependent with each other and we temporarily leave out unusual or external events, such as the discovery of a new gold mine." Or in talking about juvenile delinquency in system terms, the sociologists choose to treat the lower-class values, lack of job opportunities, ragged parental images, as interrelated with each other, in back-and-forth cause-and-effect fashion, as determinants of delinquent behavior. Or the industrial sociologist may regard the factory as a social system, as people working together in relative isolation from the outside, in order to examine what goes on in interactions and interdependencies of the people, their positions, and other variables. In our descriptions and analyses of a particular concrete system, we can recognize the shadowy figure of some such analytic model of system.

The analytic model of system demands that we treat the phenomena and the concepts for organizing the phenomena as if there existed organization, interaction, interdependency, and integration of parts and elements. System analysis assumes structure and stability within some arbitrarily sliced and frozen time period.

It is helpful to visualize a system* by drawing a large circle. We place elements, parts, variables, inside the circle as the components, and draw lines among the components. The lines may be thought of as rubber bands or springs, which stretch or contract as the forces increase or decrease. Outside the circle is the environment, where we place all other factors which impinge upon the system.

Boundary

In order to specify what is inside or outside the system, we need to define its boundary line. The boundary of a system may exist physically: a tightly corked vacuum bottle, the skin of a person, the number of people in a group, etc. But, in addition, we may delimit the system in a less tangible way, by placing our boundary according to what variables are being focused upon. We can construct a system consisting of the multiple roles of a person, or a system composed of varied roles among members in a small work group, or a system interrelating roles in a family. The components or variables used are roles, acts, expectations, communications, influence and power relationships, and so forth, and not necessarily persons.

The operational definition of *boundary* is the line forming a closed circle around selected variables, where there is less interchange of energy (or communication, etc.) *across* the line of the circle than *within* the delimiting circle. The multiple systems of a community may have boundaries that do or do not coincide. For example, treating the power relationships may require a boundary line different from that for the system of interpersonal likes or dislikes in a community. In small groups we tend to draw the same boundary line for the multiple systems of power, communications, leadership, and so on, a major advantage for purposes of study.

In diagnosing we tentatively assign a boundary, examine what is happening inside the system, and then readjust the boundary, if necessary. We examine explicitly whether or not the "relevant" factors are accounted for within the system, an immensely practical way of deciding upon relevance. Also, we are free to limit ruthlessly and neglect some factors temporarily, thus reducing the number of considerations necessary to be kept in mind at one time. The variables left outside the system, in the "environment" of the system, can be introduced one or more at a time to see the effects, if any, on the interrelationship of the variables within the system.

---

*A useful visual aid for the idea of a system can be constructed by using paper clips (elements) and rubber bands (tensions) mounted on a peg board. Shifting of the position of a clip demonstrates the interdependency of all the clips' positions, and their shifting relationships.

Tension, Stress, Strain, and Conflict

Because the components within a system are different from each other, are not perfectly integrated, or are changing and reacting to change, or because outside disturbances occur, we need ways of dealing with these differences. The differences lead to varying degrees of tension within the system. *Examples:* males are not like females, foremen see things differently from workers and from executives, children in a family grow, a committee has to work with a new chairman, a change in the market condition requires a new sales response from a factory. To restate the above examples in conceptual terms, we find built-in differences, gaps of ignorance, misperceptions, or differential perceptions, internal changes in a component, reactive adjustments and defenses, and the requirements of system survival generating tensions. Tensions that are internal and arise out of the structural arrangements of the system may be called *stresses and strains* of the system. When tensions gang up and become more or less sharply opposed along the lines of two or more components, we have *conflict*.

A word of warning. The presence of tensions, stresses or strains, and conflict within the system often are reacted to by people in the system as if they were shameful and to be done away with. Tension reduction, relief of stress and strain, and conflict resolution become the working goals of practitioners but sometimes at the price of overlooking the possibility of increasing tensions and conflict in order to facilitate creativity, innovation, and social change. System analysts have been accused of being conservative and even reactionary in assuming that a social system always tends to reduce tension, resist innovation, abhor deviancy and change. It is obvious, however, that tension and conflict are inherent in any system, and that no living system exists without tension. Whether these facts of life in a system are to be abhorred or welcomed is determined by attitudes or value judgments not derivable from system theory as such.

The identification of and analysis of how tensions operate in a system are by all odds *the* major utility of system analysis for practitioners of change. The dynamics of a living system are exposed for observation through utilizing the concepts of tension, stress and strain, and conflict. These tensions lead to activities of two kinds: those which do not affect the structure of the system (dynamics), and those which directly alter the structure itself (system change).

Equilibrium and Steady State

A system is assumed to have a tendency to achieve a balance among the various forces operating within and upon it. Two terms have been used to denote two different ideas about balance. When the balance is thought of as a fixed point or level, it is called "equilibrium." "Steady state," on the other hand, is the term recently used to describe the balanced relationship of parts that is not dependent upon any fixed equilibrium point or level.

Our body temperature is the classic illustration of a fixed level (98.6° F.), while the functional relationship between work units in a factory, regardless of the level of production, represents a steady state. For the sake of simplicity, we shall henceforth stretch the term "equilibrium" to cover both types of balance, to include also the idea of steady state.

There are many kinds of equilibria. A *stationary equilibrium* exists when there is a fixed point or level of balance to which the system returns after a disturbance. We rarely find such instances in human relationships. A *dynamic equilibrium* exists when the equilibrium shifts to a new position of balance after disturbance. Among examples of the latter, we can observe a *neutral* type of situation. *Example:* a ball on a flat plane. A small push moves it to a new position, and it again comes to rest. *Example:* a farming community. A new plow is introduced and is easily incorporated into its agricultural methods. A new level of agricultural production is placidly achieved. A *stable* situation exists where the forces that produced the initial equilibrium are so powerful that any new force must be extremely strong before any movement of a new position can be achieved. *Example:* a ball in the bottom of a goblet. *Example:* An organization encrusted with tradition or with clearly articulated and entrenched roles is not easily upset by minor events. An *unstable* situation is tense and precarious. A small disturbance produces large and rapid movements to a new position. *Example:* a ball balanced on the rims of two goblets placed side by side. *Example:* an organization with a precarious and tense balance between two modes of leadership. A small disturbance can cause a large swing to one direction and a new position of equilibrium. *Example:* A community's balance of power between ethnic groups may be such that a "minor" disturbance can produce an upheaval and movement to a different balance of power.

A system in equilibrium reacts to outside impingements in several ways. *(1)* It resists the influence of the disturbance, refusing to acknowledge its existence, or by building a protective wall against the intrusion, and by other defensive maneuvers. *Example:* A small group refuses to talk about a troublesome problem of unequal power distribution raised by a member. *(2)* It resists the disturbance through bringing into operation the homeostatic forces that restore or re-create a balance. The small group talks about the troublesome problem of a member and convinces him that it is not "really" a problem. *(3)* It accommodates the disturbances through achieving a new equilibrium. Talking about the problem may result in a shift in power relationships among members of the group.

The concepts of equilibrium (and steady state) lead to some questions to guide a practitioner's diagnosis.

1. What are the conditions conducive to the achievement of an equilibrium in this case? Are there internal or external factors producing these forces? What is their quality and tempo?

2. Does the case of the client system represent one of the typical situations of equilibrium? How does judgment on this point affect intervention strategy? If the practitioner feels the situation is tense and precarious, he should be more cautious in intervention than in a situation of stable type.

3. Can the practitioner identify the parts of the system that represent greatest readiness to change, and the greatest resistance to and defense against change? Can he understand the functions of any variable in relation to all other variables? Can he derive some sense of the direction in which the client-system is moving, and separate those forces attempting to restore an old equilibrium and those pushing toward a new equilibrium?

Feedback

Concrete systems are never closed off completely. They have inputs and outputs across the boundary; they are affected by and in turn affect the environment. While affecting the environment, a process we call output, systems gather information about how they are doing. Such information is then fed back into the system as input to guide and steer its operations. This process is called feedback. The "discovery" of feedback has led to radical inventions in the physical world in designing self-guiding and self-correcting instruments. It has also become a major concept in the behavioral sciences, and a central tool in the practitioner's social technology. *Example:* In reaching for a cigarette we pick up tactile and visual cues that are used to guide our arm and finger movements. *Example:* Our interpersonal communications are guided and corrected by our picking up of effect cues from the communicatees. *Example:* Improving the feedback process of a client system will allow for self-steering or corrective action to be taken by him or it. In fact, the single most important improvement the change agent can help a client system to achieve is to increase its diagnostic sensitivity to the effects of its own actions upon others. Programs in sensitivity training attempt to increase or unblock the feedback processes of persons, a methodological skill with wider applicability and longer-lasting significance than solving the immediate problem at hand. In diagnosing a client system, the practitioner asks: What are its feedback procedures? How adequate are they? What blocks their effective use? Is it lack of skill in gathering data, or in coding and utilizing the information?

Open and Closed Systems

All living systems are open systems—systems in contact with their environment, with input and output across system boundaries. What then is the use of talking about a closed system? What *is* a closed system? It means that the system is temporarily assumed to have a leak-tight boundary—there is relatively little, if any, commerce across the boundary. We know that no such system can be found in reality, but it is sometimes essential to analyze a system as if it were closed so as to examine the operations of the system as affected "only by the conditions previously established by the environment and not changing at the time of analysis, plus the relationships among the internal elements of the system." The analyst then opens the system to a new impact from the environment, again closes the system, and observes and thinks out what would happen. It is, therefore, fruitless to debate the point; both open and closed system models are useful in diagnosis. Diagnosing the client as a system of variables, we have a way then of managing the complexity of "everything depends upon everything else" in an orderly way. Use of system analysis has these possibilities: (a) Diagnosticians can avoid the error of simple cause-and-effect thinking; (b) they can justify what is included in observation and interpretation and what is temporarily excluded; (c) they can predict what will happen if no new or outside force is applied; (d) they are guided in categorizing what is relatively enduring and stable, or changing, in the situation; (e) they can distinguish between what is basic and what is merely symptomatic; (f) they can predict what will happen if they leave the events undisturbed and if they intervene; and (g) they are guided in selecting points of intervention.

Intersystem Model

We propose an extension of system analysis that looks to us to be useful for the problems confronting the change agent. We urge the adoption of an intersystem model.

An intersystem model involves two open systems connected to each other.* The term we need to add here is *connectives*. Connectives represent the lines of relationships of the two systems. Connectives tie together parts (mechanics) or imbed in a web of tissue the separate organs (biology); connectives in an industrial establishment are the defined lines of communication, or the leadership hierarchy and authority for the branch plants; or they represent the social contract entered into by a therapist and patient; or mutual role expectations of consultant and client; or the affective ties between family members. These are conjunctive connectives. But we also have conflicts between labor and management, teenage gang wars, race conflicts, and negative emotional responses to strangers. These are disjunctive connectives.

Why elaborate the system model into an intersystem model? Cannot we get the same effect by talking about "subsystems" of a larger system? In part we can. Labor-management conflicts, or interpersonal relations, or change

---

*A visualization of an intersystem model would be two systems side by side, with separately identified links. Two rubber band–paper clip representations can be connected with rubber bands of a different color, representing the connectives.

agent and client relationships can each be treated as a new system with subsystems. But we may lose the critical fact of the autonomy of the components, or the direct interactional or transactual consequences for the separate components when we treat the subsystems as merely parts of a larger system. The intersystem model exaggerates the virtues of autonomy and the limited nature of interdependence of the interactions between the two connected systems.

What are some of the positive advantages of using intersystem analysis? First, the external change agent, or the change agent built into an organization, as a helper with planned change does not completely become a part of the client system. He must remain separate to some extent; he must create and maintain some distance between himself and the client, thus standing apart "in another system" from which he rerelates. This new system might be a referent group of fellow professionals, or a body of rational knowledge. But create one he does and must. Intersystem analysis of the change agent's role leads to fruitful analysis of the connectives—their nature in the beginning, how they shift, and how they are cut off. Intersystem analysis also poses squarely an unexplored issue, namely the internal system of the change agent, whether a single person, consultant group, or a nation. Helpers of change are prone at times not to see that their own systems as change agents have boundaries, tensions, stresses and strains, equilibria, and feedback mechanisms that may be just as much parts of the problem as are similar aspects of the client systems. Thus, relational issues are more available for diagnosis when we use an intersystem model.

More importantly, the intersystem model is applicable to problems of leadership, power, communication, and conflict in organizations, intergroup relations, and international relations. *Example:* Leadership in a work group with its liaison, negotiation, and representation functions is dependent upon connectives to another group and not solely upon the internal relationships within the work group. Negotiators, representatives, and leaders are parts of separate systems each with its own interdependence, tensions, stresses, and feedback, whether we are thinking of foreign ministers, Negro-white leaders, or student-faculty councils.

In brief, the intersystem model leads us to examine the interdependent dynamics of interaction both within and between the units. We object to the premature and unnecessary assumption that the units always form a single system. We can be misled into an utopian analysis of conflict, change agent relations to client, and family relations if we neglect system differences. But an intersystem model provides a tool for diagnosis that retains the virtues of system analysis, adds the advantage of clarity, and furthers our diagnosis of the influence of various connectives, conjunctive and disjunctive, on the two systems. For change agents, the essence of collaborative planning is contained in an intersystem model.

DEVELOPMENTAL MODELS

Practitioners have in general implicitly favored developmental models in thinking about human affairs, while social scientists have not paid as much attention to these as they have to system models. The life sciences of biology and psychology have not crystallized nor refined their common analytic model of the development of the organism, despite the heroic breakthroughs of Darwin. Thus, we are forced to present only broad and rough categories of alternative positions in this paper.

Since there is no standard vocabulary for a developmental model, we shall present five categories of terms that we deem essential to such models: direction, states, forces, form of progression, and potentiality.

The Major Terms

Developmental Models

By developmental models we mean those bodies of thought that center around growth and directional change. Developmental models assume change; they assume that there are noticeable differences between the states of a system at different times, that the succession of these states implies the system is heading somewhere, and that there are orderly processes that explain how the system gets from its present state to wherever it is going. In order to delimit the nature of change in developmental models we should perhaps add the idea of an increase in value accompanying the achievement of a new state. With this addition, developmental models focus on processes of growth and maturation. This addition might seem to rule out processes of decay, deterioration, and death from consideration. Logically, the developmental model should apply to either.

There are two kinds of "death" of concern to the practitioner. The first, death, is loss of some part or subvalue, as a constant concomitant of growth and development. Theories of life processes have used concepts such as katabolic (destructive) processes in biology, death instincts in Freud's psychology, or role loss upon promotion. On balance, the "loss" is made up by the "gains," and thus there is an increase in value. The second kind of death is planned change for a group or organization—the dissolution of a committee or community organization that has "outlived its purpose and function," and the termination of a helping relationship with deliberateness and collaboration of participants is properly included as part of a developmental model.

Direction

Developmental models postulate that the system under scrutiny—a person, a small group, interpersonal interactions, an organization, a community or a society—is going "somewhere," that the changes have some direction. The direction may be defined by *(a)* some *goal* or end state (developed, mature), *(b)* the *process* of becoming (developing, maturing), or *(c)* the degree of achievement *toward* some goal or end state (increased development, increase in maturity).

Change agents find it necessary to believe that there is direction in change. *Example:* Self-actualization or fulfillment is a need of a client system. When strong directional tendencies are present, we modify our diagnosis and intervention accordingly. A rough analogy may be helpful here. A change agent using a developmental model may be thought of as a husbandman tending a plant, watching and helping it to grow in its own natural direction of producing flowers. He feeds, waters, and weeds. Though at times he may be ruthless in pinching off excess buds, or even in using grafts, in general he encourages the plant to reach it "goal" of producing beautiful flowers.

Identifiable State

As the system develops over time, the different states may be identifed and differentiated from one another. Terms such as "stages," "levels," "phases," or "periods" are applied to these states. *Example:* psychosexual definition of oral and anal stages, levels of evolution of species, or phases of group development.

No uniformity exists in the definition and operational identification of such successive states. But since change agents do have to label the past, present, and future, they need some terms to describe successive states and to identify the turning points, transition areas, or critical events that characterize change. Here, system analysis is helpful in defining how parts are put together, along with the tensions and directions of the equilibrating processes. We have two polar types of the shifts of states: *(a)* small, nondiscernible steps or increments leading to a qualitative jump (*Example:* black hair gradually turning gray, or a student evolving into a scholar); *(b)* a cataclysmic or critical event leading to a sudden change (*Example:* a sickness resulting in gray hair overnight, or an inspirational lecture by a professor). While the latter type seems more frequently to be externally induced, internal factors of the system can have the same consequence. In other words, the internal disequilibration of a balance may lead to a step-jump of the system to a new level. Personality stages, group stages, and societal phases are evolved and precipitated from internal and from external relations.

Form of Progression

Change agents see in their models of development some form of progression or movement. Four such forms are typically assumed. First, it is often stated that once a stage is worked through, the client system shows continued progression and normally never turns back. (Any recurrence of a previous state is viewed as an abnormality. Freudian stages are a good example;

recurrence of a stage is viewed as regression, an abnormal event to be explained.) Teachers expect a steady growth of knowledge in students, either in a straight line (linear) or in an increasingly accelerating (curvilinear) form.

Second, it is assumed that change, growth, and development occur in a *spiral* form. *Example:* A small group might return to some previous problem, such as its authority relations to the leader, but now might discuss the question at a "higher" level where irrational components are less dominant.

Third, another assumption more typically made is that the stages are really phases which occur and recur. There is an oscillation between various states, where no chronological priority is assigned to each state; there are cycles. *Example:* Phases of problem solving or decision making recur in different time periods as essential to progression. Cultures and societies go through phases of development in recurrent forms.

Fourth, still another assumption is that the form of progression is characterized by a branching out into *differentiated* forms and processes, each part increasing in its specialization and at the same time acquiring its own autonomy and significance. *Example:* Biological forms are differentiated into separate species. Organizations become more and more differentiated into special task and control structures.

Forces

First, forces or causal factors producing development and growth are most frequently seen by practitioners as "natural," as part of human nature, suggesting the role of genetics and other inborn characteristics. At best, environmental factors act as triggers or releasers, in which case the presence of some stimulus sets off the system's inherent growth forces. For example, it is sometimes thought that the teacher's job is to trigger off the natural curiosity of the child, and that growth of knowledge will ensue. Or the leadership of an organization should act to release the self-actualizing and creative forces present in its members.

Second, a smaller number of practitioners and social scientists think that the response to new situations and environmental forces is a coping response that gives rise to growth and development. Third, at this point it may be useful to remind ourselves of the earlier discussion of the internal tensions of the system, still another cause of change. When stresses and strains of a system become too great, a disruption occurs and a set of forces is released to create new structures and achieve a new equilibrium.

Potentiality

Developmental models vary in their assumptions about potentialities of the system for development, growth, and change. That is, they vary in assumptions about the capabilities, overt or latent, that are built into the original or present state so that the necessary conditions for development may be typically present. Does the "seed"—and its genetic characteristics—represent potentialities? And are the supporting conditions of its environment available? Is the intelligence or emotional capability or skill-potential sufficient for development and change in a social and human process?

Change agents typically assume a high degree of potentiality in the impetus toward development, and in the surrounding conditions that help actualize the potential.

Utility to Practitioners

The developmental model has tremendous advantages for the practitioner. It provides a set of expectations about the future of the client system. By clarifying his thoughts and refining his observations about direction, states in the developmental process, forms of progression, and forces causing these events to occur over a period of time, the practitioner develops a time perspective which goes far beyond that of the more here-and-now analysis of a system model, which is bounded by time. By using a developmental model, he has a directional focus for his analysis and action and a temporal frame of reference. In addition, he is confronted with a number of questions to ask of himself and of his observations of the case: Do I assume an inherent end of the development? Do I impose a desired (by me) direction? How did I establish a collaboratively planned direction? What states in the development process may be expected? What form of progression do I foresee? What causes the development? His diagnoses and his interventions can become strategic rather than merely tactical.

THE CHANGE AGENT AND MODELS

The primary concern of this paper has been to illustrate some of the major kinds of analytic models and conceptual schemata that have been devised by social scientists for the analysis of change and of changing human processes. But we need to keep in mind that the concern with diagnosis on the part of the social scientist is to achieve understanding, and to educe empirically researchable hypotheses amenable to his methods of study. The social scientist generally prefers not to change the system but to study how it works and to predict what would happen if some new factor were introduced. So we find his attention focused on a theory of change, of how the system achieves change. In contrast, the practitioner is concerned with diagnosis: how to achieve understanding in order to engage in change. The practitioner, therefore, has some additional interests; he wants to know how to change the system, he needs a theory of changing the system.

A theory of changing requires the selection or the construction, by theoretically minded practitioners, of thought models appropriate to their intended purpose. This has to be done according to explicit criteria. A change agent may demand of any model answers to certain questions. The responses he receives may not be complete nor satisfactory since only piecemeal answers exist. At this period in the development of a theory of changing, we ask four questions as our guidelines for examining a conceptual model intended for the use of change agents.

The first question is simply this: Does the model account for the stability and continuity in the events studied at the same time that it accounts for changes in them? How do processes of change develop, given the interlocking factors in the situation that make for stability? Second, where does the model locate the source of change? What place among these sources do the deliberate and conscious efforts of the client system and change agent occupy? Third, what does the model assume about how goals and directions are determined? What or who sets the direction for movement of the processes of change? Fourth, does the model provide the change agent with levers or handles for affecting the direction, tempo, and quality of these processes of change?

A fifth question running through the other four is this: How does the model "place" the change agent in the scheme of things? What is the shifting character of his relationship to the client system, initially and at the termination of relationship, that affects his perceptions and actions? The questions of relationship of change agent to others needs to be part and parcel of the model since the existential relationships of the change agent engaged in processes of planned change become part of the problem to be investigated.

The application of these five questions to the models of systems and models of development crystallizes some of the formation of ingredients for a change agent model for changing. We can now summarize each model as follows:

A system model emphasizes primarily the details of how stability is achieved, and only derivatively how change evolves out of the incompatibilities and conflicts in the system. A system model assumes that organization, interdependency, and integration exist among its parts and that change is a derived consequence of how well the parts of the system fit together, or how well the system fits in with other surrounding and interacting systems. The source of change lies primarily in the structural stress and strain externally induced or internally created. The process of change is a process of tension reduction. The goals and direction are emergent from the structures or from imposed sources. Goals are often analyzed as set by "vested interests" of one part of the system. The confronting symptom of some trouble is a reflection of difficulties of adaptability (reaction to environment) or of the ability for adjustment (internal equilibration). The levers or handles available for manipulation are in the "inputs" to the system, especially the feedback mechanisms,

TABLE 1. Assumptions and Approaches of Three Analytic Models

	Models of Change		
Assumptions and Approaches to:	System Model	Developmental Model	Model for Changing
1. Content			
Stability	Structural integration	Phases, stages	Unfreezing parts
Change	Derived from structure	Constant and unique	Induced, controlled
2. Causation			
Source of change	Structural stress	Nature of organisms	Self and change agent
Causal force	Tension reduction		Rational choice
3. Goals			
Direction	Emergent	Ontological	Deliberate selection
Set by	"Vested interests"		Collaborative process
4. Intervention			
Confronting symptoms	Stresses, strains, and tensions	Discrepancy between actuality and potentiality	Perceived need
Goal of intervening	Adjustment, adaptation	Removal of blockages	Improvement
5. Change Agent			
Place	Outside the target system	Outside	Part of situation
Role	External diagnoser and actor	External diagnoser and actor	Participant in here and now

and in the forces tending to restore a balance in the system. The change agent is treated as separate from the client system, the target system.

The developmental model assumes constant change and development, and growth and decay of a system over time. Any existing stability is a snapshot of a living process—a stage that will give way to another stage. The supposition seems to be that it is natural that change should occur because change is rooted in the very nature of living organisms. The laws of the developmental process are not necessarily fixed, but some effects of the environment are presumably necessary to the developmental process. The direction of change is toward some goal, the fulfillment of its destiny, granting that no major blockage gets in the way. Trouble occurs when there is a gap between the system and its goal. Intervention is viewed as the removal of blockage by the change agent, who then gets out of the way of the growth forces. Developmental models are not very sharply analyzed by the pure theorist nor formally stated, usually, as an analytic model. In fact, very frequently the model is used for studying the unique case rather than for deriving laws of growth; it is for descriptive purposes.

The third model—a model for changing, is a more recent creation. It incorporates some elements of analyses from system models, along with some ideas from the developmental model, in a framework where direct attention is paid to the induced forces producing change. It studies stability in order to unfreeze and move some parts of the system. The direction to be taken is not fixed or determined, but remains in large measure a matter of choice for the client system. The change agent is a specialist in the technical processes of facilitating change, a helper to the client system. The models for changing are as yet incompletely conceptualized. The intersystem model may provide a way of examining how the change agent's relationships, as part of the model, affect the processes of change.

We can summarize and contrast the three models as in Table 1. We have varying degrees of confidence in our categories, but, as the quip says, we construct these in order to achieve the laudable state of "paradigm lost." It is the reader's responsibility to help achieve this goal!

THE LIMITATIONS

It is obvious that we are proposing the use of systematically constructed and examined models of thought for the change agent. The advantages are manifold and—we hope—apparent in our preceding discussion. Yet we must now point out some limitations and disutility of models.

Models are abstractions of concrete events. Because of the high degree of selectivity of observations and focus, the fit between the model and the actual thought and diagnostic processes of the change agent is not close. Furthermore, the thought and diagnostic processes of the change agent are not fixed and rigid. And even worse, the fit between the diagnostic processes of the change agent and the changing processes of the actual case, is not close. Abstract as the nature of a model is, as applied to the change agent, students of the change agent role may find the concepts of use. But change agents' practices in diagnosing are not immediately affected by models' analyses.

Furthermore, there are modes of diagnosing by intervening, which do not fall neatly into models. The change agent frequently tries out an activity in order to see what happens and to see what is involved in the change. If successful, he does not need to diagnose any further, but proceeds to engage in further actions with the client. If unsuccessful, however, he may need to examine what is going on in more detail.

The patchwork required for a theory and model of changing requires the suspension of acceptance of such available models. This paper has argued for some elements from both the system models and the developmental models to be included in the model for practitioners, with the use of a format of the intersystem model so as to include the change agent and his relationships as part of the problem. But can the change agent wait for such a synthesis and emerging construction? Our personal feeling is that the planning of change cannot wait, but that the change agent must proceed with the available diagnostic tools. Here is an intellectual challenge to the scientist-scholar of planned change that could affect the professions of practice.

Arnold M. Rose

A Systematic Summary of Symbolic Interaction Theory

Much of existing psychological theory is grounded on assumptions about vertebrate behavior in general and has sought confirmation in research on animals other than man—whether these be the rats studied by the behaviorists or the apes studied by the Gestaltists.* The result is that we know a good deal about man's behavior insofar as the principles governing his behavior are also applicable to other animals. When psychologists of the behaviorist and Gestaltist schools have studied man's behavior, they have either limited their study to those aspects of man's behavior which he shares with the other animals, or they have substituted middle-range theories in the place of large-scale theories. The frustration-aggression theory of the Yale neobehaviorists, and the group-influence theory of the "group dynamics" Gestaltists are examples of such middle-range theories. Insofar as these excellent researches and theories can be linked up to large frameworks of theory they make no reference to man's distinctive characteristics which make his behavior different from that of the other vertebrates.

It would seem valuable to have a social psychological framework of theory—as distinct from a general psychological theory—grounded on assumptions about man's distinctive characteristics and on researches dealing with man himself. This would not be in opposition to the behaviorist and Gestaltist theories, but supplementary to them. Both psychoanalytic and symbolic interactionist theories seek to do this. The present essay seeks to set forth symbolic interactionist theory in a systematic fashion as grounded on

From Rose, A (ed): Human Behavior and Social Processes. An Interactionist Approach. Boston, Houghton Mifflin, 1962. Courtesy of the author and the Houghton Mifflin Co.
*This statement has benefited from the criticism of Herbert Blumer, Caroline Rose, Gregory Stone, and Sheldon Stryker, but they did not always agree with the author or with one another.

man's distinctive characteristics. The attempt is made to state the theory in terms that will fit the framework of reference of the behaviorist or Gestaltist so as to make it more generally understandable. (It is not suggested that the theory is reducible to behaviorists or Gestaltist proportions.) Only assumptions, definitions, and general propositions are presented here; specific hypotheses deduced* from the theory are set forth in other contributions to *Human Behavior and Social Processes.*

Assumption 1 *Man lives in a symbolic environment as well as a physical environment and can be "stimulated" to act by symbols as well as by physical stimuli.*

A *symbol* is defined as a stimulus that has a learned meaning and value for people, and man's response to a symbol is in terms of its meaning and value rather than in terms of its physical stimulation of his sense organs.† To offer a simple example: "chair" is not merely a collection of visual, aural, and tactile stimuli, but it "means" an object on which people may sit; and if one sits on it, it will "respond" by holding him up—and it has a value for that purpose. A *meaning* is equivalent to a "true" dictionary definition, referring to the way in which people actually use a term in their behavior. A *value* is the learned attraction or repulsion they feel toward the meaning. A symbol is *an incipient or telescoped act,* in which the later stages—involving elements of both meaning and value—are implied in the first stage. Thus, the symbol "chair" implies the physical comfort, the opportunity to do certain things which can best be done while sitting, and other similar "outcomes" of sitting in a chair. It should be understood, as Mead points out, that "language does not simply symbolize a situation or object which is already there in advance; it makes possible the existence or the appearance of that situation or object, for it is a part of the mechanism whereby that situation or object is created" (Strauss, 1956).

Practically all the symbols a man learns he learns through communication (interaction) with other people, and therefore most symbols can be thought of as common or shared meanings and values‡. The mutually shared character

---

*The term "deduced" is used here in a hopeful, rather than a rigorous, sense. Ideally, the specific hypotheses ought to be logically deducible from the theory. Actually, the theory has not yet been elaborated to the point where the hypotheses used in research are rigorously deducible, and the most we can say is that they are logically consistent with the theory. Similarly, the general propositions ought to be deduced, but in fact they are merely logically consistent. (General propositions differ from hypotheses in that they are too broad to be empirically testable.)

‡Common values may be considered in two categories: *(1) norms,* which are direct guides to actual positive or negative actions; *(2) ideals,* which are what the individual says or believes he would like to do, and which may coincide sometimes with the norms but at other times have only an indirect and remote relationship to actual behavior. Values have degree, and strong common norms have the character of mobilizing collective sanctions when they are breached. Even when ideals do not coincide with norms, they provide guides to behavior in the sense of being remote goals, which are to be reached indirectly. When considering the values from a subjective aspect—that is, from the standpoint of the individual—we call them *attitudes.* Attitudes thus also may be considered to have two categories, the normative and the idealistic, and the difficulty of

of the meanings and values of objects and acts give them "consensual valida-tion," to use a term of Harry Stack Sullivan (although it must be recognized that the consensus is practically never complete). "Meaning is not to be conceived as a state of consciousness," says Mead, ". . . the response of one organism (or object) to the gesture of another in any given social act is the meaning of that gesture, and also is in a sense responsible for the appearance or coming into being of the new object—or new content of an old object—to which the gesture refers through the outcome of the given social act in which it is an early phase." (Strauss, 1956).

Man has a distinctive capacity for symbolic communication because he alone among the animals (a) has a vocal apparatus which can make a large number and wide range of different sounds, and (b) has a nervous system which can store up the meanings and values of millions of symbols. Not all symbols are words or combinations of words that are transmitted through hearing—symbols are also transmitted through sight, such as gestures, mo-tions, objects. But for most individuals and for men as a species, sound symbols precede sight symbols. In other words, man is distinctive in having language, which is based (in the necessary not the sufficient sense of causation) on certain anatomical and physiological characteristics such as a complex brain and vocal apparatus, and this permits him to live in a symbolic environment as well as a physical environment.

Assumption 2 *Through symbols, man has the capacity to stimulate others in ways other than those in which he is himself stimulated.*

In using symbols man can evoke the same meaning and value within himself that he evokes in another person but which he does not necessarily accept for himself. We may oversimplify and say that a man communicates to another in order to evoke meanings and values in the other that he "intends" to evoke.*
Studies indicate that communication among other animals is based on obser-vation of the body movements or sounds of another, and *invariably* evokes the same body response in the observer as in the stimulator. Following Mead,

---

distinguishing between these two is one of the main sources of difficulty in using attitude research to predict behavior. Some sociologists and psychologists use the term "values" in the same, more restrictive, sense in which I use the term "ideals." Talcott Parsons (1963), for example, says: "By the values of the society is meant conceptions of the desirable type of society, not of other things the valuations of which may or may not be shared by its members." Everyday usage of the term "values," as well as the usage of most economists and some sociologists and psychologists, is the broader meaning which I use here. In any case, a term is needed to cover the valuational aspects of both what people say they would like to do and what people actually do, and "values" is as good a term for this as any.

*This is oversimplified in many respects, among which we may note: (a) that the meaning evoked is seldom absolutely identical for two persons, but is merely similar; (b) that the meaning evoked is not necessarily the one intended by the evoker; (c) that the meaning may be only partial and anticipatory of communication of further meanings.

we may say that man's communication can involve *role-taking*—"taking the role of the other" (also called empathy)—as well as more spontaneous expression that happens to evoke in the other a feeling tone and body response that are present in himself. The learned symbols that require role taking for their communication Mead called *significant symbols,* as distinguished from *natural signs,* which instinctively evoke the same body responses and feeling tones in the observer as in the original expresser. An animal expresses natural signs whether another animal is around or not, but the human individual does not express significant symbols unless another person is around to observe them (except when he wishes to designate a meaning or value to himself or to a spiritual force imagined to be present); yet both signs and symbols are means of communication.

In communication by natural signs, the communicator *controls* the behavior of the attender, whether by intention or not, for the body of the attender invariably responds in a specific way to the impact of stimuli on his sense organs. In communication by significant symbols, on the other hand, the communicator may *influence* the behavior of the attender, but he cannot control it for the symbol communicates by its content of meaning and value for the attender. While the communicator emits the sound or the visible gesture, it is the attender who ascribes the meaning and value to the sound or sight. Thus the symbolic communication is a social process, in which the communicator and attender both contribute to the content of the communication as it impinges on the nervous system and behavior of the attender. This is true even when the attender appears to be perfectly passive, and it does not become more true when the attender responds with a new communication directed to the original communicator.

For example, a bee that has discovered a source of honey wriggles in a kind of rhythmic dance. Other bees, observing this, tend to follow the wriggling bee to its discovery and so aid in carrying the honey to the hive, but each bee discovering a source of honey will wriggle whether other bees are around to observe it or not. The tension in the body of one animal, usually occurring in the presence of presumed danger, will transmit itself to observing animals of the same species; and we note in man also the tendency for emotion expressed in the manner or voice of one individual to be transmitted to other individuals. These are examples of natural-sign communication, and may have had the original biological function of alerting the observing individual, or otherwise preparing him to act quickly in response to dangers in the environment or to attack from the emotion-emitting individual. Communication by means of significant symbols, on the other hand, involves words or gestures intended to convey meaning from the communicator to the observer. It is not the noise of the words or the physical movement of the gesture itself which communicates, but the meaning for which the noise or physical movement stands as a symbol. Both the communicator and the observer have had to learn the meaning of the words or gestures in order to communicate symbolically, but the communication by natural signs takes place instinctively and spontaneously.

Role taking is involved in all communications by means of significant symbols; it means that the individual communicator imagines—evokes within himself—how the recipient of his communication understands that communication.* Man can take the role not only of a "single other," but also of a "generalized other"—in which he evokes within himself simultaneously the diverse behaviors of a number of persons acting in concert in a team, a group, a society.

Assumption 3 *Through communication of symbols, man can learn huge numbers of meanings and values—and hence ways of acting—from other men.*

Thus, it is assumed that most of the modern adult's behavior is learned behavior, and specifically learned in symbolic communication rather than through individual trial and error, conditioning, or any other purely psychogenic process. Man's helplessness at birth—his "need" to learn from others—as well as the relatively lengthy proportion of his life in which he is immature are biological facts which also aid this learning process. It is to be noted that this social learning process, while slow in the young infant, becomes extremely rapid. Through tests with readings or lectures using new material, it has been found that a normal, alert person can learn over a hundred new meanings within the space of an hour, and that most of this new learning can be retained for weeks without reinforcement. In most human learning involving trial and error (except for learning manual skills), it has been found that only one failure is enough to inhibit the false response, and usually one success is enough to fix the correct response—unlike trial-and-error learning among other animals, where many failures and successes are necessary to fix the new correct response.

All this is another way of saying that man can have a *culture*—an elaborate set of meanings and values shared by members of a society—which guides much of his behavior.

General Proposition (Deduction) 1 *Through the learning of a culture (and subcultures, which are the specialized cultures found in particular segments of society), men are able to predict each other's behavior most of the time and gauge their own behavior to the predicted behavior of others.*

This general proposition is deduced from the previous assumptions about role

---

*There is a methodological implication here that the investigator should view the words through the eyes of the actor and not assume that what he—the investigator—observes is identical with what the actor observes in the same situation. Mead was emphatic in distinguishing between his own concept of "empathy" and Charles H. Cooley's concept of "sympathy"—defined as the process in which one imagines himself in the same situation as another.

taking with common symbols, as the predictions are based on *expectations* for behavior implied in the common meanings and values. A society can be said to exist only when this proposition is true. In this sense and only in this sense, society is more than a collection of individuals; it is a collection of individuals with a culture, which has been learned by symbolic communication from other individuals back through time, so that the members can gauge their behavior to each other and to the society as a whole.*

There is thus no need to posit a "group mind" or "folk soul" to explain concerted behavior or social integration, as some psychologists (William McDougall and Willhelm Wundt and others) have done. There is also no need to posit a "tendency" for society to have functional integration as some sociologists and anthropologists of the functionalist school have done.

Assumption 4 *The symbols—and the meanings and values to which they refer—do not occur only in isolated bits, but often in clusters, sometimes large and complex.*
The evocation of a lead meaning or value of a cluster will allow fairly accurate prediction of the rest of the meanings and values that can be expected to follow in the same cluster. Different terms have been used to refer to these clusters, but we shall use the following two terms:

1. The term *role* will be used to refer to a cluster of related meanings and values that guide and direct an individual's behavior in a given social setting; common roles are those of a father, a physician, a colleague, a friend, a service club member, a pedestrian. A person plays one of these roles in each social relationship he enters. A person is thus likely to play many roles in the course of a day, and role playing constitutes much of his behavior.
2. The term *structure* will be used to refer to a cluster of related meanings and values that govern a given social setting, including the relationships of all the individual roles that are expected parts of it. Structures may be fairly small or temporary ones, such as a conference committee, or a large and "permanent" one, such as a state or a society.

A structure and the roles that are related in it are two aspects of the same thing, one looked at from the standpoint of the individual, the other looked at from the standpoint of the social setting.

General Proposition (Deduction) 2 *The individual defines (has a meaning for) himself as well as other objects, actions, and characteristics.*
The definition of himself as a specific role player in a given relationship is what Mead calls a "me." William James observed that each of us has as many

*Whether this be in cooperation or in conflict is unimportant in this context.

selves as there are groups to which we belong; or—in Mead's terminology—we have a defined "me" corresponding to each of our roles (i.e., "me" and role are the same thing, the first viewed from the subjective aspect and the second viewed by another person or persons). Some roles may have more positive value associated with them than do others; the "groups" or relationships in which we play these more highly valued roles are called reference groups.* An individual's various "me's" are seen by him not only as discrete objects; he may perceive all of them at once and in a hierarchy according to the degree of positive attitude he holds toward them. This perception of himself as a whole Mead called the "I" or "self-conception."† Once defined, the self-conception takes on characteristics and attributes which are not necessarily part of its constituent roles. That is, the self-conception acquires a purely personal aspect once the individual establishes a relationship to himself. Mead (Strauss, 1956) distinguished the "I" and "me" as follows: "The 'I' is the response of the organism to the attitudes of the others; the 'me' is the organized set of attitudes of others which one himself assumes. The attitudes of the others constitute the organized 'me,' and then one reacts toward that as an 'I.'" In sum, the individual has parts of himself which are reflections of his relationships with others, and which others can take the role of and predict fairly accurately how the individual is going to behave in the relationship. There is another part of the individual—his self-conception—the attitudes of which may be, in part, assigned by the individual to himself and which are not necessarily expected in the culture. This personal self-conception may be conformist as well as deviant, and while it is always subject to change, it is often stable enough for another person to predict fairly accurately what behavior the individual will engage in even aside from the cultural expectations

---

*I would prefer calling them reference relationships rather than reference groups, since the term "group" usually refers to a number of individuals, whereas a "relationship" can be to only one other person or to oneself alone. Also, the term "group" is sometimes confused with a collectivity or agglomeration of individuals in which no relationship is involved, such as all people aged 10–20, an audience in a darkened theater, or the observers of a given advertisement. A relationship occurs when—and only when—role taking is involved among the persons in the group.

While I have said that a reference relationship is one which is valued highly, the term is obviously relative; except for the very lowest one, every reference relationship is higher than some other one. We must think of reference relationships as forming a continuum from high to low with some of the low ones possibly even having a negative value. Negative reference relationships seem typically to occur when a person is forced into having the relationship against his personal values, and is obliged to act in accord with the expectations for one in the relationship as in the case of a Negro who hates being a Negro but is obliged by his Negroness to act in accord with the expectations for Negroes' behavior.

Mead used the terms "significant other" and "significant others," but these do not allow for the "other" to be oneself, nor do they imply that there are degrees of significance. The concept of reference relationship seems best because it permits the "other" to be a single individual, a group, or even oneself in the case of a narcissistic individual. It also permits one to have degrees of "reference" or "significance" in the relationship, even down to a negative value.

†It is not clear whether Mead equated the "self-conception" with the "I" or the "me," but the author of this article finds it more consistent and otherwise preferable to equate the conception of self with the "I."

for his roles. The "I," while personal, is by no means independent of cultural expectations, since it is built on the individual's "me's," and since the individual always sees himself in relation to the community.

Assumption 5 *Thinking is the process by which possible symbolic solutions and other future courses of action are examined, assessed for their relative advantages and disadvantages in terms of the values of the individual, and one of them chosen for action.*

Thinking is strictly a symbolic process because the alternatives assessed are certain relevant meanings, and the assessment is made in terms of the individual's values. In thinking, the individual takes his own role to imagine himself in various possible relevant situations. Thinking is a kind of substitute for trial-and-error behavior (which most animal species engage in) in that possible future behaviors are imagined (as "trials") and are accepted or rejected (as "successes" or "errors"). Thought can lead to learning, not through hedonistic rejection of errors or reinforcement of successful trials, but through drawing out deductively the implications of empirical data already known. Thinking is generally more efficient than actual trial-and-error behavior in that (a) imaginative trials usually occur more rapidly than behavioral trials, (b) the individual can select the best solution (or future course of action) known to him rather than merely the first successful solution, and (c) he takes less risk in experimenting with trials that are likely to be dangerous. Through thinking, man brings the imagined or expected future into the present, so that present behavior can be a response to future expected stimuli, and courses of action can be laid out for quite some time into the future. For example, a college freshman, in choosing a future occupation, engages in immediate behavior intended to get him into that occupation and lays out future actions for himself that will probably get him into that occupation. In much the same way that the future is brought into the present during the process of thinking, so is the past. The individual imagines the past symbolically—not only his own past experience but the past experiences of anyone he knows about, including people who lived thousands of years ago. Present and future courses of action may be selected in terms of what the individual knows, or thinks he knows, about the past.

The presentation of symbolic interaction theory thus far has been analytic in terms of its major concepts and their assumed interrelationships. The presentation can also be genetic—that is, in terms of the process of socialization of the individual child. This approach will now be presented in brief form.

Assumption 1 *Society—a network of interacting individuals—with its culture—the related meanings and values by means of which individuals interact—precedes any existing individual.*

The implication of this assumption is that the individual is expected to learn the requirements for behavior found in the culture and to conform to them most of the time. Robert E. Park (1915) put this in epigrammatic form: "Man is not born human. It is only slowly and laboriously, in fruitful contact, cooperation, and conflict with his fellows, that he attains the distinctive qualities of human nature," in which the word *human* stands for conforming to expected patterns of man's behavior.

While this statement puts the cultural expectations foremost, it does not mean a cultural determinism for several reasons:

1. Some of the interaction between individuals is on a noncultural or natural-sign level, so that some learned behavior is universally human and independent of specific cultures.
2. Most cultural expectations are for ranges of behavior rather than for specific behaviors. The expectations that people will wear clothes, for example, sets limits for permissible coverings for the human body, but leaves room for considerable choice within those limits.
3. Most cultural expectations are for certain roles rather than for all individuals, and for certain situations, rather than all situations, and the individual has some freedom of choice among the roles and situations he will enter. Different occupations, for example, require different clothing, and the process of entering a given occupation is not culturally determined.
4. Some cultural expectations are for variation rather than conformity. The scientist and the fashion designer, for example, are culturally expected to be innovators in certain ways, and their innovations are not predictable from the culture.
5. The cultural *meanings* indicate possibilities for behavior, not requirements or "pressures" for a certain kind of behavior (as the cultural *values* do). The fact that a chair is an object to be sat on, for example, does not mean that a chair is only to be used for sitting or that one must always sit when a chair is available.
6. The culture, especially our culture, is often internally inconsistent, and one may move from one culture or subculture to another, so that there are conflicting cultural expectations for an individual. This does not mean solely that the individual has a choice between the two conflicting patterns of behavior he is exposed to, or can make a synthesis of them, but also that he can—within the limits permitted by the culture—define for himself somewhat new patterns suggested by the variation among the old ones.
7. To extend the last point somewhat, whenever the individual is "blocked" in carrying on behavior expected within the society, he has some possibility of innovating—within the limits of cultural tolerance—to devise new behavior patterns that will take him around the block. The self—Mead's "I"—is a creative self (the nature of thinking in symbolic interaction theory has already been indicated).

8. Finally the symbolic interactionist does not exclude the influence of biogenic and psychogenic factors in behavior, even though he does not incorporate them into his theory.

These eight important qualifications to a cultural determinism do not nullify the importance of the basic assumption that all men are born into an ongoing society and are socialized in some significant degree into behavior that meets the expectations of its culture.

Assumption 2 *The process by which socialization takes place can be thought of as occurring in three stages.*

The first stage, in the young infant, is learning through some psychogenic process—such as conditioning, trial and error, or any process found also among other animals—so that the infant is "habituated" to a certain sequence of behaviors and events. When a blockage arises in this habit—for example, the mother does not appear when the infant is hungry—the image of the incompleted act arises in the mind of the infant; this is the second stage. By designating the image with a word or words (perhaps not at first part of the common lanugage but later so modified), he is in the future capable of calling up the image mentally even when he is not blocked. The image in our example is that of the mother feeding him, and through numerous similar events he is able to differentiate "mother" as an object designated as a symbol.

The world of the infant is at first a motley confusion of sights, sounds, and smells. He becomes able to differentiate a portion of this world only when he is able to designate it to himself by means of a symbol. Initially, the infant acts in a random fashion, and a socialized other responds to the random gestures in a meaningful way, thus giving a social definition to the random gesture of the infant. Once the infant understands the meaning of its gesture (e.g., a cry, a wave of the arm), through a combination of his imagining the completion of his act and of others' defining by their behavior the completion of the act for him, that gesture has become a symbol for him. Socialized others complete the act which the infant's gesture suggests to them and thus make a meaningful symbol out of the gesture for him. The symbol may remain fixed in meaning and value or take on increments of meaning and value, depending on subsequent experiences. In the third stage as the infant acquires a number of meanings, he uses them to designate to others as well as to himself what is in his mind. In the increasing communication, very slowly at first but with growing frequency, he learns new meanings (and later values) through purely symbolic communication from others. The new meaning is transmitted through combinations of, and analogies with, existing meanings. This is not to say that there is no further psychogenic learning, but as the fund of vocabulary increases, the child is able to learn by means of symbolic communication with ever increasing rapidity. The amount of such learning can increase throughout life, although typically the child reaches a level of socialization after a while and so does not try to learn much more, or there is not much more to be learned unless he moves into another culture or subculture. The *rate* of such learning reaches an insurmountable level which is a function of the intelligence and time limitations available to the child. Except for rare spurts, probably no child actually learns as rapidly as he is capable of learning once he achieves an adequate vocabulary, so intelligence limits are never a barrier to socialization except for the feebleminded child. There are, however, emotional and external barriers to socialization, as Rose (1960) has pointed out.

Assumption 3   *The socialization is not only into the general culture but also into various subcultures.*
A society has not only a culture expected to be learned by all, but also distinctive groups with their own subcultures. By his interactions within these groups, the child learns their subcultures at the same time as he learns the general culture. Through adult life, he may change his group affiliations and so continue to be socialized into subcultures, even though he may already be adequately socialized in terms of the general culture. Some group affiliations are typically dropped as the individual matures, whereas others are characteristically retained. Thus, socialization continues throughout life as society and its members are constantly creating new meanings and values. Social change results as these newer aspects are learned and some of the old ones are discarded.

Assumption 4   *While "old" groups, cultural expectations, and personal meanings and values may be dropped, in the sense that they become markedly lower on the reference relationship scale, they are not lost or forgotten.*
Symbolic interaction theory shares with psychoanalytic theory the assumption that man never forgets anything.* But this memory is not simply a retention of discrete "old" items; there is an *integration* of newly acquired meanings and values with existing ones, a continuing modification. In this integrative sense, man's behavior is a product of his life history, of all his experiences, both social and individual, both direct and vicarious through communication with others. The long-neglected concept of the nineteenth-century psychologist J. F. Herbart—"apperceptive mass"—would be valuable here if it is understood that it applies to all behavior and not merely to perception.

The integrated, cumulative, and evaluated character of experience—

---

*Mead would recognize that it is possible for a person not to recall something he once knew. That is, he cannot guide himself by the recollection because it is not a specific object for him. In the text we are pointing to the fact that the unremembered object still influences his behavior because it has been incorporated into the meanings of other objects.

symbolic learning—in symbolic interaction theory gives it certain aspects which are not found in other theories. We may consider the following characteristics of human experience as deductions from symbolic interactionist assumptions on a genetic level. In the first place, the relation of experience and behavior is seen as highly complex. While it is feasible to conceive of developing an automatic machine that can learn as an animal does, without symbolic learning—the "mechanical mouse" that learns to run a maze as efficiently as a live mouse—it is as yet beyond knowledge how to invent a machine that can learn and behave symbolically. It is not inconceivable theoretically to invent such a social machine, but the necessary knowledge is not nearly at hand, and the anthropomorphic machines optimistically or fearfully promised by certain scientists and engineers are a function of their behaviorist theories of man's psychology more than a function of their present knowledge.

Second, a *group* composed of individuals learning by means of symbols according to symbolic interaction theory, has a culture with a history. Thus there is no pure (i.e., uncultured) group that can serve as a universal control group in group-dynamics experiments. When Bales (1950) sought to measure the characteristics of such a "universal control group" he soon found the characteristics of the group changing and he had to collect new individuals periodically. Symbolic interactionists would interpret this to be partly a result of the individuals' getting to know each other and acting partly in terms of their increasingly informed expectations for each other's behavior. But, since each individual's behavior is a function of his cultural and subcultural experience in one degree or another, and since therefore he "knows" the other individuals as co-members of the society or subsocieties, they cannot form a "pure" group even before they come to know each other as individuals.

Third, because a person can never "unlearn" something—although he can drastically modify the learning ("relearn" it)—and because the conception of self is the most important meaning for man's behavior, a conception of self once learned affects an individual's behavior throughout his life. If an individual, for example, once conceives of himself as an alcoholic, a drug addict, a criminal, or whatever, he will never completely eliminate that self-conception, and—even if he were to be "cured" by learning new self-conceptions—a temptation to take a drink or drugs or steal something will have a challenging meaning for such an individual that it does not have for another individual who has never defined himself as an alcoholic, a drug addict, or criminal. The psychogenic "habit" may be broken, but the self-conception is never forgotten, and the ensuing behavior is an outcome of a struggle between an old self-conception and newer ones.

The symbolic interaction theory of human behavior has been stated above in outline form, without all the nuances and qualifications which its proponents would add. Mead's posthumously published *Mind, Self, and Society* is a far more complete and satisfactory, although in some ways obscure, statement of the theory. Yet the very starkness and simplicity of our statement has advantages for comprehension by those trained to think in other theoretical frameworks. Subsequent chapters in this work will develop selected aspects of the theory or will illustrate uses of the theory in empirical research.

REFERENCES

Bales RF: Interaction Process Analysis. Reading, Addison-Wesley, 1950
Park RE: Principles of Human Behavior. Chicago, The Zalaz Corp., 1915
Parsons T: Toward a healthy maturity. J Health Soc Behav 1:163, fall 1960
Rose AM: Incomplete socialization. Social Soc Res 44:244 March-April, 1960
Strauss A (ed): The Social Psychology of George H. Mead. Chicago, U. of Chicago
    Press, 1956

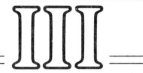

Developmental Models for Nursing Practice

Developmental Models are those that are based on theories of growth. They focus on growth and development, maturation, and socialization. Peplau is one author of a developmental model. Her model is described in Chapter 5 by Blake. For Peplau the person is an organism, living in an unstable equilibrium, who has the ability to learn and develop skills for solving problems and adapting to the tensions created by his needs. The goal of nursing action, according to Peplau, is the forward movement of the personality and other ongoing human processes in the direction of creative, constructive, productive, personal and community life. In the course of nursing intervention, the patient with a felt need seeks the assistance of a nurse. The patient and the nurse then begin to go through the phases and roles of the interpersonal process described by Peplau. Focus is always on the growth of patient and nurse. After Blake's chapter introduces the Peplau model, Nordal and Sato provide an application of the model to primary nursing.

The final chapter in this section was written by Chrisman and Fowler. They are respiratory clinical nurse specialists who together have developed a model that has proved serviceable for them in their practice. The framework of their model encompasses the biological, social, and personal systems in a continual process of change. Both structure and process are emphasized, with the systems constituting the structure, and development throughout life being the active process involving change. In addition to presenting the theory of their model, they describe how different levels of nursing personnel in a clinical setting can use the model. They discuss the implementation of the model utilizing the steps in the nursing process and include a comprehensive case analysis from their perspective as respiratory nurse specialists.

Mary Blake

5

The Peplau Developmental Model for Nursing Practice

This chapter explores one of the earliest nursing models to be developed, that of Hildegard E. Peplau. This significant leader in nursing presented the elements of her developmental model in her 1952 book, *Interpersonal Relations in Nursing*. The key concepts of the model will be described and then the elements of the model will be explored. Finally, Peplau's model will be applied to primary nursing in clinical practice.

KEY CONCEPTS DESCRIBED

As a framework for discussing Peplau's model, the key concepts used in the model are described below:

Interpersonal relations in nursing: the fostering of personality development in the direction of maturity.
Personality development: the dynamic interaction that occurs in early infancy and childhood at each era of development for the purpose of productive living.
Function of personality: to grow and to develop.
Nursing: an interpersonal process that aids patients to meet their present needs so that more mature ones can emerge and be met.
Need: a requirement within a person that creates tension. Tension creates energy that is transformed into some form of behavior.
Growth: the learning of more positive behaviors.
Society: culture.
Psychodynamic nursing: the ability to understand one's own behavior, to help others identify felt difficulties, and to apply principles of human relations to the problem.

Professional closeness: a special kind of involvement with a patient, client, or family that requires the nurse to observe the patient, and her own participation in the situation—the end result being a clinical judgment that would most likely benefit the patient.

Professional: those who know better than others the nature of certain matters; and know better than their clients what ails them or their affairs.

Health: conditions that facilitate forward movement of personality and other ongoing human processes in the direction of creative, constructive, productive, personal and community living.

ELEMENTS OF THE MODEL

The following discussion examines the elements of Peplau's model—the assumptions, goal of action, setting, goal of nursing, patiency and actor, source of difficulty, intervention focus, and consequences.

Assumptions

The Peplau developmental model for nursing (Peplau 1952) is based on four assumptions. The first assumption deals with man, the second with the nurse, and the third and fourth with nursing and nursing education.

Assumption 1: Man is an organism, living in an unstable equilibrium, who has the ability to learn and to develop skills for solving problems and adapting to the tensions created by his needs.

Assumption 2: The kind of person each nurse becomes makes a substantial difference in what each patient will learn as he is nursed through his illness.

Assumption 3: Fostering personality development in the direction of maturity is a function of nursing and nursing education; it requires the use of principles and methods that permit and guide the process of grappling with everyday interpersonal problems or difficulties.

Assumption 4: The nursing profession has legal responsibility for the effective use of nursing for its consequences to patients.

Goal of Action

Peplau defines nursing as an interpersonal process that focuses on the support processes, or self-repair and self-renewal. The author repeatedly stresses that the resultant experiential learning causes an evolution in both the patient and the nurse; that is, the nurse is also experiencing growth. In addition, in the learner's process of seeking healthy behaviors or in remediating unhealthy ones, the nurse can make an important difference.

The goal of action is the forward movement of the personality and other ongoing human process in the direction of creative, constructive, productive, personal, and community life. This means assisting the conditions of self-repair and self-renewal. These conditions are psychobiological in nature and are summarized in two categories: (1) physiological demands of the organism and (2) interpersonal needs of the organism. Meeting these demands and needs are part of the goal of forward movement.

Setting

The setting of nursing is everywhere—schools, clinics, hospitals, the entire community. Peplau stresses the role of the profession at all three preventive levels—primary, secondary, and tertiary—the primary being her ideal. She envisions that more individuals and communities will be able to experience health as more is known and taught about conditions that produce optimum health.

Goal of Nursing

In *Interpersonal Relations in Nursing* Peplau summarizes her concept of nursing as follows:

> Nursing is a significant, therapeutic, interpersonal process. It functions cooperatively with other human processes that make health possible for individuals in communities. In specific situations in which a professional health team offers health services, nurses participate in the organization of conditions that facilitate natural ongoing tendencies in human organisms. Nursing is an educative instrument, a maturing force, that aims to promote forward movement in the direction of creative, constructive, productive, personal and community living.

In later writings (1970, 1975, 1976) Peplau has expanded her description because she felt no definition of nursing would be complete without the idea of nursing collective action. Peplau stresses the role of nursing in the development of health plans, programs and policies, and involvement in broad and specific social issues such as the rights of women and the aging. She believes that nursing must be concerned with where nursing is, where nursing ought to be, and where nursing can be.

Patiency and Actor

Peplau's descriptions of patiency and actor presented in interpersonal terms, as each being contingent upon the other.

The patient is seen as a unique person, who is capable of new learning and positive change. While the recipient of the activity is the identified patient

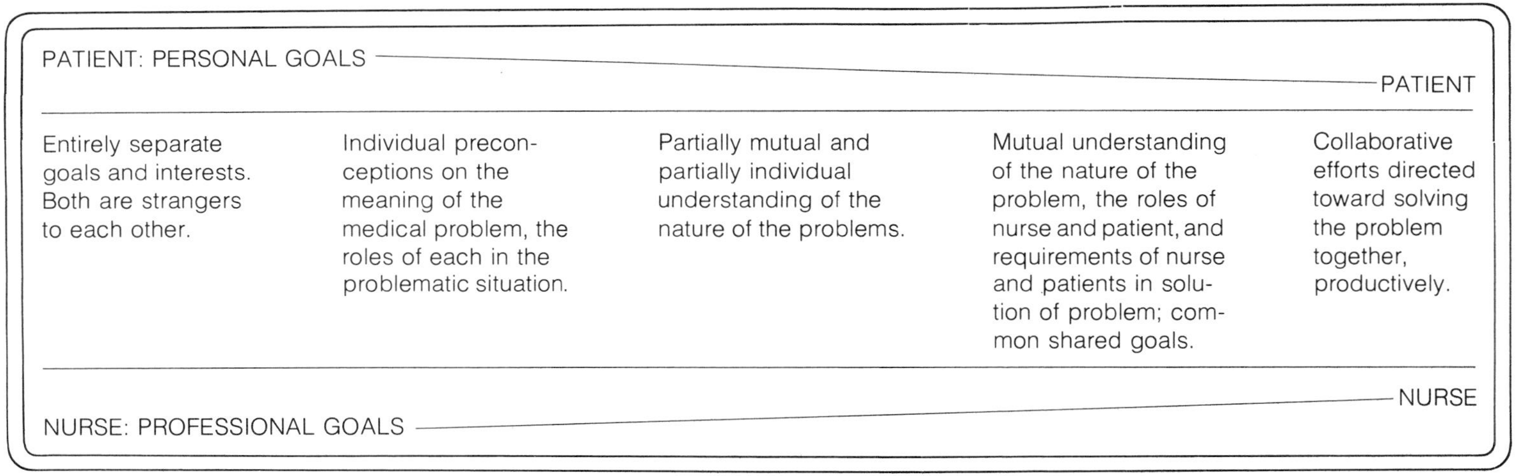

PATIENT: PERSONAL GOALS ————————————————PATIENT

Entirely separate goals and interests. Both are strangers to each other.	Individual precon- ceptions on the meaning of the medical problem, the roles of each in the problematic situation.	Partially mutual and partially individual understanding of the nature of the problems.	Mutual understanding of the nature of the problem, the roles of nurse and patient, and requirements of nurse and patients in solu- tion of problem; com- mon shared goals.	Collaborative efforts directed toward solving the problem together, productively.

NURSE: PROFESSIONAL GOALS ————————————————NURSE

Figure 1   A continuum showing changing aspects of nurse—patient relations.

in a health or illness setting, the nurse is also a participant in new learning and change. The nurse, however, has the responsibility to seek the skills that will help the patient make a positive change whenever it is possible.

The patient is a person undergoing stress, whether of a biological or a psychological origin. Stress creates tension and tension produces energy that can be used well or poorly. The nurse acts with the patient to help him define, understand, and deal productively with the problem at hand.

Figure 1 is a continuum showing the author's conception of the changing aspects of nurse–patient relations. The patient and nurse, upon meeting, may have entirely separate goals and interests. As their involvement progresses, their goals draw closer until, at the end of the continuum, there is productive collaboration.

Source of Difficulty

Source of difficulty refers to the originating point of deviations from the desired state or condition. If growth is the desired state, then what does Peplau see as inhibiting that growth? Basically, according to this model, the source of difficulty would be unmet needs, frustration, or a conflict of goals. We have seen that this meeting of needs is related to the achievement of the goal. Unmet needs, and the resulting frustration, then, are a source of difficulty. Since forward movement of the personality is goal oriented, a conflict of goals can also be a source of difficulty. Development is impeded by any of these difficulties.

Intervention Focus

Intervention begins when a patient with a felt need seeks assistance of a nurse in the hospital or community. The patient and nurse begin to go through phases and roles as they proceed with the interpersonal processes. The phases and roles are fluid in nature and tend to flow together or move backward or forward as the patient regresses or matures.

The patient goes through four phases as he moves toward health and the nurse keeps pace with him in the four corresponding steps of the nursing process (Peplau, 1952):

Patient	Nurse
Orientation Phase	Assessment
Identification Phase	Planning
Exploitation Phase	Intervention
Resolution Phase	Evaluation

In the orientation phase, the patient tries to learn the nature of his difficulty and the extent of his need for help. The nurse who is involved with the

Developmental Models for Nursing Practice

patient in the orientation phase is also learning as she uses her skills in the assessment process. The nurse must exercise critical judgment at this time because she must make an important distinction—whether the need is an emergency or whether action can be delayed until the patient can understand and collaborate and learn during the course of treatment. The patient *may* learn during the orientation phase; the nurse *must* learn as she proceeds with an attitude of professional closeness (Peplau, 1969).

The identification phase is the period in which the patient responds to persons who seem to offer the help he needs. He starts to feel as though he belongs. He identifies with the nurse. The nurse at that time is making the nursing diagnosis, formulating the nursing care plan, and identifying with the patient.

The exploitation phase occurs when the patient has identified with a nurse who can recognize and understand the interpersonal relations in the situation and the patient proceeds to make full use of the services offered to him. The nurse is intervening to help both the patient and the nurse to the mutual goal and the intended consequence—maturity.

The resolution phase is the period in which old ties and dependencies are relinquished as the patient prepares to go home or to resume independence. The nurse is doing the evaluation of the growth that occurred in both people.

As the patient goes through the four phases, he assumes the roles that are appropriate to his personality. For example, if he has not fully developed in an area during infancy, when he encounters the stress of illness he may regress. He may display the behavior of an infant or a child, even though he appeared a fully functional adult before the time of tension. The nurse responds by assuming one or several of the roles seen in Table 1, that is, counselor, if that is what the patient needs, or leadership role of technical expert. The final objective is, ideally, that the patient reach the resolution phase as an adult, mature person. The nurse, having learned from the interpersonal relationship, can also be seen in the adult role.

TABLE 1.   Phases and Changing Roles in Nurse—Patient Relationships

Nurse	Stranger	Unconditional Mother Surrogate		Counselor Resource person Leadership Surrogate Mother Sibling	Adult person
Patient	Stranger	Infant	Child	Adolescent	Adult person
		Orientation ⟶		Identification	
				Exploitation ⟶	Resolution

Consequences

The intended consequences of the model are (1) the positive use of the energy created by the person in stress in order that change and self-actualization may occur and (2) the increase of potential for intervention as knowledge about change is increased.

The unintended consequences of the model are (1) its indistinct mission for nursing and (2) the dependency of the goals of action on value systems.

Conclusion

The Peplau Model, with its attitude that both patient and nurse are capable of growth, provides an optimistic framework for nursing. It is hoped, as this most relevant of professions reaches toward a unified model, that it maintains the positive posture of Hildegard Peplau's work.

REFERENCE

Peplau HE: Professional closeness. Nurs Forum 8:4:346, 1969

Dorothy Nordal
Alice Sato

Peplau's Model Applied to Primary Nursing in Clinical Practice

A framework for nursing practice provides for the intelligent use of the nursing process. A model must be flexible, reality oriented, and applicable to the clinical unit. The purpose of this section is to apply Peplau's conceptual model to primary nursing. Utilization of the model will be explored through three patient case presentations within a primary nursing unit. For our purposes, the following definitions of key concepts are offered:

Primary nursing: The nursing care provided to the patient by one nurse who plans with the patient the type of care that is needed. The care includes coordination and integration with other health team members (Logsdon, 1973). The focus of nursing is on the developmental growth of patients and nurses.

Primary nurse: The registered nurse who is responsible for implementation of the nursing process for patients under her care from the time of admission to discharge (Hegyvary, 1977). The primary nurse plans and delegates care. She has full authority to see that the nursing care plan is followed. Lastly, she serves as a role model of professional nursing.

Associate nurse: One who cares for the patients in the absence of the primary nurse. The associate nurse may be a registered nurse or a licensed practical nurse.

Primary unit: May be a clinical floor in an acute care hospital that has primary nursing, or it may refer to a group of three to four patients under one primary nurse within the clinical setting.

PRIMARY NURSING

Primary nursing was introduced in 1970 at the University of Minnesota Hospital under the guidance of Marie Manthey. In the years since then, many hospitals across the nation have adopted primary nursing because it is patient centered, family and community oriented, and professionally satisfying to the nurses themselves, and allows for continuity of care (Scott, 1977 and Daef-fler, 1975). Also, it is more cost effective than team nursing (Marram, 1976, and Swanson, 1977). Although nurses do not like to equate money and patient care, the reality of the situation is that if a hospital cannot survive financially, it will have to cut back on services. It appears from review of the literature that primary nursing does have much to offer and is gaining in popularity. The philosophy of primary nursing and Peplau's conceptual model for nursing are very nearly congruent and homogeneous.

SIMILARITIES

Twelve similarities have been identified and will be explored.

1. The head nurse assumes many roles as the nursing care coordinator of a primary care unit. For example, she is a leader, counselor, resource person, and a staff development person. The head nurse facilitates the staff in identifying growth potentials within themselves by mutual dialogue. When a new nurse is hired, it is the head nurse's duty to provide unit inservice training for development of primary nursing skills. The head nurse assigns patients to primary nurses, keeping in mind to match the skills of a nurse with the needs of the patient (Marram, 1974). The role of the primary nurse is teacher, counselor, technical expert, resource person in her relationships with the patient and nursing staff working with her.
2. There is always a one-to-one interaction; for example, nurse to nurse, patient to nurse, nurse to health team member (Figure 1).
3. Every individual is unique. The patient and the nurse are unique in their personality development. A patient may have grown and developed his potential up until the time of his hospital admission, when a dependency need unfulfilled in the early developmental years may surface as a result of stress.
4. Concern for the total patient is stressed. One cannot deal with a physical need while ignoring psychological needs and still label the process therapeutic nursing.
5. Continuity of care is emphasized. In primary nursing, each patient has an individualized 24-hour nursing care plan. Peplau's model uses process records to ensure continuity of care.
6. Development and growth of the nurse is accented. Much like a chain reaction, in primary nursing the head nurse provides for an environment that will allow for developmental growth of her staff. The staff helps one another (Manthey, 1973). Peplau's model places the responsibility for

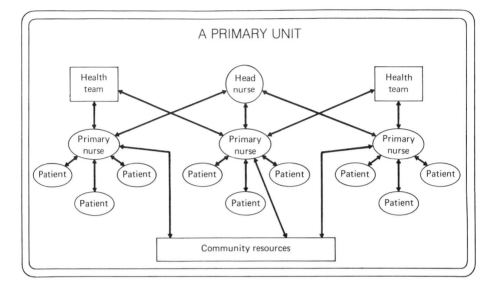

Figure 1 *Primary nursing.*

developing mature, young adults on the schools of nursing. After the student graduates, growth continues through professional contact.

7. The primary nurse is responsible for personality development towards maturity and growth for each patient. Because illness and hospitalization are oftentimes unique experiences for the patient, the nurse helps him to view the experience as a growth process.

8. Concern for the family and significant others is stressed. Peplau and primary nursing recognize the role of the family, society, culture, and the environment. The nurse dons her role as a resource person and counselor to coordinate the health care from hospital to community (Figure 1).

9. Nursing goals are set by the patient and the nurse. Peplau (1952) states that "if the nurse has a goal and the patient has a different goal, disharmony results." In the nursing process, goals are set by the patient and the nurse bearing in mind that a developmental behavior is altered positively or negatively by a felt need that may also affect the achievement of the goal.

10. A nurse is flexible, creative, and innovative in responding to the patient's felt needs. The primary nurse has the freedom to expand and grow in giving patient care because she is ultimately held responsible for each 24 hours of care. Peplau stresses the importance of being creative; for example, experiential learning in the nursing setting is a way for nurses to learn, and, in turn, to teach patients (Peplau, 1957).

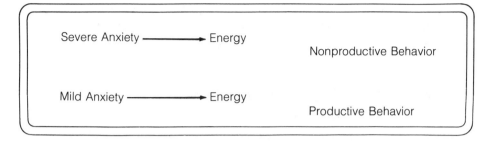

Figure 2 Anxiety levels.

11. Research to expand nursing knowledge is advocated by primary nursing and Peplau. Primary nursing enthusiasts are searching for more research to evaluate patient satisfaction, effectiveness of nursing practice, and cost effectiveness of primary nursing in comparison to team nursing. Twenty-five years ago, Peplau was advocating the role of research in nursing practice, such as in areas of interpersonal relations.

12. It is recognized that every interaction is not perfect and ideal. Stress, tension, and anxiety may be caused by personality development conflicts between the nurse and the patient. It becomes most imperative that the nurse acknowledge and identify the needs that are causing the tension. Energy expended from tension must be channeled into productive behavior or no progress will be made (Figure 2). On the other hand, a negative experience is not totally lost.

From the experience, both the patient and the nurse will grow in future similar interactions, at which point, hopefully, the experience will be a fulfilling one.

In summary, the main similarity between primary nursing and Peplau's model is that both stress the personality development and growth toward maturity of the patient and the nurse through the educative process. The process involves lifelong commitment.

Peplau's conceptual model as the basis for the nursing process is shown in Table 1.

**TABLE 1. Peplau's Conceptual Model as the Basis
for the Nursing Process**

Phases	Steps
1. Orientation	1. Assessment
2. Identification	2. Nursing Diagnosis
3. Exploitation	3. Intervention
4. Resolution	4. Evaluation

In Peplau's model of the nursing process, the patient and the nurse must be together, as for example, in a three-legged race. If the patient or the nurse falters, eventually both will fall and no progress will be made.

APPLICATION OF PEPLAU'S MODEL TO PRIMARY NURSING

In view of the many resemblences between primary nursing and Peplau's model for nursing, it is the intent of the authors to demonstrate the applicability of the model via the nursing process. A primary unit composed of three clients—a diabetic, a terminal cancer patient, and a stroke patient—is the setting. The unit is located within an acute care hospital on the medical floor.

Case Presentation 1

Mr. D. is 28 years old, single, robust, and self-assured. Mr. D was admitted via the emergency room with a diagnosis of metabolic acidosis due to insulin-dependent diabetes.

During the nursing history interview, Mr. D appeared to accept the fact that the diabetes would surely change or modify his life-style. He asked his primary nurse, Ms. Snow, many questions about diabetes, referring repeatedly to the necessity of taking insulin injections every morning—"Why can't I just take those diabetic pills instead?"

Mr. D displayed some anxiety over his health status although he tried valiantly to present a I-can-handle-anything-attitude. Ms. Snow allowed Mr. D to continue verbalizing his feelings and thoughts. Through this process Ms. Snow identified much data that was transferred from patient to nurse. (Figure 3). Through the nursing process, Ms. Snow and Mr. D arrived at the source of conflict for the client: fear of pain from insulin injections. During the nurse–patient interactions, it was revealed that as a child Mr. D had to have weekly allergy injections. Mr. D recalls that the injections were very painful and that he had much reservation about inflicting pain upon himself every morning.

Once this need was identified and resolved, Mr. D and the nurse were free to progress to other problems.

To help the reader follow the next two presentations, the authors suggest a review of Table 1 (page 63). The table is an adaptation of Peplau's model correlated with patients' phases of illness as identified by Gooding (1972).

PATIENT*	NURSE*	ACTION
Phase: Orientation The patient assesses the new environment on behavioral level. Anxiety may be present. Willingness to accept help†	Step: Assessment Allows the patient to freely express needs and feelings. Is nonjudgmental. A good listener. Many roles of the nurse surface.†	Patient's anxiety level is in a productive behavior stage. A trusting interpersonal relationship is established. Nurse gathers objective, subjective data. Checks overt and covert feelings of patient.
Phase: Identification Feels like he belongs. Identifies with a nurse on developmental level.†	Step: Nursing Diagnosis Identifies nursing problem by developmental responses of patient.†	Patient and nurse agree on a goal: lessening fear of pain from insulin injections.
Phase: Exploitation Mixed feelings of dependency vs. independency. Makes full use of the services offered to him, i.e., developmental strengths of others, other health team members.†	Step: Intervention Understands shifts in feelings. Explains all the teaching aids available.† Explains community resources that are available.	Allows patient freedom to express feelings of conflict. Patient looks at films on insulin injection techniques. Starts injecting a false arm. Discharge planning starts.
Phase: Resolution The "freeing process" begins.† Patient is independent of the nurse in giving himself insulin injections.	Step: Evaluation Goal is accomplished.†	Patient can give own insulin injections safely and comfortably.

*The patient and the nurse must be working together in the same phase or step.
†The chief characteristic of the phase or step.

Figure 3 **Peplau's conceptual model applied to the nursing process (Case 1).**

TABLE 2. Overlapping and Interconnecting of the Nurse—Patient Phases

Phases of Illness*

I	II	III	IV	V
Initial Symptom Uncertainty and Worry	Diagnosis Alarm Reaction	Initial Prescription Rationalization and Stress	Convalescence Period of Adaptation, Conflict Frustration	Rehabilitation Restoration of Equilibrium
Community ——————→		Hospital ——————→		Community
Orientation	Identification	Exploitation	Resolution	
Evaluating available community resources	Providing information regarding care processes	Continuing assessment	Assisting with goal-setting	Teaching preventative measures
Initiating and participating in programs for health education	Establishing confidence	Providing consistent approaches in care	Promoting family interaction	Communicating with community agencies
Assisting with public relations	Interpreting behavior	Identifying positive factors	Manipulating the environment	Terminating interaction
Focusing patient's energies in right direction	Assessing needs	Initiating rehabilitative plans	Teaching self-care	
		Planning for total needs	Counselling for readjustment	
		Reducing anxiety		

Orientation	Identification	Exploitation	Resolution
Seeking assistance†	Responds to help	Identifies with nurse	Terminal phase of the nurse–patient relationship
Educative needs	Problem solving	Makes full use of ser- vices	Extension of patient to future
Aid clarification	Observation	Exploits all services on basis of self-interest	Intermingling of needs and shuffling back and forth
Consent	Participation or inter- dependent relations with nurse	Explores possibilities	Strength—ability to stand alone
Understanding	Independence	More demanding	Freeing process
Expectations	Dependence, help- lessness	Self directing	
Patient observes and asks questions			

Orientation‡ ⟶ Identification ⟶ Exploitation ⟶ Resolution

*Gooding: Techniques for Utilizing Nursing Principles. St. Louis, Mosby 1972, p 59.
†Peplau E: Interpersonal Relations in Nursing, New York, 1952, Chapter Two.
‡Ibid, p 54.

Gooding illustrates the important concepts of alarm reaction (anxiety), periods of adaptation, conflicts, and frustration. Additional activities were added from Peplau (1952) under the four categories noted above. The activities and roles of the nurse and patient are stressed under phases of nurse–patient relationships, which are located at the bottom of the chart, to emphasize that the phases are flexible and move in a continuum.

Case Presentation 2

Mrs. H, a 54-year-old female with an original diagnosis of cancer of the breast, was treated with bilateral mastectomy and later, adrenalectomy. The cancer progressed to her bones. She had problems with her hips and eventually her spinal column began to disintegrate. Mrs. H's prognosis was terminal cancer. Treatment centered around emotional support and palliative measures.

Mrs. H's husband, a builder and construction worker, was very supportive. He worked in another state occasionally and could not be with his wife all of the time. Their relationship was one of strength, openness, love, and honesty. They had four children: two daughters, aged 15 and 17 years, and two sons, aged 19 and 21 years.

Resolution Phase: The Patient

Mrs. H was accepting of her diagnosis and understood the seriousness of her prognosis. Mrs. H's warmth and concern for those within her reach impressed everyone. When her doctor, an oncologist, visited, Mrs. H would look him directly in the eyes as he stood by her bedside and held her hand. The communication fluctuated between verbal and nonverbal. The interaction was very strong and positive, as if each one drew strength from the other.

Resolution Phase: The Nurse

In communicating with Mrs. H's husband, it was obvious that he had much anxiety and worry for his wife. His biggest concern was how he could make his wife's remaining days as meaningful as possible. The nurse suggested that he spend as much time as his work schedule would allow with his wife and communicate in a way that showed his interest, warmth, and concern for her well-being and desires. Mr. H accepted the suggestion. By the nursing intervention, Mr. H was able to direct his energies toward actions that would be most beneficial to his wife.

From the nurse's point of view, she must understand her feelings and beliefs about cancer and death. She must be strong enough emotionally to cope with her own feelings in order to accept the fears and doubts of another in a purposeful therapeutic interaction.

Developmental Needs of Patient and Nurse

The developmental needs of a cancer patient are recognition and acceptance, a receptive listener, individualized care, genuine concern and interest in the patient and those close to him (George, 1973).

The developmental needs of a nurse are technical competence to meet the patient's physical needs. The nurse builds the patient's self-esteem by therapeutic use of self (George, 1973).

Final Stage of Cancer

The most important aspect of helping a patient in the final stage of cancer is to allow her the opportunity to develop and grow in the time remaining. The cancer patient knows that time is limited and she will plan accordingly. Mrs. H's priority was to have a nurse write a letter to her husband because she did not have enough strength to hold a pen. Mrs. H asked her associate nurse to write the letter while Mrs. H dictated. The associate nurse could not participate in this emotionally laden activity; she sought aid from the primary nurse.

The primary nurse was able to discuss the patient's frustration at not being able to write the letter. Together the patient and the primary nurse "wrote" the letter, one dictating and one writing, both emotionally involved and tearful. The beautiful letter was completed through the joint effort of the patient and nurse. The result of this experience was not just the letter, but a sharing by two individuals of life's hopes, desires, realities, and beliefs. It was a growth process for the patient and the nurse.

The patient's last act of love was toward the development and growth of her husband primarily, but in the process the two nurses grew as professionals and human beings. In future situations with a dying patient, both nurses will have experiential background to rely on. For a schematic representation of this case, refer to Figure 4 correlating it with Tables 1 and 2.

An Addendum to Peplau's Model

Peplau states that knowledge is lacking to arrest all pathological processes or to reverse physiologic functioning in the direction of self-repair, for example, in advanced cancerous growth or extensive tuberculosis lesions. In such cases, Peplau recognizes that the patient has the right to die (Peplau, 1952). Kubler-Ross (1975), however, views death as the last stage of growth. The first step is seen as acceptance of death as the beginning of growth:

Developmental Models for Nursing Practice

Our acceptance of our own being, that is, our sensing that we are significant as a person, depends on knowing that we are accepted by someone or something larger than our individual self.

Such was the case with Mrs. H who was accepted by her husband, family, nurses and other health team members, and God. She had committed herself to awareness of her own original experience; however, she had to communicate to share that experience with others, and in turn, to appreciate and understand the original experience with others. She increasingly committed herself by dialogue,

---

Patient: Mrs. H, 54 years old
Diagnosis: Terminal cancer
Personality developmental stage of patient: Adult person*
Phase of interpersonal relations: Resolution
Nursing process step: Intervention and evaluation
Nursing problem: Patient's frustration level is high because she cannot write a final letter of love to her husband before she dies.
Role of primary nurse: Technical expert and professional leader to patient, resource person to husband, and teacher to the associate nurse.
Role of patient: Teacher to primary nurse
Role of husband: Counselor to patient, learner to primary nurse and wife, resource person to patient and primary nurse.
Nursing interventions: (1) The associate nurse tried to help the patient write the letter, but the nurse's developmental growth and maturity toward death had not been developed and she could not help Mrs. H; (2) The primary nurse allowed Mrs. H to verbalize her frustrations. Once the stress level was reduced, the patient dictated while the nurse wrote the letter.
Patient needs: Psychological—independent.   Biological—dependent. The patient could not hold the pen to write the letter. She was so weak that she could not care for herself.

*Mrs. H was in the stage of acceptance of death according to Kubler-Ross. The concept of death—the last stage of growth—has been added to this presentation.

Figure 4.   *Peplau's conceptual model applied to the nursing process (Case 2).*

letter writing, conversation, and mutual exchange with others (Kubler-Ross, 1975).

Allport (1950) sees present awareness of one's self as a major attribute of maturity. This coincides with the behavior of terminally ill persons who move toward resolution of grief. Resolution is a freeing process, but it depends for its possible success on the preceding chain of events (Peplau, 1952). Mrs. H. is an example of a patient who had arrived at acceptance and resolution. Her ultimate and final stage of growth was sharing with others.

Case Presentation 3

Mr. N, a 56-year-old male with a very recent cerebral vascular accident, was admitted to the hospital in an unconscious and comatose state (see Figure 5). The prognosis was favorable. The treatment for Mr. N centered around physical care. The family was very apprehensive and followed every movement that was made toward their father and husband.

Orientation Phase: The Patient and the Nurse

Mr. N was in a dependent stage due to his unconscious state and had to rely totally on the primary nurse at this time. Although there was no verbal communication between patient and nurse, the client's needs were met through the authoritative role of the nurse in a concrete situation (emergency) such as Mr. N's. The primary nurse will go through the orientation and identification phases. Once the patient awakens, the nurse will return to the orientation phase so the two can go through the interpersonal phases together.

Orientation Phase: The Family and the Nurse

The primary nurse recognizes that the family members must be permitted to verbally vent their tensions, apprehensions, and concerns for the patient. Assessing the developmental strengths and weaknesses of family members will give the primary nurse data on which to start the nursing care plan, incorporating family members.

Identification Phase: The Family and the Nurse

Once the family's anxiety and tension level is reduced to a working stage, the primary nurse and the family will arrive at a nursing problem: Family is experiencing stress and helplessness over patient's illness.

Patient: Mr. N, 56 years old.

Diagnosis: Cerebral vascular accident.

Personality developmental role of patient: Infant or unknown.

Personality developmental role of nurse: Stranger, unconditional mother surrogate, professional leader.

Nursing assessment: Objective data gathering.

Nursing problem 1:   Patient is unresponsive due to unconscious state.

Nursing action: The primary nurse will move through the phases of the interpersonal relations to meet the needs of the patient during the emergency state.* When the patient becomes aware of his environment the nurse and patient will go through the phases together.

Nursing problem 2:   Family members are experiencing stress because they cannot communicate with their loved one.

Family needs: Dependent. They feel helpless and stressful over the patient.

Nursing action: The primary and associate nurses will help the family grow by allowing them to verbalize their feelings. They will be shown ways to help the patient; for example, nurses will relate the patient's strengths and weaknesses and teach family members to give range of motion exercises, thereby channeling the family's tension toward positive outlets.

Patient needs: Psychological—may be dependent or independent contingent upon prior developmental growth. Status will be evaluated when the patient awakens. The biological need is dependent.

*With the nurse as the only participant, typically she will proceed to identification phase. Physical care or concrete care can occur without the nurse–patient relationship in an authoritative situation (emergency).

Figure 5   *Peplau's conceptual model applied to the nursing presentation (Case 3).*

Exploitation Phase: The Family and the Nurse

The primary nurse is aware of the need to channel the energies of the family into productive outlets. To accomplish this in Mr. N.'s case, she demonstrated to the family how to give range of motion exercises to Mr. N and stressed the importance of such exercises on a regular basis. Because they had an avenue to physically help the patient, the family's helplessness was reduced. The primary nurse has helped the family in their developmental growth through the educative process.

Resolution Phase: The Family and the Nurse

The nurse directed the family's tension into positive action. She continued to counsel and guide the family as they encountered new problems during Mr. N's hospitalization.

CONCLUSION

We have shown similarities between Peplau's conceptual model and primary nursing. Both stress the developmental growth and maturity of the patient and the nurse through the educative process. Applicability of Peplau's model in a primary nursing unit was demonstrated by three case presentations emphasizing the importance of interpersonal relations among patient, nurse, and family in implementing the nursing process. Identification of tension, frustration, or anxiety in individuals as the source of energy transferred to nonproductive behavior is a high priority within clinical practice based on Peplau's model.

REFERENCES

Allport G: The Nature of Personality, Addison Wesley, Cambridge, Mass, 1950

Daeffler R: Patients' perception of care under team and primary nursing. J Nurs Admin March–April 1975, pp. 24–26

George M: Long term care of the patient with cancer. Nurs Clin North Am 8:4:631, 1973

Gooding M: Techniques for Utilizing Nursing Principles. St Louis, Mosby, 1972

Hegyvary ST: Foundations of primary nursing. Nurs Clin North Am: 12:2:192, 1977

Kubler-Ross E: Death, the Final Stage of Growth. New Jersey, Prentice-Hall, 1975

Logsdon A: Why primary nursing? Nurs Clin of North Am 8:2:284, 1973

Manthey M: Primary nursing is alive and well in the hospital. Am J Nurs 73:1:83, 1973

Marram G: The comparative costs of operating a team and primary care unit, J Nurs Admin: May 1976, p 24

Marram GD, Schelegel M, Bevis EO: Primary Nursing: A Model for Individualized Care. St. Louis, Mosby, 1974

Peplau HE: Interpersonal Relations in Nursing. New York, Putnam's, 1952

Peplau HE: What is experiential teaching? Am J Nurs 57:886, 1957

Peplau HE: ANA's new executive director states her views. Am J Nurs 70:1:84, 1970

Peplau HE: Midlife crisis. Am J Nurs 75:10, 1975

Peplau HE: Nurses need new image as intellectual, inquiring professionals. AORN Journal 24:2:218, 1966

Peplau HE: Professional closeness. Nurs Forum 8:4:346, 1969

Marilyn K. Chrisman
Marsha D. Fowler

The Systems-In-Change Model for Nursing Practice

Applying nursing models to nursing practice is not an easy task. However, models can provide a standard for optimal patient care, regardless of setting or the health problems encountered. Both direct technical and nontechnical nursing care require a patient-centered frame of reference that can be operationalized through the nursing process. Models discussed elsewhere in this text include systems and developmental theories, adaptational concepts and stress. Both the systems and developmental models emphasize structure and analyze human characteristics and variables from their respective viewpoints. The adaptation and stress concepts are process oriented. They interpret human behavior according to those theoretical frameworks and propose a corresponding nursing approach to health problems.

These concepts are valid, theoretically sound, and pertinent to nursing activities. However, there are two major areas in which their utility is compromised: (1) applicability to clinical practice and (2) comprehensiveness and flexibility. In an attempt to incorporate the above theories and to overcome these obstacles, the following model was developed. Furthermore, this model was designed to meet the practical demands of clinical practice, integrating them within a comprehensive and easily understood framework.

THE SYSTEMS-IN-CHANGE MODEL

The purpose of the systems-in-change model is to provide a framework for practice and a conceptual approach to the nursing process. Both structure and process are emphasized. The framework refers to biologic, social, and personal systems in a continual process of change. It encompasses a broad philosophic base that brings together assumptions, values, and ethical principles pertinent to nursing.

Since nursing has an impact upon the lives of individuals and society, the professional beliefs, values, and presuppositions that underlie this perspective of "man as a system in change" should be reviewed. The following statements describe underlying nursing beliefs and values in this model:

1. Professional nursing functions and activities are directed by a therapeutic purpose.
2. Underlying all nursing activity is a genuine caring and concern for the welfare of the patient.
3. Critical analysis of the patient-client and his condition is accompanied by respect for him as an individual whose dignity is always to be maintained.
4. The patient is an integral part of all planning and decision making.
5. The nurse is the patient's advocate when he cannot be his own.
6. The nurse supports and promotes health and the quality of life. According to a definition adapted from the World Health Organization, health means complete physical, personal, and social well-being, not solely the absence of disease or infirmity.

The model framework includes the following assumptions:

1. Man can be viewed as three dynamic systems interacting with each other and with the environment, along a developmental continuum.
2. The status of each system and its interactions influence health.
3. An individual moves through time gradually from one developmental stage to another. Information and effects from the past are stored and may be incorporated into the present and utilized in the future.
4. Change is inherent in life and growth.

The structure of this model is an organized way to analyze interdependent aspects of any given patient situation. The process refers to changes that influence the growth and equilibria of the systems. Changes include those taking place within and among the individual systems and along the developmental continuum. The patient problems that are identified can be explored and can suggest implications for nursing intervention. The model framework and its implementation are discussed below.

THE STRUCTURE: SYSTEMS

At any point man can be viewed as interacting biologic, social, and personal systems that are open to the environment and to each other. These systems have an internal organization yet are interdependent and interact with each other as an integrated whole. Feedback among the systems and with the environment is a crucial aspect of the interactional process. Changes inside or outside the systems may produce stress, which disturbs the tendency of the systems to achieve a state of equilibrium. Each of the systems must be examined for its state of equilibrium (integrity of functional status). Each should also be examined for the presence, absence, or alteration of those compensatory or regulatory mechanisms that help the individual system achieve, restore or maintain its optimal integrity.

Systems can be studied in the present while at the same time the input of the patient's past and the potential for his future are considered. For example, in the biologic system past illnesses and risk factors hold implications for present and future care and must be considered with the patient's present situation.

THE PROCESS: CHANGE

Birth, growth, maturation and dying are integral parts of life. The nurse deals with the patient anywhere along this life continuum. To a greater or lesser extent the patient's present always consists of a past and a potential future. His development includes genetically and environmentally directed change that affects all systems. Stages of development range from the prenatal period, infancy, childhood, adolescence, young adulthood, adulthood, and middle age through advanced age. In all stages, development is an active process involving change.

In assessing developmental change two questions must be asked: (1) What do I observe, measure, or otherwise detect that identifies the developmental stage of this patient's biologic, social, and personal systems? (2) Considering the patient's chronological age and sociocultural milieu, what developmental stages (and consequent observations) should I expect?

Comparing the answers to these two questions, the nurse will be able to establish a general developmental assessment that will influence systems assessment, therapeutic goals, and the selection of interventions. If a serious and deficit discrepancy between observed data and expectations exists in one or more systems, then specific assessment tools should be utilized to delimit and identify the developmental problem.

In addition to developmental changes, the systems are continually undergoing change as they process input and deal with ever-changing internal and external environments (see Figure 1).

The model framework should encourage the nurse to systematically examine the multitude of variables that may affect the patient at any point. A variety of concepts and theories are available to the nurse for application in any clinical setting. For example, theories of stress may be most applicable to the intensive care setting, while adaptation theories may be better suited to long term or rehabilitative nursing. Both of these theories or other concepts

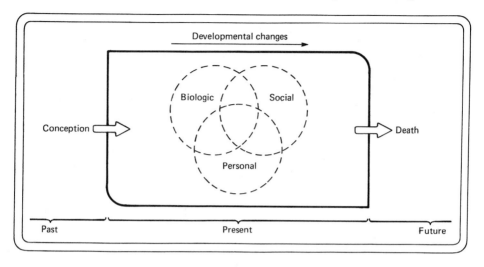

Figure 1. *Diagrammatic representation of the systems-in-change model.*

can be incorporated within an open framework of systems and change. This model should be considered to have a flexible framework and should assist the nurse in understanding clinical phenomena. One or more components of the model may be emphasized to meet the exigencies of the clinical situation or the perspective of the nurse. For example, one parochial school of nursing that adapted the model incorporated their school's spiritual emphasis by placing man's systems and environment within a theistic context. Despite changes in emphasis, however, all systems should be assessed and included in nursing care.

THE CLINICAL SITUATION

An applied model should be congruent with the variety of nursing activities that make up nursing practice. What does the nurse do? Most nurses who deal in direct nursing care to patients are engaged in both technical and nontechnical activities. Furthermore, since nursing has established divisions of labor among levels of nursing personnel, it is important to question how the model can relate to different nursing positions. Some suggestions follow.

The Nursing Assistant
The focus of supervised activities for the nursing assistant is on monitoring and detecting major signs of physical problems and patient feelings. The

nursing assistant's actions are aimed at implementing directed monitoring, safety, comfort measures, and selected therapies. Activities are present oriented, and the surrounding physical environment is considered in giving care.

The Licensed Vocational/Practical Nurse

The LVN helps to plan, effect, and direct safety and comfort measures. The LVN administers directed medical and nursing therapy. Nursing care is oriented to the present, and the surrounding physical space is considered in giving care. The LVN can use the model to examine prominent physical, social, and personal changes and to apply appropriate knowledge and skill.

The Registered Nurse

The nursing focus is the interplay of changes in the biologic, social, and personal systems in relation to the environment and the patient's developmental stage. Nursing assessment examines the patient's past and present and projects future change. The RN administers directed medical therapy and independent nursing therapy.

The Clincal Nurse Specialist

The CNS employs the same focus as the RN. He/she focuses on the interplay of each of the systems in relation to the patient's environment and developmental stage. The CNS also assesses the patient with respect to his past, present and future. In addition, the CNS may deliver care in a variety of health-delivery settings. The systems-in-change framework serves to guide the CNS as a practitioner, community health advocate, consultant, change agent, and researcher.

THE NURSING PROCESS

As a problem-solving approach, the nursing process examines the care the nurse delivers by its component parts: assessment, diagnosis and/or problem identification, goal setting, interventions, and evaluation (see Appendixes A and B).

Assessment

Nursing assessment is an organized information-gathering process with a therapeutic purpose. Any mode of data collection such as records, observations, interaction, interviews, self-reactions, physiologic or psychologic measurements are appropriate.

As discussed above, the major elements of nursing assessment in this model include examination of the following:

1. Status of each system: biologic, social, personal
   a. Functional baseline
   b. Compensatory and/or regulatory mechanisms
   c. Signs and symptoms of dysfunctional changes
2. Developmental variables: observations and expectations
3. Environmental variables

In patient assessment, systems and change are examined simultaneously. This examination includes the determination of the patient's usual baseline, including his developmental level. Assessment also involves an examination of (1) the current status of function of each of the systems, (2) signs and symptoms of dysfunctional changes within each system, and (3) the environment as it influences the systems. The systems can be analyzed according to areas that traditionally have been studied and written about in the literature and confronted in the clinical setting. The systems are described below in more detail. The implications derived from medical care and the care of other health disciplines must be considered as assessment variables for each system.

The biological system of man may be analyzed in the following subsystems:

1. Physical
   a. General health
   b. Skin, hair, and nails
   c. Head, face, and neck
   d. Breast
   e. Respiratory
   f. Cardiovascular and lymphatic
   g. Abdomen and gastrointestinal
   h. Renal and urinary
   i. Sexual and reproductive
   j. Skeletomuscular
   k. Neurosensory
   l. Endocrine
   m. Hematopoietic
   n. Immunologic
2. Activities of daily living and habits
   a. Nutrition and hydration
   b. Sleep and rest
   c. Exercise
   d. Hygiene
   e. Sex
   f. Work

Of course, the above categorization has built-in limitations, such as arbitrary anatomic and functional divisions, but it can provide a useful guide to physiologic problems as well as medical diagnostic categories. In addition, the biologic systems are congruent with many major health system specialties.

The social subsystems identify social variables and their interplay with biologic and personal systems. These subsystems include the areas listed below. Social development should be considered as an assessment variable, particularly with items three and four.

1. Culture
2. Socioeconomic influences
3. Roles
   a. Sexual
   b. Occupational
   c. Familial
   d. Affiliative
   e. Communal
   f. Religious
4. Play
   a. Developmental work
   b. Recreation
5. Situation
   a. Immediate context
   b. Current life events and circumstances

The personal subsystems relate to the personal self. They are never seen directly but are always felt and reacting. Subsystems include the following:

1. Philosophical vlaues and beliefs and moral development
2. Spiritual view
3. Self-concept
   a. Body image
   b. Self-awareness
   c. Self-esteem
   d. Self-ideal
   e. Sexuality
4. Personality characteristics, e.g., dependency/independency
5. Intelligence/education

By establishing a thorough assessment baseline, with ongoing revisions as new data is obtained, sufficient basis is provided for the formulation and/or substantiation of nursing diagnoses or problem identification.

Nursing Diagnosis/Problem Identification

A nursing diagnosis or a nursing problem is a descriptive statement of actual or potential dysfunction in one or more of the systems. The diagnosis/

problem should be patient centered, problem oriented and substantiated by subjective and/or objective data. It must be noted that there is considerable controversy surrounding the identification of nursing diagnoses. For the purposes of this model, and at this time, a nursing diagnosis is considered to be a comprehensive and well-substantiated statement of dysfunction in the biological, social, or personal system, over which the nurse has province. A nursing problem, on the other hand, may take either of two forms. It may be a variable that has implication(s) for health care, for example, inadequate transportation to clinic visits. A nursing problem may also be a component part of a nursing diagnosis, for example, when depression is tentatively identified as a dysfunction in the personal system. Subsequent data reveal that the depression is a component of this patient's grief reaction. "Grief reaction" is the nursing diagnosis, while "depression" is a component problem. In some situations depression may stand alone as a diagnosis.

Diagnoses can be drawn from the rich variety in nursing literature, which includes a diversity of subjects, e.g., anxiety, sleep deprivation, and malnutrition. There are several approaches to the development of nursing diagnoses. One major approach involves comprehensive and exhaustive data collection. This subsequently progresses to the generation of diagnoses. Another approach begins at the point of identifying the chief problem, symptom, or concern. Data are then collected to identify related variables and shared characteristics. From this data, diagnoses are identified. Whatever the approach to data collection, certain precautions must be observed. Whenever an hypothesis is generated, clinical liabilities may include (1) possible bias caused by the tentative diagnosis, (2) premature weighting of findings, and (3) inflexibility of data interpretation.

When the nursing diagnosis has been clearly defined and substantiated by data, goals and objectives may then be formulated.

Goals and Objectives

A nursing goal reflects the direction of change that is required by the nursing diagnosis. Goals are general patient-centered statements of therapeutic outcomes. An attempt should be made to formulate specific outcome objectives congruent with the goal. Outcome objectives help to gauge progress toward a goal, identifying the component steps toward that goal. Objectives identify short-term and long-term priorities. Both goals and objectives assist the nurse in selecting specific nursing interventions.

Intervention

The nursing intervention selected must be congruent with nursing goals and objectives, the patient's situation, and the nurse's skills. The nurse is accountable for the identification of patient problems and for the interventions employed to deal with those problems. The mode of intervention includes therapeutic use of social self, transactions with others, techniques, or the therapeutic use of the environment. Throughout the nursing process and particularly subsequent to intervention, the entire nursing process must be subjected to evaluation.

Evaluation

Within the nursing process, evaluation is directed toward both process outcomes and therapeutic outcomes. Evaluation should proceed both concurrently with care and as a retrospective analysis of care. The nurse should be able to identify through evaluation the thoroughness and appropriateness of the implementation of each phase of the nursing process. Furthermore, evaluation identifies the efficiency and effectiveness of the use of the nursing process, that is, to what degree the desired therapeutic outcome has been achieved.

Evaluation can be a sensitive indicator of the dynamic nature of the nursing process and the System-in-Change model. It serves to provoke continuous remobilization of the nursing process and reflection on systems analysis and the process of change.

Appendix C is a sample case analysis that utilizes the nursing process as described above. While the analysis has been altered to protect patient privacy, it reflects an authentic patient situation.

CONCLUSION

In order to utilize the nursing process in the complex reality of the clinical situation, it is necessary to have systematic guidelines for nursing care. The Systems-in-Change model provides these guidelines as drawn from the collective experience of nursing practice. It is based upon two observations: first, that the patient is the prime source of clinical information which will direct nursing care and second, that nothing is static or unchanging, neither patients nor nursing practice.

APPENDIX A
Assessment Guidelines

The following is an outline of assessment categories and variables that may be pertinent to an adult patient in a medical-surgical setting utilizing the systems-in-change model. It is a fairly inclusive assessment, although questions, exams, and tests related to specific patient problems will need to be added. This guideline is offered only as an example of considerations that may be significant for any given patient in a specific setting. It may be useful for nursing students to review several patients in depth in order to learn prioritization of assessment items. The practicing nurse or clinical nurse specialist will be more selective in the degree of detail in the assessment. Assessment guidelines for pediatrics, obstetrics, psychiatry, and other specialties will of course vary considerably. However, each system (biologic, social, personal) should be assessed for each patient. The assessment could be further condensed in time-limited emergency situations. It is important to note, here, that the nurse reviews medical diagnostic tests, examinations, and laboratory data to assess patient function. That is, the nurse utilizes medical data and skills, not to make medical diagnoses, but rather to determine their implications for nursing practice.

Systems are categorized into subjective (review of systems and symptomatology) and objective (physical exam and/or observations and/or lab data/bedside measures) data. This assessment guideline lists topics for data collection; it is *not* an assessment tool. Interview questions should be developed based upon the guideline and should follow accepted interviewing techniques (e.g., beginning with nonthreatening factual questions, progressing to more intimate questions, and ending the assessment with a comfortable, even emotional level). Appropriate open-ended and closed questions should be integrated into the interview. As a general rule, the interview and the physical exam should be conducted separately, the interview immediately preceding the exam.

This assessment guideline is based upon the gathering of data that will enable the nurse to conduct (a) health screening and preventive health maintenance programs, (b) monitoring of system disequilibrium, and (c) baseline and change-from-baseline data collection upon which to deduce or induce nursing problems and appropriate therapeutic goals, interventions, and evaluations.

Finally, it should be noted that the laboratory test section is very abbreviated. Tests such as culture and sensitivity of selected specimens, serum electrolytes, SGOT, SGPT, LDH, BUN, alkaline phosphatase, etc. should be reviewed and may be pertinent to a variety of biologic subsystems.

Systems-In-Change Model: Assessment Guideline

Identifying Data

Name
Address
Phone
ID no.
Date admitted

Date discharged
Age   Race
Sex
Birthplace, area reared
Parent's birthplace

Marital status
Children
Income
Religious preference
Medical diagnoses

(Developmental assessment should be included in the history and exam of each system if appropriate)

Review of Systems and Symptomatology	Physical Exam and Observations	Bedside Measures and Lab Data

I. Biologic System
A. Physical subsystems
  1. General Health
    Previous illness, hospitalizations, surgeries treatments, accidents, allergies, immunizations, travels, history of family's health, current medications, treatments, general sense of well-being, frequency of physical exams, doctor visits
	Overall appearance	Height, weight, apparent level of energy

2. Skin, Hair, Nails Changes, itching, rashes, bruising/bleeding, growths, sweating	Color, texture, temperature, turgor, moisture, hair distribution, shape/condition of nails	

3. Head and Neck
    Headache, dizziness, trauma, convulsions, vertigo, syncope, nasal obstruction, colds, allergies, sinus problems, epistaxis
    Dental history, voice changes, dysphagia, bleeding/sore gums, last dental exam, neck stiffness
    Eyes: diplopia, pain, refractive errors, hemianopsia, blurring, photophobia, color blindness, acuity, visual changes, last eye exam
	Inspect: configuration
	Eyes: visual acuity, conjuctivae, sclerae, visual fields, pupillary reactions, funduscopic exam of lens, discs, retinal vessels
	Ears: auditory acuity, otoscope exam	

(continued)

85

Systems-In-Change Model: Assessment Guideline (*continued*)

Review of Systems and Symptomatology	Physical Exam and Observations	Bedside Measures and Lab Data
Ears: aches, tinnitus, infections, deafness discharge Disturbances in smell, taste, swallowing, chewing, facial weaknesses, parethesias	Nose: nasal inspection Mouth: inspect teeth, gums, tongue, tonsils, pharynx, note odor Neck: inspect and palpate thyroid and trachea, auscultate trachea, palpate cervical and epitrochlear nodes, observe ROM.	Serum PBI radioactive iodine uptake T_3, T_4 uptake
4. Breasts History of trauma, lumps, pain, discharge, changes, frequency and skill in self-breast exams	Inspect for nipple retraction, fissures, discharge. Inspect breast for dimpling, color, texture, swellings. Palpate for nodules, masses, auxillary lymph nodes.	
5. Respiratory Subsystem History of chest pain, SOB, DOE, wheezing, sputum, hemoptysis, early morning headache, asterixis, weakness, fatigue, fever, orthopnea, night sweats, cough	Inspect: configuration of chest, spine, PMI. Note rate, pattern of respirations, use of respiratory muscles. Palpate: bilateral expansion, tenderness, spinal alignment. Percuss: normal areas of reasonance, diaphragmatic excursion. Ausculate: breath sounds, adventitious sounds.	Chest X-ray PFT's ABG's Hb/Hct Sputum C and S amount Certain dx studies, e.g., ventilation/perfusion scans

6. Cardiovascular and Lymphatic Subsystems History of chest pain, palpitations, cyanosis, night sweats, edema, paroxysmal, nocturnal dyspnea, weakness, SOB, nocturia exertional dyspnea, orthopnea, syncope, hypertension, intermittent claudication, phlebitis, skin changes. Enlargement, pain or draining from lymph nodes	Inspect for skin color, integrity, capillary filling, venous integrity/distension, PMI. Palpate pulses: carotids, brachial, radial, femoral, dorsalis, pedis, posterior tibial precordial heave thrills, rubs. Auscultate: heart sounds, murmurs, clicks, rubs, bruits. Palpate lymph nodes for size, tenderness, mobility, texture, margins. Inspect lymph nodal areas for red streaking, edema.	ECG. Chest X ray, cardiac enzymes, cholesterol, triglicerides, invasive studies, e.g., angiography. Invasive monitoring, e.g., pulmonary capillary wedge pressure, cardiac output. Noninvasive studies, e.g., echocardiograph.
7. Abdomen and Gastrointestinal History of appetite, food intolerance, dysphagia, nausea, vomiting, pain, bleeding, diarrhea, constipation, bowel habits, (date of last BM), hemorrhoids, jaundice, foods or fluids used to regulate BM's	Inspect for abdominal distension, scars, peristalsis, pulsations, masses, hemorrhoids. Auscultate for bowel sounds. Palpate for liver, spleen, distended bladder, abd. tenderness, rigidity.	X rays Occult blood in stool Liver function studies Serum amylase
8. Renal and Urinary History of dysuria, polyuria, nocturnia, urgency, frequency, hesitancy, incontinence		Intake and output Routine urinalysis Renal function tests IVP
9. Sexual and Reproductive History of sexual changes or problems Venereal disease history, potency, orgasm, complications of pregnancy, LMP, dysmenorrhea, menstrual history and changes	Inspect for normal structures swelling. Palpate for tenderness. Vaginal exam (selected settings)	Hormonal studies, e.g., estrogen, pregnanetriol

(continued)

87

Systems-In-Change Model: Assessment Guideline (continued)

Review of Systems and Symptomatology	Physical Exam and Observations	Bedside Measures and Lab Data
10. Musculoskeletal: History of muscle pain, cramps, joint pain, stiffness, limitations and changes in range of motion, swellings, weakness, how far and fast can the patient walk without discomfort	Inspect build, proportions, range of motion, muscle wasting, atrophy, fine and gross motor coordination, posture, gait.	
11. Neurosensory History of pain: location, duration, character, mode of onset, radiation, precipitating/aggravating/relieving, ameliorating factors, effect of pain on ADL, past experiences with pain Eyes Ears see Head and Neck Smell Taste Equilibrium disturbances, seizures, loss of consciousness, paresis, paralysis, tremor, nervousness, depression, anxiety, hallucinations, illusions, reaction to heat and cold, sweating, control of bowel and bladder (History of psychiatric disturbances)	Observe mood, affect, methods of reacting to stress, patterns of relationships to staff/family, memory. Note confabulation, perseveration. Test for reflex status. Test for other cranial nerve, cerebellar and neuromotor functions. Mental status: mood, affect attention, recent/past memory, reactions to stress. Verbal and math proficiency.	X-ray studies CSF tests
12. Endocrine History of temperature intolerance, dry skin/hair, polyuria, polydipsia, polyphagia, glandular problems	Inspect: body configuration, weight, hair distribution, secondary sex characteristics, sexual function, skin pigmentation. See: general health, skin, musculoskeletal system exams.	Serum glucose Urinary steroids Urinary VMA Urinary glucose Urinary acetone

13. Hematopoietic

History of anemia, bleeding, bruising, infections, blood dyscrasias — Inspect skin for color, signs of capillary fragility. — Hemoglobin / Hematocrit / CBC / PTT / Protime

14. Immunologic

History of infections, allergic reactions, skin tests, irradiation and/or therapies causing immuno-suppression — Skin tests / Allergen prick test / Serum immunoglobuli / Nasal smear for eosinophils

B. Activities of Daily Living

1. General: effects of illness/situation upon ADL
Activities with which assistance is needed

2. Nutrition and Hydration

Meals: times, location, describe typical meals/snacks in a day, who prepares meals, food preferences, foods avoided and why, appetite, special diets, reducing diets

Amount consumed per day: coffee, tea, water, liquor, other fluids, vitamins

Eating problems, e.g., with teeth or swallowing

Allergies, intolerances, reactions, nausea, anorexia, belching, fatigue knowledge of nutrition, questions — Inspect teeth, observe dental hygiene. — Calorie count / Intake and output

3. Sleep and Rest

Sleep: quantity, quality, pattern, time of day, problems, somnambulism, dreams

Rest and relaxation: relaxation habits, relaxation techniques, leisure activities, hobbies, sports — Note patient's actual activity, rest, sleep. Schedule in hospital or facility

4. Exercise: quantity, type, frequency usual activity level

5. Hygiene: dental, bath, hair, nails, douche

6. Sex: quantity, type/week, month

7. Work: type (specific activities) hours/day, week

(continued)

89

Systems-In-Change Model: Assessment Guideline (*continued*)

Review of Systems and Symptomatology	Physical Exam and Observations	Bedside Measures and Lab Data

II. Social System
  A. Culture
    Beliefs, customs, rituals, health practices, child-rearing practices, values, temporal reference (e.g., present-oriented) taboos and behavioral sanctions, male-female roles, territoriality, privacy, kinship patterns, language, health-care priorities and expectations
  B. Socioeconomic Influences
    Financial status, funds available for health care, including transportation, social class, social contacts (type and number/day, month) communication style, political beliefs
  C. Roles
    1. Sexual: history of sexual activity and functioning, dysfunctions (impotence or dyspareunia), methods of conception or contraception, sexual preferences, current level of activity
    2. Occupation: type of work, exposure to hazards, spouse's occupation and his/her exposure to hazards
    3. Familial: strength of relationships, frequency of family contacts, birth order, relations with parents. To whom does this patient turn in time of trouble or need?
    4. Affiliative: affiliative patterns
      a) Affiliative subsystem
        (1) Description of patient's and family's health, any health-care treatments at home
        (2) Any changes in personality, activities of daily living
        (3) Who will assist in patient's care at home regarding transportation, finances, equipment, diet, medications, etc.

(4) Impact upon family of the illness, hospitalization, etc.
5. Communal: membership and degree of involvement in organizations of any type
6. Religious: religious beliefs and practices especially those that deal with health related implications, membership and activity in organized religious groups; desire to receive visits from religious representatives

D. Play
1. Developmental work: use of humor, play activities
2. Recreation: see activities of daily living

E. Situation
1. Immediate context, e.g., first hospitalization
   Patient's expectations, feelings
2. Current life events and circumstances: living situation, e.g., lives alone with pet; life changes; e.g., death of loved one; retirement; changes in occupation, finances, schooling, marital status, etc

    Compare usual expectation for developmental stage, sociocultural sanctions, and patient's individual characteristics with observed behavior.

III. Personal System
A. Philosophical values and beliefs and moral development, e.g., utilitarianism, fatalism, hedonism, ethical code
B. Spiritual view: spiritual beliefs, values, especially in terms of death, conception, and relationships with other people, Self-concept, view of health and illness, resources of faith

    Note patient's personal religious practices.

C. Self-concept
1. Body image: positive and negative views about body and body parts, acceptance of handicaps, deformities, differences; hygienic practices; mode of dress; use of cosmetics
2. Self-awareness: able to describe feelings—positive and negative, aware of how he/she is perceived by others, refers to self when describing illness
3. Self-esteem, self-acceptance, self-confidence.
4. Self-ideal: personal and life goals, people admired/respected

    Body language, grooming

(continued)

Systems-In-Change Model: Assessment Guideline (*continued*)

Review of Systems and Symptomatology	Physical Exam and Observations	Bedside Measures and Lab Data
5. Sexuality: libido, importance of sex in patient's life		
D. Personality characteristics and coping style: introspection, extroversion; mood lability; dependency-independency; ways of dealing with problems or emotions, pain, tension, anger, fear, frustration, joy; suicidal thoughts		
E. Intelligence/education: highest level of education	Note patient's general ability to grasp ideas, to generalize, to simplify, to abstract, to concretize, to integrate similar concepts, verbal and math proficiency, use of logic.	
See: mental status exam under Neurosensory subsystem		
IV. Assessment of Patient's Environment		
A. General		
Effect of climate, weather, light, noise, odors, quiet, unfamiliar setting, colors		
B. Presence of sensory/perceptual stimulation		
Quality, familiarity, meaningfulness of sight, hearing, smell, touch, position, taste, temperature, time, balance, humidity		
C. Environmental safety		
1. Mechanical		
2. Chemical		
3. Electrical		
4. Thermal		
5. Pathogenic		

Guidelines for Diagnosis, Goals, Intervention, and Evaluation

Guidelines for nursing diagnosis, goals, intervention, and evaluation will emphasize the congruence of these elements with the systems-in-change model. The diagnostic process, skills and techniques of intervention, and evaluation methodology are particulars that may be gleaned from the literature. For this model there are no model-dependent/derived diagnoses or interventions.

GUIDELINES FOR DIAGNOSIS AND PROBLEM IDENTIFICATION

1. Are diagnoses or problems patient centered and descriptive of a dysfunction in a system, a developmental level, or interactions with the environment?
2. Do the data substantiate the diagnosis/problem?
3. Is the diagnosis described according to its acuity, severity, etiologic or associated variables, and progress toward resolution?
4. Are actual, tentative, and potential diagnoses/problems so identified?
5. Are diagnoses specific, concise, and easily understood by peers?
6. Are *all* diagnoses/problems listed?
7. Are all diagnoses nursing diagnoses, that is, are they potentially amenable to nursing intervention?

GUIDELINES FOR THE DEVELOPMENT OF NURSING-CARE GOALS

1. Were the goals developed with active patient participation?
2. Are the goals realistic and achievable in the light of the data base that has been established?
3. Do the goals address all the identified problems?
4. Will the goals, when met, resolve the particular problems identified?
5. Are the goals flexible enough to withstand patient change?
6. Are the goals congruent with the patient's developmental level?

7. Are the objectives, when met, sufficient to achieve the goals?
8. Will the goals, when met, constitute a gain or beneficial change in one or more systems, without adversely affecting another system?
9. Are the goals, stated in positive terms, designed to achieve optimal physical, social, and personal well-being?

GUIDELINES FOR THE SELECTION OF NURSING INTERVENTIONS

1. Are the interventions derived from the goals?
2. Are the interventions sufficient and necessary to result in the resolution of the problem(s) identified?
3. Is the plan of intervention sufficiently flexible in method or technique to accommodate patient changes?
4. Are there untoward side effects to the intervention(s) chosen?
5. In considering all systems, will the specific intervention(s) chosen to meet the goals produce the greatest benefit to the patient?
6. Does the intervention respect the patient's dignity and rights?

GUIDELINES FOR EVALUATION

1. Did the evaluation show that the steps of the nursing process were thoroughly and appropriately implemented?
2. Did the evaluation confirm the diagnosis?
3. Did the evaluation clearly determine whether the interventions were safe, appropriate, and responsible for achieving the desired therapeutic outcome?
4. How effectively and efficiently were the goals and objectives met?
5. Did the evaluation method pose no harm, no risk and no deprivation of rights to the patient?
6. Was the evaluation planned concurrently with the delivery of care as well as at the termination of nursing care?
7. Did the evaluation process identify nursing accountability?
8. Will the conclusions about nursing care derived from the evaluation serve to direct remedial action or act as a guideline for future practice?
9. Did the evaluation identify unanticipated outcomes?
10. Were each of the systems in the model included in the nursing process?
11. Were developmental stages and the environment considered as variables in the nursing process?
12. Was the concept of change included in each step of the nursing process?

Systems-In-Change Model:
Sample Case Analysis

The following case analysis is an example of how the systems-in-change model may be applied in the clinical setting. The setting and the clinical focus of the RN (CNS or general duty hospital RN, private duty RN, PHN, etc.) will greatly influence the type and depth of data collection and the direction for the plan of care.

INITIAL HOME VISIT BY RCNS

Mr. LC is a 38-year-old Caucasian male of northern European descent who was born, raised, and resides in this city. He's referred to a Respiratory Clinical Nurse Specialist (RCNS) by primary MD and RN from respiratory ICU, General Hospital.

Past Health

Reports that previous health has been excellent until four months prior to this past hospitalization. Previous medical/surgical care include cholescystectomy in 1971. No accidents, known allergies or travel. Usual childhood illnesses/immunizations. Family health negative for obesity, TBC, DM, ASCVD, MI, stroke, cancer, mental illness. Immediate family A and W.

Present Health

Admitted to RICU September 1 and discharged October 2 for Pickwickian syndrome. Was brought to ER by fire department after friend found him "blue" and unresponsive. Treated in RICU with ET tube and IPPB, O_2 for one week; diuresed 120 lbs. Medical plan upon discharge: bypass surgery after additional 200 lb loss. Patient reportedly does not want this surgery. Currently, he presents as a grossly obese man appearing older than stated age, tired, lethargic, and complaining of fatigue.

Current Situation

Lives alone in small, ground-floor apartment with two noisy dogs. Will have home health aide for 2 hrs/day for a month under MediCal coverage.

Neighbor with pickup will assist with clinical transport. Has plugged tracheostomy tube. RN from home health agency will visit three times a week and coordinate care with RCNS until home status is stable.

ADL

Illness and weight have markedly diminished ability to manage ADL. Assistance is needed for meal preparation.

Nutrition: Reports adhering to 900-calorie diet, with 12 glasses water daily. Sister is temporarily assisting with meal preparation. Patient denies food preferences or any difficulty related to eating or dieting. Taking one multivit daily. Denies alcohol or street-drug intake. In the past, he's gone on "crash diets," has lost 20 or more pounds, then quickly regained his weight by what he called "eating binges."

Sleep/rest: Sleeping three to four hours per night. Says he "can't get comfortable with this tube in." Complained of nightmares the week prior to hospitalization. Naps throughout day. Recreation includes reading and TV.

Exercise: Unable to walk more than half a block for past six months before disabled by SOB and fatigue. Sits in chair during day watching TV.

Hygiene: Disheveled appearance, but bathed, hair uncombed. Complains of difficulty bathing due to weakness and fatigue.

Work: On leave from job as bill collector (a position held for past 15 yrs). Previously was professional wrestler.

Social Status

Culture: No particular cultural variables related to health. Present oriented. Believes in superordination of males. Strong sense of territoriality and personal space. Native English speaking. Expects to be "cured" of present illness.

Socio-economic status: Current illness has depleted resources. Has applied for disability benefits through social services. Transportation is a problem as he only fits in large station wagons or pickup trucks. In lower middle socioeconomic class. No particular political beliefs affecting health.

Religious/spiritual views: Says he's "Protestant," doesn't participate in church activities, no particular resources of faith or beliefs, practices, preferences that currently affect health status.

Relationships: Divorced for ten years, no children. Sexual preference is heterosexual, but disclaims interest in sex and has had few female contacts in past three to four years. Sees parents and sister one to three times/week when not ill, more frequently recently. He is first in birth order. In one observed interaction with sister, patient was passive, acquiescing to suggestions. Has several acquaintances, but no close friends. A friendly neighbor helps with limited needs, such as occasional transportation.

Personal System

Philosophy, values, moral development: Believes "luck" plays a large part in his current situation. Pragmatic in orientation, but this may be affected by illness. Moral development oriented concretely toward adherence to civil code rather than broad principles. Feels he is "a good person who tries to live a good life."

Body image: States, "I've always been big and strong." Denies serious concern about weight. Poor attention to appearance, seemingly apart from illness. Dislikes tracheostomy, says he would like it removed as he will take his chances without it.

Self-awareness: Poorly identifies feelings. Is outwardly congenial, but says he's not close to anyone, even within family. Focuses on trach and feels that everything "will be all right when it comes out." Refers to body parts fairly impersonally.

Self-esteem/confidence/acceptance: Expresses low self-esteem. Feels he's competent in his job, but otherwise "can't do much else."

Self-ideal: Disclaims any particular short- or long-term goals other than to return to previous health and his job after trach removed and he's "stronger."

Intelligence/education: Two years junior college. Difficult to differentiate effects of hypoxia/hypercapnea from underlying intellectual capabilities.

Environmental Assessment

Home is sparsely furnished, dusty. No threats to mechanical or electrical safety noted. Patient prefers warm temperature.

Development Assessment

Personal and social development may be impaired. Will assess further. On gross examination, physical systems are developmentally intact. See biologic system review.

REVIEW OF BIOLOGIC SYSTEMS

Height: 6 feet, 2 inches
Weight: 610 lbs
Skin, hair, nails: Denies changes, rashes, growths. Complains of bruising. No bruises, petechiae observed. Skin pale, warm, dry. Intertrigenous areas dry without rashes. Ruborous, scaly ischemic changes, shiny and taut skin, nonpitting edema of both lower legs. Scanty distribution of hair on extremities. Nails WNL with normal capillary filling time.
Head and Neck: Denies dizziness, vertigo, trauma, syncope, nasal obstruction, sinus problems, colds, epistaxis. Complains of early A.M. headache. Last dental exam one year ago. Uses magnifying glass to read, otherwise denies ocular problems. Denies olfactory, auditory symptoms. Eyes clear, no corneal or lens opacities. Otoscopic and nasal exams WNL. Nares patent. Mouth without lesions. Teeth in good repair, need scaling. Sinus stereo films normal. Neck unremarkable; T3-T4 normal. Complains of mild pain around tracheostomy stoma.
Breasts: Obese, otherwise unremarkable.
Respiratory: No previous respiratory history. Denies smoking, chest pain, SOB, wheezing, sputum, hemoptysis, weakness, fatigue, fever, flu syndrome, orthopnea, cough. RR 24, unlabored, shallow. Marked DOE. Mouth breather. No retractions. Single cannula trach tube in place, plugged. Significant trach leak around tube. No drainage, but stoma is reddened. Chest symmetrical with decreased expansion. Spine straight, nontender. No CVA tenderness. Upper thorax resonant to percussion; Unable to percuss diaphragm excursion. Vesicular breath sounds LUL field with end-inspiratory rales not clearing with cough. Bronchial breath sounds RUL field. Breath sounds otherwise inaudible over lower thorax. No forced, expiratory wheeze or E-A changes. In hospital CXR uninterpretable two-degree scatter from obesity, but suggests pulmonary vascular enlargement, slight heart enlargement, bibasilar fluffy infiltrates. Bedside PFT's before D/C indicate markedly decreased VC, TV, FEV_1. Decreased FEV_1, probably secondary to effort. D/C ABG's: on room air, P_{O_2} 55; P_{CO_2}, 47; pH, 7.42; HCO_3^-, 29; SO_2, 89 percent. P_{CO_2} on admission: 86
COR and Lymphatic: Denies cardiac history, PND, palpitations, syncope, intermittant claudication, phlebitis. Moderate hypertension by history. Nocturia ×2/night. No lymph changes. Skin as noted above. PMI fifth ICS—5 cm left of sternal border. No lifts, thrills. A and R pulse, 104. BP, 150/90. DOE with 20-foot walk. Unable to palpate. Popliteal and pedal pulses. One pitting edema. Feet warm. No carotid bruits. Heart sounds distant and regular. No gallops, clicks. Short II/VI systolic plateau mur-

mur. Lymph nodes WNL. BP deferred two degrees cuff size needed. EKG shows indeterminate axis of -140 degrees, p-pulmonale, absent precordial R-wave progression and some evidence of right heart failure. Serum enzymes SGOT, SGPT, CPK, fractionated LDH—normal. Cholesterol and triglycerides normal.

Abdomen and GI: History of choleystitis and cholelithiasis treated surgically. No food intolerances, dysphagia, n and v, pain, change in bowel habits, melena or bleeding. One bowel movement every A.M. Abdomen grossly obese with striae. BS inaudible. Unable to palpate organs. No tenderness. Liver function tests and serum amylase normal. Stool guiac negative.

Renal and Urinary: History negative except for nocturia $\times 2$ which continues to be present. U/A normal.

Sexual and Reproductive: Exam deferred. Serum testosterone normal.

Musculoskelatal: History negative. Weight grossly out of proportion with build. Obesity is primarily truncal.

Neurosensory: History negative for neuro problems, depression, anxiety, loss of consciousness. Complains of nightmares prior to last admission. All special senses grossly intact, as are cerebral and cerebellar functions and cranial nerves. Unable to elicit reflexes. Some decrease in light touch sensation lower legs, feet, lower back. Mood and affect appear dull and flat. However, facial obesity masks expressions. Slow to respond verbally to questions; does answer appropriately.

Endocrine: Fractional urine negative. FBS normal.

Hematopoietic: History of bruising. None observed. No petechia. Hb 16.8, hct 58. Normal differential.

Immunologic: No known allergies. TB skin test negative six months ago. No history of infections.

Problem List:

1. Moderate to severe denial of relationship between weight and illness
2. Chronic hypoventilation (with hypoxemia and hypercapnea) associated with obesity; potential respiratory failure
3. Potential thrombosis associated with high hematocrit and (2) above
4. Potential cardiac failure associated with (2) above
5. Body-image disturbance
6. Chronic nutrition-activity imbalance
7. Chronic low self-esteem
8. Sleep disturbance associated with tracheostomy and probably hypoventilation
9. Severe reduction in ADL associated with hypoventilation and obesity

10. Tracheostomatitis
11. Noncompliance with home tracheostomy care
12. Uncorrected visual impairment

EXAMPLES OF PROBLEM ANALYSIS USING SOAP FORMAT

Problem 1:

Moderate to severe denial of relationship between weight and illness

Subjective data:

"I'll be OK as soon as they take this (trach) tube out and I can get some sleep. I can breathe better without it. All I need is to get it out."

Does not suction trach as he feels that it will be removed if he keeps it plugged.

Objective data:

He has received preliminary information re his weight and illness. Asterixis present. P_{CO_2} ± 70 with trach plugged. VC and FEV_1 markedly reduced due to obesity. Narcoleptic mid-conversation. Somnolent and lethargic. Deep breathing improves attention.

Assessment:

The denial is chronic and moderate to severe. Although the relationship between obesity and hypoventilation syndromes is complicated by CNS disorders in some patients, it can reasonably be expected in this case that the truncal obesity plays a significant role in his hypoventilation. The patient's chronic denial may be secondary to anxiety and/or related to acidosis. It is manifested by a premature and narrowed focus upon anticipated removal of trach and failure to follow trach hygiene. Lack of knowledge may play a part in his behavior since CO_2 retention does affect understanding and recall. Can expect further episodes of respiratory failure, increased disability and early mortality if positive changes in behavior do not develop.

Goal:

Mr. LC will articulate his need to control obesity and improve respiratory status by his third post-hospital visit. He will actively participate in his health-care planning and home regimen as agreed upon with him.

Plan:

The respiratory clinical nurse specialist will

1. Establish a trusting rapport with Mr. LC, facilitating his ventilation of feelings and cooperation with care.
2. Be present at clinic visits to help plan continuity of care and to assist patient with informational needs.
3. Explore in a joint session with MD and patient and RCNS, patient's goals, health-care goals, and medical/nursing-care regimen.
4. Further assess informational needs, current knowledge and comprehension of the ramifications of current health status, health beliefs, values, any feelings of threat.
5. Plan a health teaching program with the interdisciplinary team within the scope of mutual goals and the patient's emotional, intellectual and physiologic capacity relative to disease process, treatment and the incorporation of these into life-style.
6. Explore non-health personnel sources of support and assistance; assist patient to recruit these resources as appropriate and necessary.

(Note: Although this intervention plan is directed at reinforcing the realities of the patient's situation, all staff should realize that he may react with increasing anxiety, more denial and noncompliance or hostility. If we provide positive direction with goals and activities of which he is capable and give much social support and reinforcement this is less likely to happen.)

Evaluation:

Evaluate goal at third visit and reassess at that time.

Problem 2:

Chronic severe hypoventilation associated with obesity; potential respiratory failure.

Subjective data:

Complains of fatigue, DOE, weakness, early AM headache.

Objective data:

ABG's on discharge showed increased P_{CO_2} with partially compensated acidosis. Asterixis present. Diminished breath sounds with bronchial sounds over posterior LUL field and end-inspiratory rales posterior RUL field. PFT's show restrictive pattern consistent with marked obesity.

Assessment:

Unless his weight is controlled, his severe hypoventilation will probably progress. He is also prone to atelectasis and subsequent pneumonias.

Goals:

The long-term goal is for the patient to reassess his life-style plus his own goals and participate in health behaviors that will enhance his physical, personal, and social health status. Stable P_{O_2} will return close to normal. Short-term goals include patient's recognition of signs and symptoms of increasing CO_2, decreasing O_2, impending respiratory failure. He will seek medical attention with early distress and attend medical clinics.

Plan:

1. Use a weight reduction plan.
2. Design and implement a teaching plan to include chest expansion exercises with cough (to be done on cue hourly) and instruction for the patient and a significant other in the signs and symptoms of decreasing P_{O_2} and increasing P_{CO_2}.
3. Reinforce his keeping of all clinic appointments and following of medical/nursing regimen.
4. Establish with the patient a plan for contacting medical assistance when and if respiratory status worsens.
5. Explore significance of trach to patient and his failure to follow plan of trach care as taught.
6. Assess patient's respiratory status weekly.

Evaluation:

Weekly, evaluate breathing exercises, clinic visits, return demonstration of trach care, return explanation of signs and symptoms of respiratory failure.

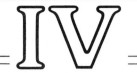

Systems Models for Nursing Practice

The initial article in this section is by Abbey. She defines FAN-CAP as a mnemonic device designed to assist student nurses in learning to give patient care. It is a framework of multidimensional concepts containing six factors and three major systems: central (physiological), proximal (psychosocial), and distal (social-environmental). The six factors are fluids, aeration, nutrition, communication, activity, and pain. As Abbey points out, the ordering of these factors has no special meaning but by the arrangement according to first letters into the acronym FANCAP the terms are more easily remembered. FANCAP is a tool for the teaching of clinical nursing. It provides a systematic structure to the student that enables her to organize the identification and resolution of patient care problems. Regardless of the theoretical model employed by the nurse, these factors will certainly be included in any consideration of the patient's total care. As such, FANCAP is one approach that is useful in introducing student nurses to conceptual frameworks for nursing practice.

The second article is by Neuman and is the first of a series that discuss the Neuman model. In the intial paper, the Neuman Health-Care System Model presents a total person approach to patient problems [As illustrated in her diagram, her model consists of three phases: primary; secondary, and tertiary prevention, any stage of which might be the point of entry of the client into the health-care system. The model focuses primarily upon stress, emphasizing how the patient reacts to stress and how the nurse can assist him in coping with it. In addition to the necessary assumptions and her explanation of the model, Neuman provides an assessment tool and an intervention plan as a guide to the practitioner.]

Following the Neuman article is a paper by Venable who offers an analysis of the Neuman model. Although the fact is not discussed in her article, Venable used the Neuman Model in an acute care setting for patients with orthopedic conditions. The fourth paper is also by Neuman and addresses itself to the subject of education for nurse administrators. The Lebold and Davis article discusses implementation of the Neuman model in a baccalaureate nursing curriculum. Craddock and Stanhope give their interpretation and recommended adaptation of this model. Finally, Beitler, Tkachuck and Aamodt illustrate the use of the Neuman model in mental health, community health, and medical-surgical nursing settings.

The Roy Adaptation Model, discussed in Chapter 15, is concerned with promoting health by assisting the patient to adapt in the areas of physiologic needs, self-concept, role function, and interdependence. Roy presents the basic assumptions of the model, and then the elements of the model in terms of values, goal of action, patiency, source of difficulty, and intervention. The earlier edition of this work gave two basic case study examples of the use of the model in practice. This text focuses on application in two areas where questions frequently arise about the use of the model. First, Starr applies the Roy model to the dying client, and then Schmitz uses the model in the wellness-oriented community setting.

A series of articles based on the Johnson model are presented in Chapters 18 through 23. The first of these is written by Dorothy Johnson. Though her early writings stimulated much of the work on nursing models done in the last twenty years, this is the first account of the Johnson model by the author herself that has been published. Johnson describes the behavioral system and each subsystem and notes the structural elements and functional requirements of the subsystems. She sees nursing's goal as to restore, maintain, or attain behavioral system balance and stability at the highest possible level for the individual.

In Chapter 19, Grubbs presents her view of the Johnson Behavioral System Model. In it, she reviews the assumptions, basic concepts, basic elements (which incorporate eight subsystems), the functional requirements or sustenal imperatives within the subsystems, the regulating and control mechanisms between the subsystems, the variables affecting the model, and how the model corresponds with the nursing process.

The articles by Holoday, Small, and Damus illustrate the use of the Johnson model in practice. Holoday and Small selected a pediatric setting in which to implement the model and both incorporate some of Piaget's theory as well. In addition, Holoday includes Erikson's theory and uses clinical case material throughout. Small's article resulted from her Master's thesis and she, thus, discusses her research and the utilization of the results in clinical practice. The article by Damus also deals with research. She worked with adult patients diagnosed as having post-transfusion hepatitis and dealt with them as inpatients and outpatients. The last article in this section is by Glennin. It is not another example of the model's use but is included because it employs the Johnson framework to formulate standards of nursing practice. This concept should be kept in mind, and perhaps such standards should be developed for any other model used in nursing practice.

Another systems model is that developed by Dorothy Orem and is presented in Chapters 24 and 25. Caley, Dirksen, Engalla, and Hennrich provide a theoretical discussion of this model. Nursing is needed, according to Orem, when the therapeutic self-care demand exceeds the assets of the self-care agency of an individual or group. The basic goals of nursing action are to accomplish the patient's self-care demand and to move the patient toward responsible action in matters of self-care. Intervention deals with the nursing agency—the partly compensatory, wholly compensatory, and educative-developmental systems that the nurse can use. These same authors illustrate the use of the Orem model in the case study of a psychiatric patient.

Coleman presents her view of the Orem model in the second of these two articles. In the first part of her paper, she summarizes Orem's self-care concept of nursing in terms of the concepts that may be useful to nursing service personnel, including the steps of the nursing process, a classification of patients, the essential techniques needed for nursing practice, and the utilization of nursing personnel. In part two, Coleman discusses the application of the Orem model as a guide for nursing activities with a hospital nursing service. She treats such topics as the nursing department's operational documents, its philosophy, goals, policies, and the position descriptions. She reviews the nursing tools, such as the admission assessment and nursing care plan, that were revised to facilitate the use of Orem's model in the department. And, finally, Coleman comments on the method of preparing nursing personnel and the process of change involved in implementing the Orem model with the nursing services.

Another popular systems model is the one that was developed by Martha Rogers. In Chapter 26, Rogers describes her science of unitary man. In considering the universe one of open systems, Rogers notes that the environment is integral to the study of unitary man. Unitary man is seen as a synergistic phenomenon whose behaviors cannot be predicted by knowledge of the parts. Rogers explains her conceptual system for unitary man and environment. Some brief comments on the implications of the model for practice conclude the chapter.

June Abbey

FANCAP: What Is It?

FANCAP is a mnemonic device that is designed and intended to assist the memory of student nurses involved in learning to give direct patient care. It exists primarily as a framework of concepts, the purpose of which is to discover patient-care problems and propose solutions for them. The student works from signs and symptoms, obtained from whatever source and augmented by considerations of the etiology of each sign or symptom. FANCAP organizes impressions, solutions, and related nursing intervention into a nursing care plan.

FANCAP, used as originally intended, deals with a person who has a recognized health problem and who is therefore a patient. The patient—as a complex of interacting physiological, psychological, and social systems—presents a series of problems as each system responds to the initial difficulty. The student concentrates his or her efforts, both in learning and in giving care, on a single individual, and this concentration permits in-depth exploration of the person, the health problem, its etiology, and its possible solutions. The solutions represent specific nursing actions or interventions that are individual to the patient.

The teacher chooses the time for evaluation and shaping. The student's plan can be assessed as a proposal for care, and so the teacher "walks through" the thinking process, pointing out the essential decision-making criteria, winnowing out the extraneous and the irrelevant, sharpening and reinforcing the ethical and idealistic aspects of care that are so often lost when the student is under pressure. But after care has been given, the plan can also serve as a model for self-evaluation. The actions taken by the student are shared, appraised, modified, and corrected by the student and the teacher. The student's care plan is studied for its intrinsic worth as a care plan and as a record of what learning progress is actually being made by the student.

At the present time, FANCAP remains a framework of concepts to be used in teaching nursing. It is a tool for the integration of cognate science content and nursing theory and care. The concepts involved are of two different types, which may be called, for clarity and differentiation, parameters and factors.

PARAMETERS

Parameters pertain to the physiological, psychological, and sociological aspects of care, which appear as recurrent themes in nursing theory (Mayers, 1972; Murphy, 1971; Byrne and Thompson, 1972; Witt and Mitchell, 1973; Roy, 1974; Bergersen, 1971). An illness or health problem in one parameter induces disturbances in all three parameters, with consequent interest and concern to nurses. Total patient care requires that attention be given to each of the parameters to a greater or lesser extent, depending upon the problem and which patient system is more profoundly affected, the course or sequence of events within the problem, and the acuity of the problem relative to the system. Problems and their ramifications are viewed, first, according to the system they affect primarily and, second, according to the disturbances of factors. The parameters are thus overall classifications or categories of problems under one parameter.

The classification of a problem under one parameter does not preclude applying its solution to a different system. Placement is determined by appropriateness. For example, a patient dying from cancer may best be helped if the nurse works with his family. Here the patient's physiological problems associated with dying need the sociological solution of the nurse, who can guide the family and help both the family and the patient psychologically as they learn to accept and deal with the inevitable. Another example is the geriatric patient who seemingly sleeps while sitting at his bedside most of the day. According to one study (Abbey, 1973), there is a consistent drop in body temperature of two to four degrees Fahrenheit when patients are sitting away from their beds. When the patients are kept warm with leggings, shawls, and lap robes, their temperatures do not fall and they remain warm and awake. In this instance, the observed problem is psychological somnolence and the effective intervention is physiological warmth.

Despite the fact that there are some instances where the problem and the solution fall into different classifications, the usual case presents problems that can be solved within the same parameter. For nursing students, the parameters afford a set of priorities. The classification of the problem indicates where the student can first consider finding an appropriate solution. Then, as the problem begins to come under control, the student can given attention to concomitant but lesser disturbances in the same or other systems.

The teacher, from the broader base of clinical expertise, directs original and additional system classification, shapes the process of selection, and rewards problem identification and relevant solution by commenting on the plan. The parameters provide the teacher with the basis for total patient-care evaluation as the student's preoccupation with any one of the systems, for either finding problems or designing care to solve the difficulty, becomes readily apparent. If the student expects not only to find and use the three parameters as aspects of care for every patient but also to be held responsible for including the increment in each of these dimensions, the process of considering the total patient becomes automatic. This fact in no way implies, however, that problems and their solutions are the same in all situations; it is the pattern for discovery that is routinized and available to the student for easy recall and application.

The parameters are intended to be broad enough to permit flexibility of study and individualized student approach. The categories are not precise. Anthropologists, surely, would have difficulty accepting the inclusion of cultural and environmental concerns in parameters that are called sociological and psychological, but this difficulty represents only a problem of refinement. FANCAP is designed for teaching and clinical care. The purpose of the categorization is to differentiate between the physical (body) characteristics, the emotional and feeling relationships, and the interactions with others, groups of others, and society in general—as all of these are presented by the patient. The parameter provides a focus for the student. By placing the problem or solution under a parameter, the student can indicate where effort is anticipated and what type of intervention and care can be given. The placement also informs the instructor about how the student views or wishes to view the problem.

FACTORS

FANCAP began as a bridging device for content integration in a curriculum based on general systems theory (Bailey *et al.,* 1971), a theory that integrated Maslow's (1954) needs and Selye's (1956) general adaptation syndrome into a problem-solving framework. Essentially, FANCAP extracted universal nursing concerns for a living, pain-free, relating human being and designated these concerns factors of care. The concerns, not surprisingly, encompass Maslow's first-level physiologic needs. The difference between Maslow's needs and FANCAP, however, becomes clearer when it is noted that Maslow lists food, air, water, temperature, elimination, rest, and pain avoidance as *needs for,* whereas FANCAP lists fluids, aeration, nutrition, communication, activity, and pain as *concerns about* or the "do-not-miss" requirements of nursing. Moreover, they are all factors that are involved with the matter of control. Normally, it is the patient himself who controls these factors, but when he is ill he surrenders this control in varying degrees. It is then the nurse who takes over the responsibility, and it is the nurse, therefore, who must be aware of needs and changes involving all of the factors. The object of the nurse's attention is to keep the patient alive and to make him as pain-free as possible, so it is essential that the nurse observe and correctly interpret signs and symptoms. There remains, however, one more element: A person is something more than a living, pain-free organism, and so some attention must also be given to the parameters of physiologic, psychologic and sociologic considerations.

The factors center attention on specific aspects of nursing care as dictated by the signs, symptoms, and etiology of each. The use of the words *signs* and *symptoms* rather than the word *manifestations,* as defined by the curriculum (Bailey et al., 1971), teaches the student to note all objective findings or signs and to ask the patient for information to discover symptoms. The two terms *signs* and *symptoms* are common in clinical situations, both in the standard history and in physical examinations, as well as in record keeping that uses the Weed Problem-Oriented Medical Record with the SOAP (Subjective, Objective, Assessment, and Plan) format. Concentration on the etiology of each sign and symptom requires the student to formulate a hypothesis about the sign or symptom—its nature, history, duration, and progress—and to note the interplay between them. The etiology often prescribes problem placement within factors while also prescribing in which parameter the solution lies.

The factors of FANCAP—fluids, aeration, nutrition, communication, activity, and pain—present the learner with concepts that are representative of the basic concern of nursing, the maintenance of a live, interacting, pain-free person. Since FANCAP was designed not as a model but as a teaching tool to be used in a curriculum resulting from a synthesis of a number of theoretical frameworks—namely, general systems (von Bertalanffy, 1968), adaptation (Selye, 1956), and self-actualization (Maslow, 1954)—formulated within a problem-solving approach, it concentrates on nursing concerns and on providing a bridge between cognate science content and the patient. The factors deal with the "here and now" because they develop directly from the signs and symptoms presented by the patient. Only as the patient's past history affects the present problem is it relative. The curriculum stressed totality of nursing care for an individual, and FANCAP therefore has focused—and focuses—on care for the individual patient.

The factors of FANCAP—the nursing concerns for care—consist of six concepts of function (the six elements of the mnemonic device) ranged along a continuum regarding each word in the device. Points on the continuum include the usually understood meaning, the precise definition, and the associative characteristics of each word. With the word *fluids,* for instance, the usually understood meaning would be "liquids capable of flowing." Refinement of the term would expand it to include a class of substances whose particles move freely among themselves; thus it would then include liquids and gases. In hospital settings, the word *fluids* may be accompanied by directives such as "force," "limit," "record," or "measure," and *fluids* may thus mean any liquids or solutions taken in or put out by whatever means by a patient. To the physiologist, the word conjures up a myriad of physical laws regarding pressure, volume resistance, viscosity, flux, gradients, concentrations, forces, compartments, and spaces. To most people, however, inherent in the meaning of the word is the concept of easy changeability or lability. Each of these interpretations of the word has relevance to patient care.

Aeration, although not so commonly used as the other terms in FAN-CAP, is readily understood as the process of "exposing to air or a gas." The word has come to have a fairly common place in everyday language, however, because of aerated bread, aerated fishtanks, and aerated swimming pools and because it is a topic in first-aid classes. In clinical situations, the word contains a variety of applications that determine interpretation. Aeration problems are generally said to consist of "pulmonary" problems where the subject has a "respiratory" condition or disease. Patient care, therefore, concentrates on getting oxygen to the alveoli and removing the accumulating carbon dioxide. But the condition can just as well occur at a cellular level as the result of a profusion or circulatory anomaly. With aeration there is implied a movement or exchange by which the supportive substance oxygen is made available and the buildup of the metabolic gaseous end products is eliminated. One aerates the lungs through ventilation or by making certain that airways are patent, that the thorax moves, and that sufficient quantities of oxygen and air are available for inhalation. The word *ventilate,* of course, derives from "to vent," to make an opening to the air. To ventilate one's feelings is to discuss them, and psychologists use the term to describe a release of feelings or emotions by "talking them out." *Aeration,* as it is used in FANCAP, pertains to all of these meanings and interpretations, to providing oxygen to the lungs or tissues, to opening things up to the air, and to the psychosocial ventilation of problems. The student selects the aspect of care from the central (physiological), the proximal (psychosocial), or the distal (social-environmental) realms of functioning.

In contrast to aeration, *nutrition* is an everyday public concern, and it is subject to a variety of uses. Through use, *nutrition* has come to mean a descriptive state, and it is therefore usually preceded by an adjective such as "good," "poor," or "inadequate." Oftentimes, the word is used as a substitute for "nutriment" or "nourishment," as in the statement "That cereal is full of empty calories and has little nutrition." In any case, when the word *nutrition* is used, the idea of nourishment is inherent in it. While the public thinks of "plenty of good, warm food," the nutritionist considers vitamins, minerals, proteins, fats, carbohydrates, roughage, and calories. The anthropologist explores and develops a compendium of significant beliefs and mores about differing cultural customs regarding eating habits and means of procuring food. The sociologist studies governmental and structural ethical systems for society's exchange practices revolving around food. World governments hold meetings about the nutritional needs of the world, both now and in the future. The concept of nutrition pervades all related disciplines and cultures, and the term flows reasonably, therefore, into other essential areas of need, along with its opposite, "deprivation." Such terms as "psychological nutrition," "cognitive nutrition," "deprivation of sensory stimulation," "cultural nutrition," and "spiritual nutrition" can be found in the sciences, arts, and religions of the world. The acts of providing, obtaining, and sharing nourishment influence and even dominate most aspects of existence. Any health problem in whatever area will consequently impinge on the nutrition of the patient.

The word *communication* signifies for the average person a document containing a message or an interchange of thoughts by speech, writing, or some type of sign. This person, if pressed, might think of a bridge or a tunnel or a road between places or compartments. To a psychologist or a psychiatrist, the word summons a whole host of ideas and ramifications, each with a significant fretwork (such as "level" or "depth") that includes such qualities as searching, defining, reaching, defending, screening, purposes represented by therapeutic information, manipulation, conversation, facilitation, sharing, and teaching. Moreover, there are the implications of the term having to do with whether communication is within the self or external to the self, whether it is a matter of perception or interpretation. The physiologist considers the impact of the sense organs and the various aspects of neurologic communication from the cellular level through the three nervous systems. The biochemist focuses on aspects of DNA and genetic communication, on hormonal controls and immunologic response to recognition of the signs of the cause of disease. When the subject is a human being and the problems are related to illness, the interpretations of the word *communication* seem infinite; possibilities involve many disciplines along with their theories, laws, and hypotheses.

Activity is another factor of FANCAP with a generalized cultural definition. In nursing, activity relates to a level or quality of doing things for oneself. On occasion, the term applies to a series of specific actions, such as the activities of daily living, which can be graded for degrees of difficulty, steps of rehabilitation, and levels of work expenditure. In addition, physicians over the years have developed a jargon specifically related to the limitation of activities. For the most part, these terms, although used nationwide, take on meanings that are operational only in particular settings, according to the dictates of the prescribing physicians. Unless instructed otherwise, however, it is the nurse who determines what a patient can do when he is limited to absolute bed rest or is allowed to ambulate. Besides physical exertion, there is another activity which has to do with the psychosocial aspects of nursing care—for example, reading, conversing, learning, writing, planning, or drawing. Basic scientists consider activity in terms of measurements, expenditures, energy levels, ergs, works, physiologic responses to increased demands, cardiac output, oxygen consumption, and temperature, to name but a few. The patient and his problem contribute to and are affected by the activities permitted, encouraged, and demanded by the health-care setting. The oft-heard complaint that a hospital is not a place to go to rest is true. Activity on the part of the patient, whether physical or mental, is constant, both for custodial and therapeutic reasons. The complex interacting systems of a hospital veritably thrive on activity, and the patient, introduced into the pulsating course of daily events there, must relate, exchange, consume, expand, and respond in order to retain his own integrity.

Pain, although not unique to the world of the ill, indicates the existence of a problem. Physiologic pain accompanies injury, stretching, and the lack of oxygen. Psychologic pain, by contrast, attends any number of types of assaults. To say that pain is "an acute discomfort of the body or mind," (*New Century Dictionary,* 1948) however, is to disregard entirely another meaning of the word that relates to assiduous attention or careful efforts, as in the expression "to take pains with." Nursing, recognizing that all patients are subject to physiologic and psychologic pain from whatever etiology, has as one of its primary concerns this second meaning of the term—to take pains with or to offset or alleviate the pain itself. Nurses as a group—because of tradition, role, area of functioning and responsibility, and setting—face pain daily without being able to withdraw, ignore, or blame without guilt. Unlike the physician, who can prescribe a medication and then go on to another ward, hospital, or office, the nurse must give and evaluate the action of the drug and assess the response of the patient. The nurse must also acknowledge the effects on pain of fear, loneliness, grief, and helplessness. He or she must deal with each of these effects (take pains, as it were, with each) to allay pain. In pain merge the strengths and frailties of mankind, the hopes and fears of life, the beliefs and dreads about death, the cacophonies of cultures, and the vulnerability of science. Pain is an ever-present concern to nurses, a concern that indicates and locates but rarely defines a problem.

The factors of FANCAP, then, are multidimensional concepts described by many disciplines, and they exist in a multiplicity of settings. They are brought together with all of their meanings and values because they are essential to patient care. Whatever the theoretical model, these factors will be among the primary concerns of nursing. All are representative of processes, of interactions, and of adjustments. All are products of circumstance, and all are bound in time. The attributes of each factor depend upon the choice of the user in the clinical situation, however. For instance, although every patient-care problem requires a concern with nutrition, the nurse has a wide range of choice for focus—from cellular amino acid transformation and all of the chemical and physiologic considerations, through local and systemic circulation, dietary preferences or cultural dictates, and therapeutic limitations or specifications, to psychologic nurturing. Each conceptual process, therefore, is complex.

The words selected to designate the concerns or processes are characteristically those found in clinical settings and used at all levels of nursing. They are simple, everyday terms used in nursing work, and they are understood, in context, by all who give care to patients. They are, moreover, relevant to the care of every patient. The factors are noted, assessed, and mentioned when nursing shifts change, when the patient is admitted or discharged, when the patient is to be treated or has been given treatment. Each word is a noun, and each word contains an inherent process that implies an interaction or exchange between the patient's system and the environment in which he functions. This balance, to put it simply, can be expressed by the two opposing terms "in" and "out." Communications are received and sent; oxygen is consumed and carbon dioxide is discharged. It is a matter of intake and output along continuums of function. The one factor that does not fit neatly into this format is pain. It is not enough, perhaps, to say that pain lies in opposition to comfort or that it represents an inhibition of function. To speak plainly, pain is an essential factor in FANCAP simply because of what it is. It is a nursing concern, a factor of patient care to be assessed and dealt with. It is one of the reasons why a patient is a patient and why he has a need for nurses.

The six factors of FANCAP represent six possible problem areas for search and assessment in any one of three major systems—central, proximal, and distal. Since FANCAP, as designed, breaks with the medical model of evaluation of each of the body's physiologic systems in order to make a diagnosis, the question must be asked: Search and assessment for what? FANCAP uses information obtained from the medical or nursing physical examination as facts from which to develop a care plan that also includes the psychosocial aspects of health and illness. FANCAP's emphasis is on nursing care, and in nursing care, medical diagnosis and treatment make up an important but not an all-inclusive part. The physiologic diagnosis may not be the cause of the entire array of signs and symptoms. An example of such a circumstance is the patient who has an asymptomatic but malignant tumor. Although the patient is psychologically under massive assault, he is nevertheless physiologically intact. Therefore, nursing care must go beyond diagnosis and treatment. An essential part of FANCAP is consideration of the etiology of the obvious objective signs and the often obscure subjective symptoms.

The etiology contributes to the categorization of the sign or symptom under one of the areas of nursing concern. There is, however, no single constantly correct placement. The user of FANCAP interprets the findings and selects the factor that is most appropriate. When FANCAP is used in this way as an assessment–intervention tool, the care plan is unique and individualized. Placement itself acts as relevant mnemonic action to "integrate information into more or less coherent organization or schema which then governs . . . judgments." (Cofer, 1973) The signs and symptoms, along with the etiology of each (called manifestations and antecedents in the Experimental Curriculum), indicate priority.

There is no magical ordering involved in the formation of the acronym. The ordering of the initial letters of the factors—fluids, aeration, nutrition, communication, activity, and pain—is not intended to offer special meaning or ideological bias. The sequencing of the letters is simply the result of student-nurse manipulation of the terms to render them easy for one to remember.

HOW FANCAP IS DESIGNED TO BE USED

FANCAP developed as a tool for teaching clinical nursing. It was intended to provide a structure for the organization of nursing concerns, to permit the integration of relevant principles from the cognate sciences into patient-care problems, and to allow for individual expression, interpretation, and creativity. The directions for its use, consequently, were nonstructured and flexible. A typical example of directions for use is "Find the signs and symptoms, consider the etiology of each, and FANCAP-off the care."

The signs, symptoms, and etiology act as reality moorings to the patient. The outcome of each, however tangential the approach to the patient problem might be, ultimately resolves into a nursing care plan that is subject to clinical testing and evaluation by the student, the patient, the teacher, and innumerable other people concerned with the patient.

Writing up a formal FANCAP nursing-care plan for complete in-depth development of patient care requires considerable work on the part of the student. The FANCAP nursing-care plan requires the application and integration of cognate science and discipline content; it is an exercise in how to solve clinical problems and set priorities, and it teaches the student to propose practical and feasible solutions. Teacher evaluation and comments give close attention to a number of levels and kinds of performance, and FANCAP permits the teacher, through shaping, to model thinking and values.

Unlike other nursing-care plans—in which a patient need or problem is locked into a classification of behavior within one of four modes (as with Roy's adaptation model, 1974) and then analyzed from that singular perspective—FANCAP permits and encourages a number of alternative views and perspectives. The teacher discovers the student's perspective by observing which factor and which parameter the student uses to begin exploration of the problem. To illustrate the wide range of FANCAP's adaptability to individual perspectives, here is an example taken from actual clinical practice that has a religious motif. The patient, a Catholic woman, was seriously ill and wanted to see a priest. The student, who was a Jewish girl, appreciated the patient's feelings of grief and loss and urgency, but on the first day she classified the priest's visit under psychologic pain. The instructor, who was Protestant, observed the student's interpretation of the problem but said nothing. On the second day, the patient was given communion, and the student classified the priest's visit under nutrition. When the instructor asked her if communication might not be a possible classification, the student replied: "But what about the sustenance and real support she got? It's more than a message. When she has him in for confession, *that's* communication—or better still, aeration!" The student classified the patient's struggles with her religious beliefs—her doubts, anger, and frustration—under fluids. The patient's search for religious truth with friends, family, and priests fluctuated in the student's mind, sometimes constituting activity, sometimes communication in the sociologic parameter. The patient's disease was long and difficult, and both the student and the instructor learned from a variety of perspectives the impact that religious beliefs can have on nursing concerns. FANCAP permitted the instructor to watch the student grow in understanding the disease process and the reactions of terminal patients, in awareness of alternative resources for care, and in comprehension of the values of other beliefs and cultures.

After gaining the student's perspective, the instructor reinforces the exploration by making suggestions and questioning the value of the placement, the supporting arguments, or the solution. Both overuse and underuse of any one factor can provide avenues for exchange between the student and the instructor, so that they can arrive at an ideal, feasible solution with minimal effort. Such an exchange demands faculty commitment as well as time and knowledge. But without faculty exchange and input, FANCAP loses part of its design and raison d'être, because clinical teaching is far more than the provision of experiences and sources of information. Written work provides not only documentation for grading but an opportunity to share the processes of problem solving, the language and argot of the profession, and the nuances of values. Correction, direction, and shaping all play significant parts in the use of FANCAP as a teaching tool.

Optimally used, FANCAP relates to a real patient in a real situation. It is, in essence, an extensive and detailed development of the patient's care problem, consisting of an in-depth analysis of the difficulty with attention given to each sign, symptom, and etiology. In this phase of the examination of the problem, all sources of relevant factual information are tapped. Library resources, physicians, textbooks, instructors, patients, other nurses, other health disciplines, peers—anything that pertains to the necessary solutions can offer potential contributions. After all of the elements derived from the problem and its cause are listed, they are organized and given priority under nursing concerns—FANCAP—and solutions are proposed. This procedure, so far, is clearly compatible with the Harms and McDonald (1966) model for teaching methodology, wherein first knowledge, theories, hypotheses, and the problems discovered lead to the basis for decision. With FANCAP, the proposed solution presents a nursing-care plan. At this stage, it is a tentative, complex, and voluminous analysis of the individual patient's problems. The plan is shared with the instructor who corrects, suggests, questions, and reinforces the student. Although many instructors prefer a face-to-face meeting with the student for this exchange, there are advantages in making written statements, which can be referred to again and again and provide a permanent record.

When the nursing care plan is made, it can be implemented in the clinical setting for "reality testing." Elaborate documentation of the plan can present practical difficulties in the clinical setting. It may be too long and too bulky, and so some method of extracting what is salient and action-oriented is necessary. For the sake of communication to others giving nursing care and as a means of checking on possible omissions or completions, simplification is required. A framework for spotting priority and emphasis based on all of the preparation is called for. Moreover, students under the pressures of a complex, stressful, ever-changing setting need something with which to jog their memories.

The factors of FANCAP—fluids, aeration, nutrition, communication, activity, and pain—provide a mnemonic device for safe comfort-giving care. The patient will be turned and helped to cough; he will be fed, talked with, looked at, and listened to; the tubes that are attached to him will be checked to make sure they are working. The patient, in short, will be made as pain-free as possible. As the factors are ticked off, the student recalls details from the extensive problem analysis. He or she does not have to grope for the twenty-first basic need, but can, instead, develop deadlines and outcomes appropriate to the individual patient, the setting, and his or her own constraints. In addition, FANCAP is compatible with most conceptual models that are developed from a problem-solving, general-systems, adaptation, or basic-need theoretical framework. In times of stress, FANCAP can be abbreviated to a check list. Under proper stimulation, the device expands to encompass man's central, proximal, and distal worlds of physiologic, psychologic, and sociologic functioning.

REFERENCES

Abbey JC: Core temperatures in the aged patient. Unpublished manuscript, 1973
Bailey JT, McDonald FJ, Claus KE: An Experiment in Nursing Curriculum at a University. Belmont, California, Wadsworth, 1971
Bergersen B: Adaptation as a unifying theory. In Murphy JF (ed): Theoretical Issues in Professional Nursing. New York, Appleton, 1971

Byrne ML, Thompson LF: Key Concepts for the Study and Practice of Nursing. St. Louis, Mosby, 1972

Cofer CN: Constructive processes in memory. American Scientist 61:5:537, 1973

Emery HG, Brewster KG (eds): New Century Dictionary of the English Language. New York, Appleton, 1948

Harms MT, McDonald, FJ: A New Curriculum Design. Nurs Outlook 14: 54, 1966

Maslow AH: Motivation and Personality. New York, Harper and Row, 1954

Mayers MG: A Systematic Approach to the Nursing Care Plan. New York, Appleton, 1972

Murphy JF: Social aspects of adaptation. In Murphy JF (ed): Theoretical Issues in Professional Nursing. New York, Appleton, 1971

Roy C: The Roy Adaptation Model. In Riehl JP, Roy C (eds): Conceptual Models for Nursing Practice. New York, Appleton, 1974

Selye H: The Stress of Life. New York, McGraw-Hill, 1956

von Bertalanffy L: General systems theory and psychiatry. In Arieti S (ed): American Handbook of Psychiatry. New York, George Braziller, 1968

Witt R, Mitchell PH: Psychosocial and mental-emotional status. In Mitchell PH (ed): Concepts Basic to Nursing. New York, McGraw-Hill, 1973

The Betty Neuman Health-Care Systems Model: A Total Person Approach to Patient Problems

The health-care delivery system of today is becoming so complex that models are emerging which seem to offer some direction toward goal unification and clarification. The health-care systems model, "total person approach to patient problems," is one attempt to provide such a framework and is also appropriate for providers of health care in disciplines other than nursing. Nursing can use this model to assist individuals, families, and groups to attain and maintain a maximum level of total wellness by purposeful interventions. These are aimed at reduction of stress factors and adverse conditions which either affect or could affect optimal functioning in a given client situation. However, an attempt will be made to relate the model specifically to nursing and provide some direction for patient assessment and intervention.

Today there exists a great need to clarify and make explicit not only the relationship of variables that affect an individual during and following an illness, but also those affecting ambulatory and high-risk groups. Since the shift in focus is increasingly toward primary prevention, an understanding of how these variables interface with those of secondary and tertiary prevention seems important. These relationships will be explored in our explanation of the following conceptual model as well as in the patient assessment format (Figure 1).

The health-care systems model is intended to represent an individual who is subject to the impact of stressors. However, the model could also be used to study the response of a group or community to stressors. The following assumptions were made by the author in developing this model:

1. Though each individual is viewed as unique, he is also a composite of common "knowns" or characteristics within a normal, given range of response.

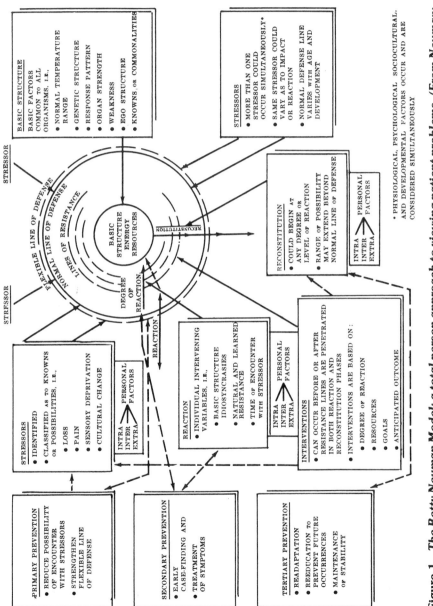

Figure 1. *The Betty Neuman Model: a total person approach to viewing patient problems. (From Neuman: Nurs Res 21:3, 1972. Copyright © 1972 American Journal of Nursing Company.)*

2. There are many known stressors. Each stressor is different in its potential to disturb an individual's equilibrium or *normal line of defense*. Moreover, particular relationship of the variables—physiologic, psychologic, sociocultural, and developmental—at any point can affect the degree to which an individual is able to use his *flexible line of defense* against possible reaction to a single stressor or combination of stressors.

3. Each individual, over time, has evolved a normal range of responses which is referred to as a *normal line of defense*.

4. When the cushioning, accordionlike effect of the flexible line of defense is no longer capable of protecting the individual against a stressor, the stressor breaks through the normal line of defense. The interrelationship of variables (physiologic, psychologic, sociocultural, and developmental) determines the nature and degree of the organism's reaction to the stressor.

5. Each person has an internal set of resistance (*lines of resistance*) factors, which attempt to stabilize and return him to his normal line of defense should a stressor break through it.

6. Man in a state of wellness or illness is a dynamic composite of the interrelationship of the four variables (physiologic, psychologic, sociocultural, and developmental) that are always present.

7. Primary prevention relates to general knowledge that is applied to individual patient assessment in an attempt to identify and allay the possible risk factors associated with stressors.

8. Secondary prevention relates to symptomatology, appropriate ranking of intervention priorities, and treatment.

9. Tertiary prevention relates to the adaptive process as reconstitution begins, and moves back in a circular manner toward primary prevention.

Nursing is seen as a unique profession in that it is concerned with all of the variables affecting an individual's response to stressors.

The aim of this model, called the total person approach, is to provide a unifying focus for approaching varied nursing problems and for understanding the basic phenomenon: man and his environment. The model is based upon an individual's relationship to stress—his reaction to stress and factors of reconstitution—and is thought of as dynamic in nature. While it is a general health-care systems model it does not seem to conflict with existing models, but rather encompasses them.

Theoretically, the model has some similarity to Gestalt theory, which suggests that each of us is surrounded by a perceptual field that is a dynamic equilibrium. Field theories endorse the molar view, which maintains that all parts are intimately interrelated and interdependent (Edelson, 1970). Emphasis is placed on the total organization of the "field." In this total person model the organization of the field considers (1) the occurrence of stressors,

(2) the reaction of the organism to stressors, and (3) the organism itself, taking into consideration the simultaneous effects of physiologic, psychologic, sociocultural, and developmental variables. Gestalt theorists view insight as the perception of relationships in a total situation.

Chardin (1955) and Cornu (1957) suggest that in all dynamically organized systems the properties of parts are determined partly by the larger wholes within which they exist. This means that no one part can be looked at in isolation but must be viewed as part of a whole. That is, just as the single part influences perception of the whole, the patterns of the whole influence awareness of the part.

AN EXPLANATION OF THE MODEL

Nursing models tend to view man as either a behavioral composite, a biologic system, an organism at a stage of development, or a part of an interaction process, but not all of these together. The result is often failure to interrelate these factors in the process of assessment and intervention. The total person model is a more comprehensive approach to this problem.

One must view the total person framework as an open systems model of two components—stress and reaction to it. The individual, represented by a series of concentric circles on the diagram, is an open system in interaction with his total interface with the environment. That is, man is a system capable of intake of extrapersonal and interpersonal factors from the external environment. He interacts with this environment by adjusting himself to it or adjusting it to himself.

By a process of interaction and adjustment the individual maintains varying degrees of harmony and balance between his internal and external environment. Selye (1950) defines stressors as tension-producing stimuli with the potential of causing disequilibrium, situational or maturational crises, or the experience of stress within an individual's life. The above interaction-adjustment process contains the variables that make up the flexible line of defense that defends against these stressors. Influencing factors would include an individual's basic physiologic structure and condition, sociocultural background, developmental state, cognitive skills, age, and sex. Moroever, it is important to view the total person concept as dealing not with one or a few of these variables, but rather all variables affecting an individual at any point in time. The wholeness concept, then, is based upon the appropriate interrelationship of variables, which will determine the amount of resistance an individual has to any stressor.

It is possible for more than one stressor to occur at a given time. According to the Gestalt theory, each stressor would at least color the individual's reaction to any other stressor. Stressors as well as reaction and reconstitution factors can be viewed as intra-, inter-, or extrapersonal in nature. An example of each follows:

1. Intrapersonal—forces occurring within the individual, e.g., conditioned responses.
2. Interpersonal—forces occurring between one or more individuals, e.g., role expectations.
3. Extrapersonal—forces occurring outside the individual, e.g., financial circumstances.

What might be classified as a noxious stressor for one individual might not be for another. Time of occurrence, as well as past and present conditions of the individual, nature and intensity of the stressor, and amount of energy required for the organism to adapt are all variables. However, one might be able to predict positive adjustment based on past healthy coping behavior in a similar situation, all factors being equal.

In keeping with today's emphasis on primary prevention in health-care delivery, it is important to focus on strengtheining the flexible line of defense to prevent a possible reaction. This process requires an assessment of what meaning an experience has to an individual in the present as well as some knowledge of his past coping patterns. An assessment tool will be presented later in the chapter to illustrate the process.

Graphically, the model is a series of concentric rings surrounding a central core. The central core consists of basic survival factors common to all members of the species. Examples are the mechanisms for maintenance of a normal temperature range, a genetic response pattern, and the strengths and weaknesses of the various body parts or organs. However, each person has certain unique or baseline characteristics within the species range of commonalities.

The series of concentric rings surrounding the core structure vary in size and distance from the center. These make up the *flexible lines of resistance*. That is, all organisms possess certain internal factors that help them to defend against a stressor. An example is the body's mobilization of white blood cells or immune response mechanisms when needed. The normal line of defense is essentially what the individual has become over time, or his so-called "normal" or usual steady state. This is a result or composite of several variables and behaviors such as the individual's usual coping patterns, life-style, developmental stage, and so forth; it is basically the way in which an individual deals with stressors while functioning within the cultural pattern in which he was born and to which he attempts to conform.

Any stressor is potentially capable of temporarily incapacitating an individual, or possibly reducing the effectiveness of his internal "lines of resistance" that protect his core structure. A stressor affects the individual's normal line of defense by reducing his ability to cope with any additional stressors at a given point. However, what constitutes a normal line of defense for one person may not for another. This state is considered to be dynamic in that it relates to the way an individual is stabilized to deal with life stresses over time.

The flexible line of defense or outer broken ring encircling the large solid ring is thought of as accordionlike in function. It is dynamic rather than stable and can be rapidly altered over a relatively short period of time. It is thought of as a protective buffer for preventing stressors from breaking through the solid line of defense. Factors such as periods of under-nutrition, loss of sleep, or multiple impact of stressors can reduce the effectiveness of this buffer system and allow a reaction from one or more stressors to occur.

Intervention can begin at any point at which a stressor is either suspected or identified. One would carry out the intervention of primary prevention since a reaction had not yet occurred, though the degree of risk or hazard was known or present. The "actor" or intervener would perhaps attempt to reduce the possibility of the individual's encounter with the stressor or in some way attempt to strengthen the individual's flexible line of defense to decrease the possibility of a reaction.

Assuming that either the above intervention was not possible or that it failed and a reaction occurred, intervention known as secondary prevention or treatment would be offered in terms of existing symptomatology. Treatment could begin at any point following the occurrence of symptoms. Optimum use would be made of the individual's external as well as his internal resources in an attempt to stablize him, or help strengthen his internal lines of resistance to reduce the reaction. Ranking of need priority can occur, within use of this model, only by proper assessment of internal as well as external resources, that is, getting at the total meaning of the experience for the individual. Should the individual fail to reconstitute, death occurs as a result of the failure of the basic core structure to support the intervention. Reconstitution can be thought of as beginning at any point following interventions related to the degree of reaction. It is well to keep in mind that reconstitution may progress beyond, or stabilize somewhat below, the individual's previous normal line of defense or usual level of wellness.

Tertiary prevention is thought of as interventions following the active treatment or secondary prevention stage where some degree of reconstitution or stability has occurred. Emphasis in tertiary prevention is therefore on maintaining a reasonable degree of adaptation. This implies proper mobilization and utilization of the individual's existing energy resources. An example of a primary goal here would be to strengthen resistance to stressors by reeducation to help prevent recurrences of reaction or regression. "Reconstitution" at this stage is seen as a dynamic state of adaptation to stressors in the internal and external environment, integrating all factors for optimum use of total resources. This dynamic view of tertiary prevention tends to lead back in circular fashion toward primary prevention. An example of this circularity would either be emphasis on avoidance of specific known stressors that are hazardous or of desensitization of the individual to them.

In summary, the total person model must be viewed as multidimensional. Its logic has to do with a consideration of all variables affecting an individual—that is, the physiologic, psychologic, sociocultural, and developmental influences—and the proper ranking of need priority at any point. Although this model is relatively new and untested, it may well prove to be a reliable system for unifying various health-related theories and thus help to clarify the relationships of variables in nursing care. Based upon this assumption, role definition at various levels of nursing practice could be clarified.

NURSING ASSESSMENT BASED ON THE MODEL

At present nursing practitioners have very little tested methodology for dealing with the complex and changing nursing situations of today. Although nurses receive training in the natural and behavioral sciences, they are expected to synthesize and conceptualize this knowledge in their own way. This may primarily account for the inadequate communications and poorly defined goals that are commonplace in nursing today. Providing meaningful definitions and conceptual frames of reference for those situations basic to nursing practice seems to be an essential beginning for establishing nursing as a science.

In developing an assessment tool related to the total person model the following three basic principles must be considered:

1. Good assessment requires knowledge of all the factors influencing a patient's perceptual field.
2. The meaning that a stressor has to the patient is validated by the patient as well as by the care giver.
3. Factors in the care giver's perceptual field that influence her assessment of the patient's situation should become apparent.

The following intermediate step (Table 1) is provided for the purpose of linking the model's conceptual framework to an operational assessment tool. Though not conclusive, this data should serve as a reference source either for using the assessment tool included in this chapter or to aid those who are interested in developing their own assessment tool based on this model.

TABLE 1. Intermediate Step in Neuman Model

Primary Prevention	Secondary Prevention	Tertiary Prevention
Stressors* Mainly covert.	**Stressors*** Mainly overt or known.	**Stressors*** Mainly overt or residual—covert factors a possibility.
Reaction Hypothetical.	Reaction Identified by symptomatology or known factors.	Reaction Hypothetical or known—residual symptoms or factors.
Assessment Based on patient assessment, experience, and theory. Data should include: 1. Risks or possible hazards to the patient based on patient/nurse perception. 2. Meaning of the experience to the patient. 3. Life-style factors. 4. Coping patterns (past-present-possible). 5. Individual differences. 6. Other.	Assessment Determine nature and degree of reaction. Determine internal/external resources available to resist the reaction. Rationale for goals—with collaborative goal setting with the patient when possible.	Assessment Degree of stability following treatment; possible further reconstitution level assessed. Possible regression factors.
Interventions Strengthen resistance to the hazard by: 1. Education. 2. Desensitization. 3. Avoidance of hazard. 4. Strengthen individual resistance factors.	Interventions Based on the following: 1. Ranking of priority of needs related to symptoms. 2. Patient strengths and weaknesses as related to the "four" variables.* 3. Shift of priorities needed as the patient responds to treatment or as the nature of stressors change. (Primary prevention needs may occur simultaneously with treatment or secondary prevention.) 4. Need to deal with maladaptive processes. 5. Optimum use of internal/external resources, i.e., conservation of energy, noise reduction, financial aid.	Interventions Might include: 1. Motivation. 2. Reeducation. 3. Behavior modification. 4. Reality orientation. 5. Progressive goal setting. 6. Optimal use of appropriate available resources. 7. Maintenance of a reasonable adaptive level of functioning.

*Assessment should include information concerning the relationship of the four variables—physiologic, psychologic, sociocultural, and developmental.

THE ASSESSMENT/INTERVENTION TOOL

The assessment/intervention tool at the end of this article is designed in such a way as to include the various aspects of the model while allowing for the inclusion or addition of other areas of information. These may relate to specific individual client needs or to those needs peculiar to a particular health-care agency. An example might be the client's age and his general situation, or the special data requirements for medicare reimbursement.

This assessment/intervention tool should be adaptable to the needs of any agency and used by care givers of various disciplines to interview clients of any age or type. A unique feature is that the kinds of data obtained from the client's own perception of his condition influence the overall goals for his care. Hence, the form itself is not to be submitted to the client but is to be used as a question guide to obtain comprehensive data.

The following format should offer a progressive total view of the facts and conditions upon which client goals are established and modified. Since all care givers can relate to this format, continuity of care should be facilitated and role relationships clarified.

AN EXPLANATION OF THE ASSESSMENT/INTERVENTION TOOL

Category A—Biographic Data

A-1 This section includes general biographic data. However, certain agencies may require additional data in this area.

A-2 Referral source and related information are important. They provide a background history about the client and make possible any contacts with those who interviewed him earlier. Requests from agencies for reciprocal relationships might be recorded in this area.

Category B—Stressors

B-1 It is important to find out from the client how he perceives or experiences his particular situation or condition. By clarifying the client's perception, data are obtained for optimal planning of his care.

B-2 The client should be allowed to discuss how his present life-style is related to past, or usual, life-style patterns. A marked change may be significantly related to the course of an illness or possible illness.

B-3 This area relates to coping patterns. It is important to learn what similar conditions may have existed in the past and how the client has dealt with them. Such data provide insight about the types of resources that were available and were mobilized to deal with the situation. Past coping patterns may be significantly related to the present situation, making possible certain predictions as to what a client may or may not be able to accomplish. For example, symptoms of present loss might be exaggerated following unresolved past losses.

B-4 The area of client expectations is important in planning health-care interventions. Goals for care could be inappropriate if not based on clarification of how the client perceives his situation or condition. For example, a client might erroneously think his case is terminal all the while that the care giver attempts to prepare him for living.

B-5 If the extent of the client's motivation to help himself can be learned, available internal and external resources can be more wisely used in his behalf.

B-6 The health-care cost factor can often be a source of stress for the client. Sufficient data should be obtained from the client about health-care services he feels he needs. However, the practitioner should bear in mind that the client frequently requires help in determining what services are realistic for him.

Category C—Stressors

That care givers have a perspective different from that of the client is considered a positive factor. Yet this fact may cause some distortion of reality in assessment/intervention. Education, past experiences, values, personal biases, and unresolved personal conflicts may get in the way of the care giver's clear conception of the client's actual condition. Category C was included to reduce this possibility. Questions one through six are essentially the same as those in category B so that the client's own perception can be compared with the care giver's. The interviewer should know the basis for his own perceptions as well as the client's so that the reality of the client's situation or condition can be fairly accurately described in a "Summary of Impressions."

Categories D, E, and F

These categories deal with the intra-, inter-, and extrapersonal factors illustrated on the model diagram. In order to assess an individual's total situation or condition at any point, it is necessary to know the relationship among internal factors, factors between the individual and his environment, as well as peripheral factors which are affecting the individual or could affect him. This set of questions attempts to clarify these relationships so that goal priorities can be established. It is well to keep in mind that the nature and priority of goals will probably change as changes occur in the relationship of factors or variables.

Category G

A clear statement of the problem requires the reconciliation of perceptual differences between client and caregiver. All other aspects of the data must be ordered in rank file according to priorities.

Category H—Summary of Goals with Rationale

Once the major problem has been defined in relation to all factors affecting the client situation or condition, further classification is needed. A decision must be made as to what form of intervention should take priority. For example, if a reaction has not yet occurred and the client has been assessed as being in a high-risk category, intervention should begin at the primary prevention of treatment level. Moreover, one should be able to state the logic or rationale for the intervention. If a reaction is noted on assessment (that is, symptoms are obvious), intervention should begin at the secondary prevention level (treatment). When assessment is made following treatment, intervention should begin at the tertiary prevention level (follow-up after treatment).

By relating all factors affecting the client, it is possible to determine fairly accurately what type of intervention is needed (primary, secondary, or tertiary) as well as the rationale to support the stated goals. At whatever point interventions are begun, it is important to attempt to project possible future requirements. This data may not be readily available on initial assessment, but should be noted when possible to provide a comprehensive and progressive view of the client's total condition. It is important to relate this section of the assessment/intervention tool to the intervention (worksheet) plan that follows.

Category I—Intervention Plan to Support Stated Goals

This portion of the assessment/intervention tool is a form of worksheet which provides progressive data as to the type of intervention given and when. Goals are listed and ranked by priority. The types of interventions, and their results, are noted. The comment section might include data useful for future planning, such as shift in goal priority based upon changes in the client's condition or responses, and success or failure of present interventions. This format classifies each intervention in a consistent, progressive, and comprehensive manner to which any care giver can meaningfully relate. This

H. Summary of Goals with Rationales

	Primary Prevention (Prevention of Treatment)	Secondary Prevention (Treatment)	Tertiary Prevention (Follow-up after Treatment)
Immediate Goals: 1. 2. 3. Rationale:			
Intermediate Goals: 1. 2. 3. Rationale:			
Future Goals: 1. 2. 3. Rationale:			

I. Intervention Plan to Support Stated Goals

Primary Prevention	Secondary Prevention	Tertiary Prevention
Date_____		
Goals:*	Goal:*	Goal:*
1.	1.	1.
2.	2.	2.
3.	3.	3.
Intervention:	Intervention:	Intervention:
Outcome:	Outcome:	Outcome:
Comments:	Comments:	Comments:

*Goals are stated in order of priority.

system of classifying data over time allows one to see the relationship of the parts to the whole, that is, to view the client in total perspective, thereby reducing the possibility of fragmentation of care and possibly cutting its cost.

REFERENCES

de Chardin PT: The Phenomenon of Man. London, Collins, 1955, pp 109–112

Cornu A: The Origins of Marxian Thought. Springfield, Thomas, 1957, pp 12–17

Edelson M: Sociotherapy and Psychotherapy. Chicago, U of Chicago Press, 1970, pp 225–231

Selye H: The Physiology and Pathology of Exposure to Stress. Montreal, ACTA, Inc., 1950, pp 12–13

An Assessment/Intervention Tool Based Upon the Betty Neuman Health-Care Systems Model: A Total Approach to Patient Problems

A. *Intake Summary*
    1. Name _____
       Age _____
       Sex _____
       Marital _____
    2. Referral source and related information.
B. *Stressors*
   Identified by and based on the *patient's perception* of his circumstances.
   (If patient is incapacitated, secure data from family or other resources.)
    1. What do you consider your major problem, stress area, or areas of concern? (Identify problem areas)
    2. How do present circumstances differ from your usual pattern of living? (Identify life-style patterns)
    3. Have you *ever* experienced a similar problem? If so, what was that problem and how did you handle it? Were you successful? (Identify past coping patterns)
    4. What do you anticipate for yourself in the future as a consequence of your present situation? (Identify perceptual factors, i.e., reality versus distortions-expectations, present and possible future coping patterns)
    5. What are you doing and what can you do to help yourself? (Identify perceptual factors, i.e., reality versus distortions-expectations, present and possible future coping patterns)
    6. What do you expect care givers, family, friends, or others to do for you? (Identify perceptual factors, i.e., reality versus distortions-expectations, present and possible future coping patterns)
C. *Stressors*
   Identified by and based on the *care giver's perception* of the patient's circumstances.

1. What do you consider to be the major problem, stress area, or areas of concern? (Identify problem areas)
2. How do present circumstances seem to differ from the patient's usual pattern of living? (Identify life-style patterns)
3. Has the patient ever experienced a similar situation? If so, how would you evaluate what the patient did? How successful do you think it was? (Identify past coping patterns)
4. What do you anticipate for the future as a consequence of the patient's present situation? (Identify perceptual factors, i.e., reality versus distortions-expectations, present and possible future coping patterns)
5. What can the patient do to help himself? (Identify perceptual factors, i.e., reality versus distortions-expectations, present and possible future coping patterns)
6. What do *you think* the patient expects from care givers, family, friends, or other resources? (Identify perceptual factors, i.e., reality versus distortions-expectations, present and possible future coping patterns)

Summary of Impressions

Note any discrepancies or distortions between the patient's perception and that of the care giver related to the situation.

D. *Intrapersonal Factors*
   1. *Physical* (Examples: degree of mobility; range of body function)
   2. *Psycho-sociocultural* (Examples: attitudes, values, expectations, behavior patterns and nature of coping patterns)
   3. *Developmental* (Examples: age, degree of normalcy, factors related to present situation)
E. *Interpersonal Factors*
   Resources and relationship of family, friends, or care givers that either influence or could influence Area D.
F. *Extrapersonal Factors*
   Resources and relationship of community facilities, finances, employment, or other areas which either influence or could influence Areas D and E.
G. *Formulation of the Problem*
   Identify and rank the priority of needs based on the total data obtained from the patient's perception, the care giver's perception, and/or other resources, i.e., laboratory reports, other care givers, or agencies.

   With this format, reassessment is a continuous process and is related to the effectiveness of intervention based upon the stated goals.

   Effective reassessment would include the following as they relate to the total patient situation:
   1. Changes in nature of stressors and priority assignments
   2. Changes in intrapersonal factors

3. Changes in interpersonal factors
4. Changes in extrapersonal factors

In reassessment it is important to note the change of priority of goals in relation to the primary, secondary, and tertiary prevention categories.

An assessment tool of this nature should offer a current, progressive, and comprehensive analysis of the patient's total circumstances or relationships of the four variables (physical, psychologic, sociocultural, and developmental).*

*This assessment tool is currently being tested by a comprehensive home health-care agency in California.

Janet F. Venable

10

The Neuman Health-Care Systems Model: An Analysis

A theoretical framework is imperative as a basis for nursing practice. Such a framework must be both understandable and practical in the work setting. For these reasons I chose the Neuman Health-Care Systems Model (discussed in the previous article). To make this decision it was necessary to analyze the utility of the model as well as its implications for nursing. This article presents one way in which such a task can be accomplished. The format will be (1) description of the model; (2) definition of terms; (3) analysis by structure, substance, and acceptability; (4) summary and critique.

DESCRIPTION OF THE MODEL

This health-care systems model is a multidimensional, total unit approach that can be used to describe an individual, a group, or an entire community. As such, the model can be applied equally well to the study of individual patient problems or problems of an organization. In this article, the model will be discussed in terms of individual patient problems.

The Neuman model is basically an open systems model of stress and reaction. The patient (represented by the concentric circles on the diagram in Neuman's article) is viewed as an open system in interaction with his environment. Mechanically, the model is fairly simple. Stressors, which are comprised of intra-, inter-, and extrapersonal factors, impinge upon the patient's *flexible line of defense* where they generate varying degrees of response. If the flexible line of defense gives way and a reaction to a stressor occurs, then the response of the patient is either toward death, when penetration of the basic structure occurs, or toward reconstitution. Examples of stressors resulting in death would be (1) irreversible cardiac arrest in which an overwhelming stressor yields rapid and permanent penetration of the basic structure, and

(2) leukemia, in which the stressor may be slowed by the *lines of resistance* and some temporary reconstitution is made, but ultimately penetrates the basic structure causing death. Stressors other than pathophysiology may cause death, e.g., suicide. When an individual's response to a stressor is toward reconstitution, the degree of reaction is dependent upon intrapersonal factors (forces occurring within the individual), interpersonal factors (forces occurring between one or more individuals), and extrapersonal factors (forces occurring outside the individual). Each of these three factors include physiologic, psychologic, sociocultural, and developmental variables. Examples of each of these factors are given below.

Intrapersonal—anger is a force within the individual whose expression is influenced by age (developmental), peer group acceptability (sociocultural), physical abilities (physiologic), and past experience with anger (psychologic).

Interpersonal—mother-child role expectations are forces occurring between individuals that are influenced by local child-rearing practices (sociocultural), age and development of child and mother (developmental and physiologic), and feelings about the role (psychologic).

Extrapersonal—unemployment is a force occurring outside the individual that is influenced by peer group acceptability (sociocultural), personal feelings toward, or past experience with, unemployment (psychologic), ability to perform a job (physiologic, developmental, psychologic).

Other factors influencing reaction and reconstitution of the system are number and strength of the stressor(s), length of encounter, and meaningfulness of the stressor to the individual.

In assessing and intervening, nurses enter this system as an interpersonal factor. According to the structure of the model, the nurse may intervene at the primary, secondary, or tertiary prevention level. Primary prevention deals with the system before an encounter with a stressor occurs. The goal of primary prevention is to prevent the stressor from penetrating the *normal line of defense* or to lessen the degree of reaction by reducing the possibility of encounter with the stressor, reducing its strength, and/or strengthening the flexible line of defense. Secondary prevention deals with the system after an encounter with a stressor has occurred and is concerned mainly with early case finding and treatment of symptoms. Tertiary prevention accompanies and follows reconstitution and is concerned with reeducation to prevent future occurrences, readaptation, and maintenance of stability.

These levels of intervention are interrelated and are somewhat circular in nature. The goals of tertiary prevention are sometimes similar to the goals of primary prevention.

DEFINITION OF TERMS IN THE MODEL

A thorough understanding of terms is prerequisite to the use of any model. The following terms for this model are defined by the author.

Normal line of defense—state of wellness; adaptational state over time that is considered "normal" for the individual.

Flexible line of defense—dynamic state of wellness; individual's current, immediate state, which is particularly susceptible to situational circumstances, e.g., amount of sleep, hormone level.

Stressor—any problem, condition, etc., capable of causing instability of the system by penetration of the normal line of defense; intra-, inter-, extrapersonal in nature.

Degree of reaction—amount of system instability caused by penetration of the stressor through the normal line of defense.

Lines of resistance—internal resistant forces encountered by a stressor which act to decrease the degree of reaction, e.g., increase of leukocytosis to eradicate invading organisms.

Reconstitution—resolution of the stressor from the deepest degree of reaction back toward the normal line of defense; may reconstitute to a level higher or lower than prepenetration.

Primary prevention—interventions initiated before or after an encounter with a stressor; includes decreasing the possibility of encounter with stressors and strengthening the flexible line of defense in the presence of stressors.

Secondary prevention—interventions initiated after encounter with a stressor; includes early case finding and treatment of symptoms following a reaction to a stressor.

Tertiary prevention—interventions generally initiated after treatment; focuses on readaptation, reeducation to prevent future occurrences, and maintenance of stability.

Intrapersonal factor—force occurring within the individual.

Interpersonal factor—force occurring between one or more individuals.

Extrapersonal factor—force occurring outside the individual.

ANALYSIS OF THE MODEL

The Neuman Health-Care Systems Model was analyzed according to Johnson's "Requirements of an Effective Model for Nursing" (Johnson, 1971). These requirements are concerned with the structure, the substance, and the acceptability of the model. The structure of a model must include the assumptions that the model makes, its value system, and its major units.

Structure

Table 1 presents the assumptions, value system, and major units that constitute the foundation of the Neuman model.*

The assumptions shown in the table provide an adequate base for the concepts embodied in the major units, which are clearly specified and observable in actual care and are consistent in their interrelationships. The value system is objective and is in keeping with both the values of society and the responsibilities of the nursing profession.

Substance

In reviewing the substance (or function) of a model, the following areas must be considered: the model's scope of action, its projection of a unique role for nursing, and its ability to account for change in the events that occur. Each of these points are discussed below.

The total person approach to viewing patient problems lends itself well to nursing practice in all areas under a wide variety of conditions. Any patient, group, or community can be considered to be in interaction with the stressors in the environment. The modes of intervention are sufficiently broad to encompass a wide variety of interventive techniques and styles while retaining sufficient structure to organize care.

This model does not readily assign unique roles to nursing and other health workers. Its strength is in the fact that it does not fragment the person (or group and community) into "disciplines" (nursing care, medical care, physical therapy care, etc.), but considers him within a "total person" framework. The model is, therefore, an interdisciplinary approach to patient care. It is compatible with our present health-care delivery system in that it pulls together the goals and foci of the many disciplines concerned with patient care. While at this point the nurse may function within certain legally and traditionally defined roles in providing nursing care, this model will increase awareness of the "total person," i.e., aspects of care currently defined as nonnursing, as well as provide a base for the expanding role of the nurse (e.g., the nurse practitioner whose role is developing to encompass pathophysiologic assessment as well as nursing care).

The model must also account for stability as well as change in the events being considered. The *basic structure* and *normal line of defense,* as described in the model, account for stability. Change comes in response to reaction to stressors and is reflected in the *flexible line of defense.* Thus the entire system is seen to be in a dynamic, adaptational balance over time.

---

*In the article by Newman, the presentation of the health-care systems model included a discussion of the model, statement of assumptions, and definitions of terms. For the purposes of analysis, this author restates many of the assumptions. The basic concepts remain the same, although in some cases they have been grouped differently or presented as definitions.

TABLE 1. Beliefs About Nursing and Its Practice

1. Nursing is concerned with the total person.
2. Nursing can intervene in patient's responses to stress at three levels: preencounter (primary prevention), encounter (treatment), and reconstitution.
3. Nursing and medicine are complementary in nature.

Assumptions
A. About Man
   1. Man may be viewed as a total person encompassing all aspects of the human being and the multiplicity of variables that may affect behavior.
   2. Man is an open system in contact with his environment.

B. About the Model
   1. Each individual has a basic structure of energy resources whose compromise is incompatible with life.
   2. Each individual has a normal line of defense, which is a dynamic state of adaptation that the individual has maintained over time.
   3. Each individual has a flexible line of defense, which is constantly changing in response to the influence of changing physiologic, psychologic, sociocultural, and developmental variables.
   4. Many stressors are universal and known; others are stressors only in relation to their meaning to the patient.
   5. Stressors are intra-, inter-, and extrapersonal in nature. They are dynamic with the possibility of causing priority needs to change at any point.
   6. The degree of reaction depends upon the resistant forces encountered by the stressor.
   7. Reconstitution in response to stress may begin at any level of reaction and proceed to any higher level of reaction with the possibility of a new level of wellness established above or below the previous normal line of defense.
   8. Interventions can occur before or after resistance lines are penetrated in both reaction and reconstitution phases.

Value System of the Model
1. There is no absolute, "acceptable" level for the normal line of defense. Rather, acceptability is relative to the potential for that individual system.
2. Nurses have the obligation to seek the highest potential level of stability for the individual patient system.
3. Nurses cannot impose their judgments upon the patient especially as regards the meaning of stressors and acceptable levels for the normal line of defense.

Major Units of the Model
Goal:	System stability.
Patiency:	An open system (individual, group, or community) whose boundary is its flexible line of defense, which is in interaction with the stressors (actual and potential) in its environment.
Actor's Role:	To regulate and control the systems response to stress through primary, secondary, and tertiary prevention.
Source of Difficulty:	Actual or potential penetration of the flexible line of defense (system instability).
Intervention Focus:	Actual or potential penetration of the flexible line of defense.
Mode:	Primary, secondary, tertiary prevention.
Consequences Intended:	Increased resistance to stress; decreased degree of reaction and increased maintained level of wellness.
Unintended:	None.

Acceptability

Acceptability of the model encompasses three areas: social congruence, social significance, and social utility.

Social Congruence

Society's expectation of nursing is probably most closely tied to the actions of secondary prevention in acute care settings. Primary prevention is more frequently seen as a nursing role in public health and community nursing. Tertiary prevention is traditionally viewed in limited settings and through limited roles, e.g., physiologically oriented rehabilitation centers and extended care facilities, or psychologically oriented mental health "halfway house" facilities. Primary and tertiary prevention are, however, important aspects of care in all nursing settings and will have more social congruence as the role of the nurse expands and society's awareness of it increases.

Social Significance

Stability of the system, which is stability of the person, group, or community in contact with a stressor, is significant in that the alternative is instability (illness) and death. The large sums of money spent annually by individuals in seeking assistance to maintain stability is one indication of the value and significance of system stability.

Social Utility

The social utility of the Neuman model can be discussed within three contexts—practice, research, and education.

Practice   The model is universal in its applicability to nursing. Perhaps its greatest strength is the clear direction that it gives for interventions through primary, secondary, and tertiary prevention.

Research   The model asks many researchable questions. Among these are the following: What are the universal stressors? What tools can be developed for measuring degrees of reaction? What are the significant stressors of certain age or cultural groups? What are some specific interventions for each prevention category?

Education   The educational process need no longer be segmented into the learning of psychosocial skills, which are considered "nursing" (interviewing, support, modification of environment), and pathophysiologic skills, which are considered "medicine" or physician assistance (monitoring vital signs, collection of specimens). As the model places physiologic variables and stressors as well as behavioral variables and stressors within the realm of the nurse, all skills can be seen as interventive tools used by the care giver through a total patient approach.

Insasmuch as the model emphasizes a total person approach, it seems to transcend the nursing model and become a health-care model. As a health-care model it would have implications for all health-care education. Some of these implications are increased joint education of health-care workers, and trends toward levels of health-care workers rather than the separate specialties of nursing, medical, and paramedical work.

SUMMARY AND CRITIQUE

This article has presented an analysis of the Neuman Health-Care Systems Model utilizing Johnson's "Requirements of an Effective Model for Nursing." The model was described, its terms defined, and it was analyzed for its structure, substance, and acceptability.

The author believes that the utility of this model lies in its simplicity and flexibility as a stimulus-response systems model. Such simplicity readily lends itself to use in a wide variety of nursing situations.

Neuman (in the previous article) states that this model may provide a unique role for nursing. This author is not convinced. However, since the total person approach of the model is so useful, the lack of a unique role for nursing is not seen as a detriment but rather as a call for reexamination of traditionally defined roles assigned to health-care workers in general.

This model is relatively new and has great potential. The major purpose of this paper is to assist in laying the groundwork for the operationalization and incorporation of this model into nursing practice.

REFERENCES

Johnson D: Requirements of an effective conceptual model for nursing, unpublished, UCLA School of Nursing, class material N203, 1971

Neuman B, Young RJ: A model for teaching total person approach to patient problems. Nurs Res, 21:3:264, 1972

Betty Neuman
Margaret Wyatt

11

The Neuman Stress/ Adaptation Systems Approach to Education for Nurse Administrators

Little research data exist concerning the unique problems and processes of nursing administration. In fact, nursing administration education is generally considered a "functional" area of a particular clinical specialist program. Few master's programs offer nurses majors in nursing administration.

In the United States, less than 20 percent of nursing service administrators have master's degrees of any kind, and another 22 percent have only baccalaureate degrees. A great need exists for highly competent leaders in nursing administration to influence major decisions being made in the health-care field, particularly since nurses represent the largest single health care discipline. A high level of management skill is needed if nursing is to meet successfully today's challenges in areas such as labor relations, the communication of nursing's goals, role, and methods to consumers and other health professionals, and advancement toward goals defined by professional nursing. A synthesis of nursing and management is mandatory if nursing is to regain leadership in administrative positions within the health care system. Control systems relating health outcome to the nursing process represents one step toward such a synthesis.

Stevens (1978) states that "adaptation of management techniques in nursing is clearly in an early development state, and the synthesis, creating management tools specific to the needs of nursing, must have a high priority in nursing administration and the education of the nurse administrator." She also believes that the problems of nursing administration, and education for nursing administration, are critical, and that nursing administration education programs need to be rebuilt to prevent loss of input from professional nurses in management decisions and overall health care planning.

In response to needs in the academic world, a growing number of nurse administrators are forming independent groups for mutual problem-solving and informal education, or are turning to programs in health care administration.

The dearth of adequately prepared nurse administrators in the southeast Ohio area of rural Appalachia is generally reflected in low morale within nursing service. Thirty master's-prepared nurses of various specialities serve a population of 765,000. In the entire state of Ohio only 45 nurse administrators (9 percent) graduated from master's programs with administration as a functional area. In addition, many qualified nurse administrators either leave the state or do not migrate to the rural areas.

In an attempt to resolve the southeast Ohio rural Appalachian dilemma, the Ohio University School of Nursing in the College of Education at Athens, Ohio, is currently developing a master's program in nursing administration. It is hoped that graduates will remain in the area to accept the existing challenges and opportunities for professionalism.

In the development of the Nursing Service Administration program it was recognized that, in the field of nursing service administration, a variety of nursing models could be used. The impact of today's environmental subsystems upon the traditional nurse administrator's role dictates a dynamic systems approach for the curriculum—one with significantly broad, general concepts to assure future relevance in educating nurse administrators.

In the Ohio University School of Nursing program, the Neuman Nursing Administration Stress/Adaptation Systems Model* will be used as the foundation for the master's level program in nursing service administration. The model lends itself well to development of strategies to meet future vast changes in the social order. The Neuman model will introduce students to the multiple concepts and constructs of nursing administration, thereby facilitating a rational approach to the study of nursing management problems.

The Neuman nursing administration model, which will act as a general guide for curriculum planning (see Figure 1), represents a synthesis of nursing and management as applied in any organization/health-care setting. Organizations and social units, as well as individuals, vary in their ability to deal effectively with change and its results. Nursing administrators should initiate and respond to changes pertinent to the health both of organizations and of clients at different levels of health care delivery, management, and interdisciplinary concerns. Nursing service function is portrayed as multidimensional, occurring in a complex environment necessitating adaptation for achievement of the ultimate goal of optimal provision of health care.

The first dimension of nursing administration is a stress/adaptation intervention system that provides a flexible, dynamic concept for nursing practice. It encompasses the entire spectrum of nursing practice while addressing various levels and degrees of health concerns.

A second dimension of nursing administration is the nurse administrator/ health manager role, through which nursing management is accomplished.

---

*The model was adapted from the original Betty Neuman model (1974).

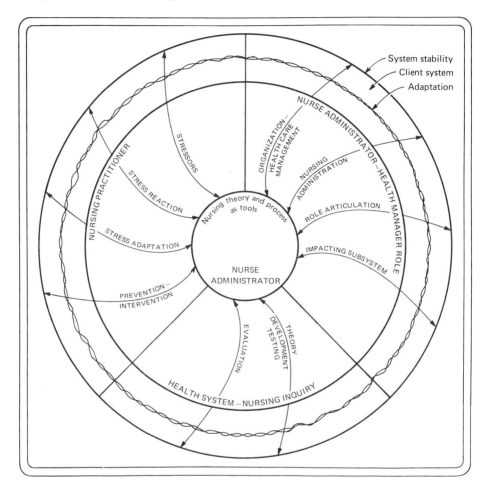

Figure 1 *The Neuman Nursing Administration Stress/Adaptation*
Systems Curriculum Model.

This role comprehends the structures, processes, content, and managerial goals of administration. "Structures" refers to the managerial job itself and the organization of the nursing service department and its parent agency; it represents the organizing framework in which nursing management takes place. "Processes" are the component events that occur within the nursing service department, i.e., the events that move through the more stable, ongoing structure. "Content" refers to human and material resources. "Goals" refers to achievement of quality control through nursing service and desired organizational outcomes.

A third dimension of nursing administration is applied research or inquiry.

While delivery of quality nursing practice is the ultimate goal of nursing management, it is recognized that practice advances only as nursing theory is developed, and nursing theory advances only as the research questions implicit in nursing theory are tested and confirmed. The field of nursing is viewed as a dynamic area within the health care system.

A fourth dimension of nursing administration is "a total view of man": the study of nursing needs of adult clients in the health care system. The Neuman model (see Figure 2) provides a comprehensive framework for viewing and organizing diverse phenomena inherent in wellness and illness across this age group. The broad framework offers a consistent base for both examining man's response to existing phenomena and for giving direction to restitution.

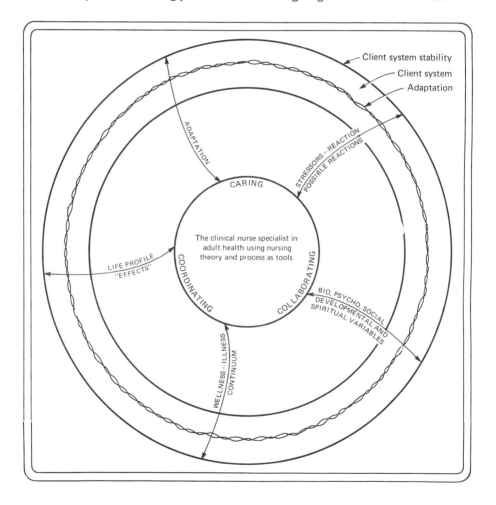

Figure 2   *The Neuman Model's Total View of Man.*

An adult health clinical focus was selected for developing professional nurses with expertise in a specialized area of clinical nursing practice. This adult population forms one arena for the application of nursing administration principles.

A fifth dimension of nursing administration is the dynamic interaction between nursing theory and practice. These two are viewed as nursing "tools" with which is effected stability or adaptation to stress in the client system. The client system includes individuals, families, groups/organizations, and/or community. Outcome data from interventions provide a feedback loop to validate or invalidate nursing theory and practice. As this dimension is pervasive, threading through all other dimensions of nursing administration, it becomes a unifying factor for the curriculum model.

This stress/adaptation systems model for nursing administration implies selected use of nursing theory and processes for intervention in stressors affecting individuals, groups/organizations, and impacting environmental subsystems. The model synthesizes nursing and management as they occur in the organizational setting, which is best described by its multiple, diverse, acting, and interacting systems. This synthesis of nursing and management is a prerequisite for successful nursing administration. Management technology cannot simply be applied, without adaptation, to the field of nursing. Management itself is changed by the nature of the nursing field to which it is applied. Martin reminds us of its impact on quality assurance in the nursing service setting.*

The master's program as a generalist program, acquaints the student with all facets of the model. The intersections of the model provide loci for student and faculty research and study.

The general curriculum approach will provide students with (1) a conceptual frame of reference within which nursing management problems can be analyzed and resolved, (2) management theory and practice applied to health service settings, and (3) management theory and practice correlated with that of nursing.

A broad conceptual stress/adaptation systems approach to nursing administration problems will be taken as follows:

1. Assessment of nursing administration problems will take place in one or more of the intra-, inter-, and extrapersonal systems to be known as nursing organization entities, fields, or client systems.†
2. Intervention in nursing administration problem areas will take place at three levels of adaptation to stress—primary, secondary, tertiary‡—using

---

*Comments made by Ruby Martin at the Advisory committee meeting for the proposed program at the Ohio University School for Nursing 2/9/79.

†These are aspects of the total nursing system as well as aspects of the surrounding environments—organizational, community, state, federal, professional, etc.

‡That is, before system imbalance, during system imbalance, and following restoration.

a prevention/intervention modality. The systems stress/adaptation prevention/intervention approach is broad enough to encompass traditional nursing theory and approaches to problem solving and yet allow needed flexibility for creative problem solving with today's complex social systems. Adaptation theory and process will thread through all administrative nursing functions and serve as an organizing curriculum theme as well as an integrating factor for both nursing administration and organizational theory and process throughout the program. Major focus will be on teaching the nursing administration student to develop skill in matching the stress/adaptation systems concept to the nature of the problems addressed.

Using nursing theory and organizational theory and processes, the nurse administrator intervenes by preventing maladaptation, restoring adaptation, or maintaining adaptation following restoration in order to effect client-system stability in one or more organizational systems at any given time. The ultimate goals for the nurse administrator are to provide optimal health-care delivery for clients, improve nursing practice, and refine nursing theory through inquiry.

The environment or client system in which nursing administration takes place is conceptualized as consisting of multiple, diverse, and interacting systems. These systems represent sites of events and interactions, and include legal, educational, logistic, political, professional-technical, social, and economic systems. Their interrelationships act as organizing centers for managerial tasks. These systems constantly influence intra-, inter-, and extra-nursing organizational entities; that is, they must be dealt with as aspects affecting the total nursing system as well as the surrounding environments—organizational, community, etc.

The nursing administration student will learn theories, processes, and techniques for smooth interface and/or integration of these systems into the nursing organization system.

The curriculum model reflects the distribution of the Neuman stress/adaptation systems conceptual framework for nursing administration. It describes the major organizing themes or principles rather than the sequence or option of courses. The curriculum plan for the master's program is described in five modules, each of which consists of one or more courses built around a set of principles or organizing themes. Interdisciplinary learning will be maximized in this scheme.

Total curriculum organization is based on the following five modules (see Curriculum Grid, page 148).

1. Dimension I focuses on nursing theory and managerial theory essential for nursing administration.
2. Dimension II focuses on nursing practice as it relates to organization and

Curriculum Grid

Dimension	Subject Matter	Means	Principles
I	Nursing management; Health services— organizational management	Structure/process/ content and goals	Systems, role, relations, decision, task
II	Nursing practitioner	Personnel compliment, nursing theory and process, adaptation, systems intervention/ prevention, role articulation	Client system, problem solving, systems, role, change
III	Subsystems	Impacting subsystems analysis and interven- tion, nursing organiza- tion entities	Stress/adaptation systems
IV	Adult health nursing	Nursing process, client education	Client, problem solving, adaptation, wellness/illness
V	Clinical inquiry	Research process	Evaluation, quality assurance

management plans for health-care delivery. The systems stress/ adaptation concept is used as a comprehensive nursing theory base for planning, implementing, and evaluating health care.

3. Dimension III focuses on the effects of impacting subsystems in relation to nursing administration and organizational systems.

4. Dimension IV focuses on adult health as the clinical component for study and promotion of adaptive processes of clients in the health care system toward advancement of nursing practice and refinement of nursing theory.

5. Dimension V focuses on nursing research in relation to evaluation of nursing theory and practice, health policies, programs, and "professionalization" of nursing.

Courses are sequenced in four phases with course limits of 25 students and each laboratory section limited to 9 students:

Curriculum Design—Master of Science—Emphasis in Nursing Administration

Phase I—Theoretical Aspects of Nursing Administration

	Credit
Nursing Administration I	2
Laboratory	2
Research—EdRe 501	4

Concepts of Health Care—Transdisciplinary	2
Theoretical Basis for Nursing Practice	4
Laboratory	2

Phase II—Functional Aspects of Nursing Administration

	Credit
Nursing Administration II	2
Laboratory	2
Clinical Inquiry	4
Laboratory	2
Concepts of Health Care—Transdisciplinary	2
Elective (select one)	3–5
Mgt. 500, 520, 525, 535	
Educ. EDGS 570, EDAD 631	
Inco 545	
Philosophy 520	

Phase III—Multidisciplinary Aspects of Nursing
Administration

	Credit
Nursing Administration III	2
Laboratory	2
Clinical Inquiry	4
Laboratory	2
Concepts of Health Care—Transdisciplinary	2
Elective (select one)	3–5
Business Law 500	
Pol. Sc. 511, 512, 513	
Sociology 532, 533, 565	
Philosophy 540	

Phase IV—Integrative Aspects of Nursing Administration

	Credit
Nursing Administration IV	2
Laboratory	2
Thesis or field project	8
Elective (select one)	3–5
Mgt. 540, 545, 550	
Bus. Adm. 560	
Pol. Sc. 514	
Eng. 540	

Graduates of the Ohio University nursing administration program will have benefited from a unique blend of theory and practice in nursing and health services management which will serve as a foundation for competent, creative nursing administration. Nursing content is designed to assist the student in making sound decisions for planning, implementing, and evaluating nursing services according to a nursing stress/adaptation systems model. Health services and organizational management content provide decision-making tools for organizing and coordinating resources in the delivery of health care to the public. The optimal blend of nursing and management content in interdisciplinary education will enable the nurse administrator to function both as a vital member of the management team and as an advocate for the profession of nursing.

REFERENCES

Drucker PF: Management: Tools, Responsibilities, Practices. New York, Harper and Row, 1974, p 553.

Neuman B: The Betty Neuman Model: a total person approach to viewing patient problems. In Riehl JP, Roy C: Conceptual Models for Nursing Practice. New York, Appleton, 1974, p 100.

Stevens BJ: Education in nursing administration. Newsletter of American Nurses Association.

Mary Lebold
Lucille Davis

12

A Baccalaureate Nursing Curriculum Based on the Neuman Health Systems Model

Professional nursing programs prepare nurses who are accountable and responsible for health care in a dynamic, pluralistic society. Nurses must be educated to assume current nursing roles and to adapt to future health needs. As a consequence, nursing programs are challenged to develop creative and flexible curriculum designs which are consistent with emerging roles and evolving health care requirements.

The challenge of meeting today's and tomorrow's realities, coupled with the rapid proliferation of knowledge and technology, necessitates a curriculum design that is not only specific, but also integrative and innovative. Such a design needs to be built on a flexible conceptual framework which provides for logical movement through the curriculum, identification of content, learning experiences and processes. The design should also facilitate role induction into the profession, be adaptive to future trends and facilitate curricular decision-making and evaluation.

This paper describes how a baccalaureate program operationalized the Neuman Model (Neuman, 1974) as a basis for its conceptual framework. The Neuman Model was selected because it provides a theoretical and comprehensive foundation for a holistic curriculum (Stevens, 1979) which is consistent with a system's perspective of individuals, health and nursing. The latter perspective is expressed in the School of Nursing's philosophy which views individuals as biological-psychological-social-spiritual beings in dynamic, reciprocal interaction with their internal and external environments. Nurses provide health care to individuals, families, and communities across the life cycle and the health-illness continuum. They are responsible for promoting maximum health at whatever point the individual, the family, or the community is on the continuum. Nursing care is provided within three separate but interrelated categories: primary, secondary, and tertiary prevention.

Nurses function in multiple systems through collaborative relationships with clients and other health team members.

Through analysis of the philosophy, objectives, conceptual framework, and Neuman's Model, eight curriculum strands are identified: (1) leadership, (2) research, (3) systems, (4) teaching, (5) nursing, (6) communications, (7) health continuum, and (8) life cycle. Leadership, research, systems, and teaching are vertical strands which are developed through each level of the curriculum. Life cycle is a horizontal strand which is repeated at each level. Due to the complex interrelation of their components, the other strands— health continuum, communication, and nursing—are seen as both horizontal and vertical strands. These concepts are presented in their entirety at each level with a special focus on a component of the concept. For example, the entire concept of the Nursing Process is presented on the sophomore level with a focus on assessment. (See Chart 1.) Using Bloom's *Taxonomy* as a guide, the strands are developed into objectives for various courses. The level objectives progress in complexity, moving from comprehension to application and analysis, and to synthesis and evaluation (Bloom, 1956).

Nursing courses are not considered in isolation, but rather as a component of a program of professional studies. The professional component is introduced at the sophomore level and builds on introductory liberal arts and sciences courses. The liberal arts and sciences courses are integral to the curriculum design and are taught throughout all four years of the program.

THE LIBERAL ARTS AND SCIENCES COMPONENT

Leadership and communication, two of the major vertical threads in the curriculum, have their base in the liberal arts and sciences courses. These courses offer a foundation for personal and professional development by providing a framework for critical thinking and reasoning. Students are introduced to the scientific method and the influences of history on society. In the humanities, the students are given opportunities to explore the concepts of self and humanity, along with experiences in various modes of expression and communication. This knowledge is not only important for leadership and communication, but it is also necessary for the understanding of clients and their needs.

Courses supportive to the nursing major are selected and designed in conjunction with other departments to provide a theoretical body of knowledge outside of the nursing framework that can be drawn on for application in nursing. These supportive courses, which enhance self-development and provide a broader base for problem-solving, either precede or are taught concurrently with the nursing courses in our curriculum. Electives are taken in the liberal arts, sciences, and nursing courses (see Chart 2).

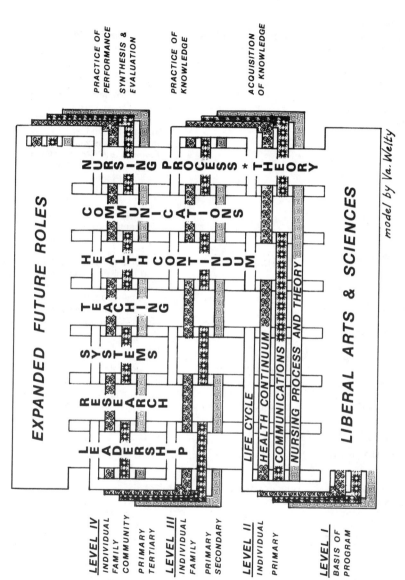

EXPANDED FUTURE ROLES

PRACTICE OF PERFORMANCE

SYNTHESIS & EVALUATION

PRACTICE OF KNOWLEDGE

ACQUISITION OF KNOWLEDGE

NURSING PROCESS * THEORY

COMMUNICATIONS

HEALTH CONTINUUM

LEADERSHIP

RESEARCH

SYSTEMS

TEACHING

LIFE CYCLE
HEALTH CONTINUUM
COMMUNICATIONS
NURSING PROCESS AND THEORY

LIBERAL ARTS & SCIENCES

model by Va. Welty

LEVEL IV
INDIVIDUAL
FAMILY
COMMUNITY

PRIMARY
TERTIARY

LEVEL III
INDIVIDUAL
FAMILY

PRIMARY
SECONDARY

LEVEL II
INDIVIDUAL

PRIMARY

LEVEL I
BASIS OF
PROGRAM

CHART 1

CHART 2. Program Design

Liberal Arts and Sciences Courses	Supportive Courses	Nursing Courses
Senior Year		Independent Study Issues in Professional Nursing

Philosophy
Theology
		Nursing Process with Individual,
		  Families, and Communities in
		  Tertiary Health Care Systems
		Nursing Process with Individual,
		  Families and Communities in Pri-
		  mary Health Care Systems
		Research Process in Nursing

Junior Year		Issues in Professional Nursing
		  (Present), Professional Issues, and
		  Delivery of Nursing Care in Acute

Philosophy Theology		Care Systems

	Pathophysiology	↔ The Nursing Process with Individual
		  and Families in Secondary Health
		  Care Systems
		The Nursing Process and Health Pro-
		  motion with Individuals and
		  Families Throughout the Life Cycle

Sophomore Year	Health Systems Abnormal Psychology	↔ Issues in Professional Nursing (Historical Forces)
Humanities Theology Social Science	Bacteriology Human Physiology Sociology of the Family Nutrition	↕ The Nursing Process and Health Assessment with Individuals
Freshman Year		
English Psychology Humanities Social Sciences Biology	Chemistry Human Anatomy Growth and Development	

The health systems thread is begun on the sophomore level in a supportive course, "Health Systems: A Socio-Political Perspective." This course
introduces students to health systems in a broad perspective, emphasizing the
sociopolitical processes that influence and shape the context of the health
care, client systems, care givers, and treatment modalities. It provides a
theoretical base for future collaborative clinical relationships and practice and

gives the students a framework for analysis of various types of health care systems.

THE PROFESSIONAL COMPONENT

The concept of primary, secondary, and tertiary prevention, as described by Neuman, is an organizing principle for the nursing courses. These three levels of prevention are presented in relation to increasingly complex systems, moving from the individual to groups, families, and communities. Primary prevention is taught on all three levels, since the faculty believes that primary prevention is more difficult than secondary prevention. This belief is based on the fact that the former includes identification of covert stressors and requires strategies of nursing intervention that involve more sophisticated and comprehensive levels of knowledge and skills than are involved in secondary prevention. Also, since health promotion is a significant characteristic of professional nursing practice, it needs to be covered more extensively in a baccalaureate program.

At the sophomore level, the first nursing course focuses on health assessment of individuals at various stages of the life cycle. The emphasis is on identification of potential stressors as they relate to physiological, psychological, sociocultural, developmental, and spiritual factors that pose a risk or possible hazard to the state of health. Supervised clinical experiences in relation to health assessment are provided in the nursing laboratory and community settings.

A concurrent seminar course, "Issues in Professional Nursing," is designed to facilitate role induction by focusing on the student's personal and professional self-concept, clarification of personal values and ethical perspectives. The concepts for this seminar flow from the health systems course and include the historical forces and professional issues related to nursing history, leadership, standards of practice, professional organization, and nursing research. Discussion of these concepts leads to an understanding of the development of nursing as a profession and the role of the nurse in the health care delivery system.

The concept of primary prevention is expanded in a two-semester junior level course in which the students work with individuals, families, and groups in the community to provide health assessment and health teaching. In the secondary prevention course, which is also introduced on the junior level in another two-semester sequence course, students apply the nursing process to individuals and families who have symptoms due to an encounter with stressors. Students assist individuals and families to use external and internal resources in order to bring about stabilization and strengthen the internal lines of resistance and reduce reactions. Clinical experiences are provided in the nursing laboratory and acute care settings. A pathophysiology course is taken concurrently with the secondary prevention course.

Experiences in acute care settings are introduced early on the junior level for a number of reasons. Professional socialization and motivation to learn are facilitated in these settings because (1) they are congruent with lay expectations of students, (2) they provide students with opportunities to identify and work with overt stressors and symptoms, and (3) skills and knowledge acquired in these settings can be used and expanded in primary and tertiary prevention.

The junior level seminar, "Issues in Professional Nursing," expands the socialization processes by having students analyze current intra- and interprofessional issues and roles that influence nursing care in secondary care systems. Within the seminar, the interpersonal process is facilitated by having students form peer support groups and negotiate independent projects. Content of the seminar includes principles of research, leadership, values, clarification, assertiveness, and change theory.

On the senior level, the course, "The Nursing Process with Individuals, Families, and Communities in Primary Health Care Systems," offers opportunities for the students to practice primary prevention in multiple community systems with individuals, families, and communities. A special focus is placed on the childbearing and child-rearing family. Students assume leadership roles in providing health screening, teaching, referral, and counseling.

Tertiary prevention is developed in another senior level course in which the student applies the nursing process to maximize and maintain optimum wellness for individuals, families, and community systems who have experienced life crisis events and in which some degree of restitution or stability has occurred. Interventions focus on readaptation and reeducation to prevent future occurrences and to foster maintenance of stability. In this course students have the opportunity to analyze various roles and communication patterns within health care settings in the community. The clinical component consists of experiences in outpatient, long-term, rehabilitation centers, community, and community mental health settings.

Primary and tertiary prevention are presented on the senior level because nursing intervention in these practice areas both requires a synthesis of knowledge from biological, behavioral, and nursing sciences, and the use of sophisticated and complex skills which are the basis for future professional practice.

The seminar course, on the senior level, "Issues in Professional Nursing," focuses on evaluation of the influences and interfaces of social, political, economic, and professional issues on the delivery of nursing care in primary and tertiary care systems. Content includes the application and evaluation of principles of leadership in effecting change in primary and tertiary health systems and the identification of future nursing roles, client systems, and health needs.

The research thread is expanded in the senior nursing courses, "The Research Process in Nursing" and "Independent Study." In the research course students use skills learned on sophomore and junior levels (i.e., literature survey and communication skills) to critique nursing research and develop research questions. Independent study is a synthesis course in the last semester of the senior year in which students have the opportunity for in-depth exploration of clinical areas of interest. In consultation with the faculty, students develop objectives, an evaluation methodology, and resources to implement the selected learning experiences.

SUMMARY AND CONCLUSIONS

The Neuman Model was operationalized as the basis for a conceptual framework for a baccalaureate program in nursing. This framework supported the development of a holistic curriculum that focuses on primary, secondary, and tertiary prevention of individuals, families, and communities in multiple and diverse systems. The resultant curriculum design facilitates learning and role induction into the profession, by providing students with a structure for integrating new knowledge and skills during the program and upon its completion.

REFERENCES

Bloom BS (ed): Taxonomy of educational objectives: The classification of education goals. Handbook I. Cognitive domains. New York, Longmans, Green, 1956

Chioni RM: A curriculum model for preparing tomorrow's nurse practitioners. Challenge to nursing education: Preparation of the professional nurse for future roles. New York: National League for Nursing, Pub. No. 15-1420, pp. 8–13, 1971

DeTornyay R: Teaching-learning strategies for baccalaureate nursing education. Teaching-learning strategies in baccalaureate nursing education. New York, National League for Nursing, Pub. No. 15-1622, 1976

Hodgman EC: A conceptual framework to guide nursing curriculum. Nurs Forum 12:2:110–131, 1973

Leavitt HR, Clark EG: Preventive medicine. New York, McGraw-Hill, 1958

Neuman B: The Betty Neuman health care systems model: A total person approach to patient problems in Riehl JP, Roy C (eds): Conceptual Models for Nursing Practice. New York, Appleton, 1974

Riehl JP, Roy C: Conceptual models for nursing practice. New York, Appleton, 1974

Roy C: Relating nursing theory to education: A new era. Nurse Educator, 41:2:16–21, 1979

Torres GJ: The implications for curriculum of changes in the health care system. Faculty-curriculum development. The process of curriculum development. New York, National League for Nursing, Pub. No. 15-1521, pp. 35−40, 1974

Torres GJ, Yura H: Today's conceptual framework: Its relationship to the curriculum development process. New York, National League for Nursing, Pub. No. 15-1529, 1974

Steven BJ: Nursing Theory. Boston, Little, Brown, 1974

Ruth B. Craddock
Marcia K. Stanhope

The Neuman Health-Care Systems Model: Recommended Adaptation

Given the complexity of the health-care system today, a model that reflects an interdisciplinary approach to health-care delivery is one that should be given careful consideration for adoption as a framework for the future direction of nursing research, education, and practice.

Neuman's total person approach to health care is a model that should be considered. This model was developed to demonstrate how all health professionals can utilize their own assessments to interact with one another in order to provide the level of care—primary, secondary, or tertiary—necessary to meet the needs of the consumer.

Neuman (1974) presents a conceptual model derived from Gestalt theory, field theory, systems theory, and Selye's stress adaptation theory. Briefly, Gestalt and field theories emphasize the person's perceptual field as a state of dynamic equilibrium. Tension in the field is created by a problem, which then results in a disturbance of the equilibrium. The disequilibrium is seen to serve as a source of motivation for interaction with the environment. Field and systems theories describe the interrelationship and interdependence of the component parts of the individual or the society (health-care system). Selye (1976) indicates that it is the stressors in the environment that produce the stimuli (tension) that cause the individual (whole) to interact with his environment.

Taking the above postulates from the theories, Neuman presents an approach for viewing man and his interaction with his environment based upon man's perception of the stressors affecting the "parts" of the whole individual. An overview of the model is presented in Table 1. Neuman does not identify a unique role for nursing in the model. It is stated, however, that nursing is concerned with the total person and could intervene in the clients responses to stress at any level of care—preencounter (primary prevention),

TABLE 1. Betty Neuman Health-Care Systems Model

I. Derivation
   A. Gestalt Theory
   B. Field Theories
   C. Systems Theory
   D. Selye's Stress Adaptation Theory

II. Observations
   A. The evolving complexity of health-care delivery system
   B. The shift in health-care focus to primary prevention
   ⁻C. The number of nursing models viewing man as a system part or as an interactive process

III. Position Statement
   Nursing is a unique profession.

IV. Postulate
   Nursing's concern is with all of the environmental variables affecting an individual's response to stress.

V. Major Constructs
   A. Man: a dynamic composite of the interrelationship of four variables (physiologic, psychologic, sociocultural, and developmental), which are always present
   B. Stressor: any problem, condition, capable of causing instability of the system by penetration of the normal line of defense

VI. Categories of Stress
   A. Intrapersonal: forces occurring within the individual
   B. Interpersonal: forces occurring between one or more individuals
   C. Extrapersonal: forces occurring outside the individual

VII. Supporting Constructs
   A. Normal line of defense: state of wellness considered normal for the individual.
   B. Flexible line of defense: dynamic state of wellness; individual's current state particularly susceptible to situational circumstances.
   C. Degree of reaction: amount of system instability caused by the stressor's penetration of the normal line of defense.
   D. Lines of resistance: internal resistant forces faced by a stressor that acts to decrease the degree of reaction
   E. Reconstitution: resolution of the stressor from the depths of reaction to the normal line of defense
   F. Primary prevention: interventions initiated before or after an encounter with a stressor
   G. Secondary prevention: interventions generally initiated after encounter with a stressor
   H. Tertiary prevention: interventions initiated after treatment

VIII. Beliefs: Nursing
   A. Nursing is concerned with the total person.
   B. Nursing can intervene in client responses to stress at three levels: preencounter, encounter, and reconstitution.
   C. Nursing and medicine are complementary.

IX. Beliefs: Man
   A. Man is viewed as a total person encompassing all aspects of the being and the number of variables that may affect behavior.
   B. Man is an open system in contact with his environment.

X. Assumptions
   A. Each individual has a basic structure or energy resources whose compromise is incompatible with life.
   B. Each individual has a normal line of defense.

TABLE 1.—Continued

    C. Each individual has a flexible line of defense constantly changing in response to the interrelating variables.
    D. Many stressors are known to be universal and others hold meaning only to the client.
    E. Stressors are dynamic and may cause priority needs to change at any point.
    F. The degree of reaction depends upon the resistant forces encountered by the stressors.
    G. Reconstitution may begin at any level of reaction and proceed to a new level of wellness above or below the previous level of the normal line of defense.
    H. Interventions can occur before or after resistance lines are penetrated.
 XI. Values
    A. The level for the normal line of defense is not the same for every individual.
    B. Nurses have the obligation to seek the highest potential level of stability for an individual system.
    C. Nurses cannot impose their judgment upon the client.

XII. Major Model Units
    A. Goal of action: system stability
    B. Target of action: an open system whose boundary is its flexible line of defnese, in interaction with the stressors (actual and potential) in its environment
    C. Actor's role: regulate and control the system's response to stress
    D. Source of difficulty: actual or potential penetration of the flexible line of defense
    E. Intervention focus: actual or potential penetration of the flexible line of defense
    F. Intervention mode: primary, secondary, tertiary prevention
    G. Consequences: increased resistance to stress, decreased degree of reaction, and increased level of wellness

---

encounter (treatment), or reconstitution. Neuman believes that nursing and medicine share complementary roles.

MODEL INTERPRETATION

Practice

Neuman presents man as the center of her model interacting with the health-care system according to perceived need. She recognizes changes in the health-care system today with an increasing emphasis on primary care. This model lends itself to a multiprofessional method of assessing clients' needs; one professional can benefit from the assessment and services offered to the client by another. This method of assessment has been found to reduce the time (economics) element in initially assessing a client's health status and in providing that client the necessary health care he needs and wants. As indicated earlier, Neuman states her belief that nursing and medicine are complementary. Perhaps, in lieu of the changing health-care scene, one should state further that the roles of all health professionals are complementary and that each should bring and share knowledge and skills in order to assist others in providing for the health/illness needs of the client.

From the belief in interdisciplinary, complementary role relationships it is anticipated that future client triage will be based on the following premise: The client will receive primary care from the health professional who can best meet the client's needs for the least cost. Given this premise it would seem that the nurse's role has the potential for evolving into more of an independent one, providing increasing opportunity for her intervention and manipulation of the client's environment. If, in fact, this does not occur the nurse must become an endangered species because in the present health-care system the nurse's functions have been parcelled out to other professionals and to paraprofessionals; the nurse's distinctive contribution is obliterated.

Education

If such a model is chosen as an approach for health-care delivery, nursing curricula would need to reflect the conceptual framework of the model and emphasize health promotion, illness prevention, and control; primary care, cost control, the use of protocols for care delivery, the health-team approach to delivery; and the theories upon which the model is based.

With the attitude in the federal government that there is an adequate supply of nurses in the country and with the proposed changes in future nursing education funding, nursing should begin to note the possibility that the only educational programs to receive the funding in the future may be the programs with curricula aimed at preparing nurses to meet the health needs of the society in a given health care delivery framework.

Research

A framework for education and practice should not be presented until the data's viability and practicality for the practice of nursing have been substantiated. The Neuman conceptual model's practicality or viability for directing the future of nursing has not yet been proven. The model deserves further testing since it does reflect many of the concepts found in today's national health policy.

APPLICATION OF THE MODEL

To date the literature does not reflect extensive application of this model. One example appears in the literature of the model's testing. In 1974 Pinkerton related the use of the Neuman model in a home health-care agency in San

Diego, California. The assessment tool provided by Neuman was used to assess the level of care required by the clients of the agency. Pinkerton described plans to implement a study to compare the use of the model to more traditional approaches to care. This study has not appeared in the literature. A staff nurse of the same agency, Balch (1974), reported the successful use of the Neuman assessment tool for identifying levels of client-care needs. She reported some difficulty in utilizing the questions of the tool as they are worded.

ADEQUACY/INADEQUACY OF THE MODEL FOR GUIDING PRACTICE

During a three-month period, a study was implemented at a private, nonprofit home health-care agency to test the usefulness of the Neuman model in nursing practice. The agency was composed of a client population of 600. There were essentially two major objectives of the study: (1) to test the model/assessment tool to determine its usefulness as a unifying method of collecting and analyzing data for identifying client problems; (2) to test the assessment tool for its usefulness in the identification of congruence between the clients perception of stressors and the care givers perception of client stressors.

For the study in the home health-care agency, a population of registered nurses and clients was chosen. The nurses each chose clients from their caseloads. One author served as a participant in the study, assessing each of the clients through the use of the Neuman assessment tool and interviewing each of the nurses to compare perceptual differences between the client and the nurse providing care concerning client problems.

The results of the study in the home health-care agency indicated that the model has the potential for guiding decision-making and the categorizing of data for assessing and planning client care. It also provides a mechanism for using input from other health professionals in the assessment of the client situation. In this study as in the study by Balch (1974) there was some concern about the reliability of the questions as worded in the assessment tool.

At this writing a similar study is being conducted by one of the authors in a primary nursing unit of a 300-bed private, nonprofit hospital. The objective of this study is to test the following portion of the Neuman assessment/intervention tool to identify congruence between the client's perception of stressors and the care giver's perception of the client's stressor:

STRESSORS
Identified by and based on the *patient's perception* of his circumstances. (If patient is incapacitated, secure data from family or other resources.)

What do you consider your major problem, stress area, or areas of concern? (Identify problem areas.)

How do present circumstances differ from your usual pattern of living? (Identify life-style patterns.)

Have you ever experienced a similar problem? If so, what was that problem and how did you handle it? Were you successful? (Identify past coping patterns.)

What do you anticipate for yourself in the future as a consequence of your present situation? (Identify perceptual factors, i.e. reality versus distortions-expectations, present and possible future coping patterns.)

What are you doing and what can you do to help yourself? (Identify perceptual factors, i.e., reality versus distortions-expectations, present and possible future coping patterns.)

What do you expect care givers, family, friends, or others to do for you? (Identify perceptual pfactors, i.e., reality versus distortions-expectations, present and possible future coping patterns.)

STRESSORS

Identified by and based on the *care giver's* perception of the patient's circumstances.

What do you consider to be the major problem, stress area, or areas of concern? (Identify problem areas.)

How do present circumstances seem to differ from the patient's usual pattern of living? (Identify life-style patterns.)

Has the patient ever experienced a similar situation? If so, how would you evaluate what the patient did? How successful do you think it was? (Identify past coping patterns.)

What do you anticipate for the future as a consequence of the patient's present situation? (Identify perceptual factors, i.e., reality versus distortions-expectations, present and possible future coping patterns.)

What can the patient do to help himself? (Identify perceptual factors, i.e., reality versus distortions-expectations, present and possible future coping patterns.)

What do you think the patient expects from care givers, family, friends, or other resources? (Identify perceptual factors, i.e., reality versus distortions-expectations, present and possible future coping patterns.)

Although this study has not been completed, it has been found that it is possible to utilize the questions as stated in the assessment tool. This finding differs from the home health-care study previously described and the study by Balch (1974). Clients have responded well to the questions and a wealth of information has been obtained.

It has also been found that there is a lack of congruence between the client's perception of his stressors and those identified by the primary nurses on the unit. This finding is in agreement with the study in the home health-care setting.

It is believed that the six questions presented by Neuman in her assessment/intervention tool can be utilized easily by nurses in any setting to quickly identify discrepancies between the client's perception of his stressors and those identified by the care giver.

The following assessment utilizing Neuman's six questions was carried out with a 70-year-old male client, admitted to the primary-care unit. The client was diagnosed as having metastatic carcinoma. The client's physician and his primary nurse had discussed his condition with him, and he was well informed about his diagnosis and his plan of treatment. At the time of this assessment the client identified his major problem, or area of concern, as the pain in his right hip, which he attributed to an injury he received when he was repairing the roof of his home. When asked what he expected from his care givers he replied, "Relief from the pain in my right hip." He felt that the cobalt treatments would surely take care of his cancer. Although this client was a highly educated man, he did not believe that the pain in his right hip was related to his metastatic carcinoma.

The primary nurse identified the client's main stressor as the metastatic carcinoma and was very surprised to learn that Mr. J did not relate the pain in his hip to the metastatic disease.

Most nurses believe that the client should participate and have a voice in planning his health care. However, how often do they assess the client's perception of his problems and give the client an actual opportunity to express his expectations from the health care providers? Neuman's assessment tool offers a quick and efficient mechanism for gaining vital information needed to plan total patient care.

Although the authors' findings differ on the ability of the clients and/or nurses to understand the questions as stated in the assessment/intervention tool, one could conjecture that the interpretations of the questions by the clients are influenced by the preventive stage (primary, secondary, tertiary,) in which the clients find themselves. The nurses' interpretation of the questions could be influenced by the client-care focus they develop by working in a specific preventive care setting. Further research needs to be done to justify these suppositions.

In reviewing the above studies one recognizes that the assessment tool of the model has been tested for its utilization in establishing a plan of nursing care. The strength of this assessment tool lies in its ability to identify discrepancies between the client's and the care giver's perceptions of stressors.

The model needs now to be tested for its usefulness in evaluating client outcomes as related to the implemented plan of care. However, it seems to be a time-effective method of obtaining an initial assessment of the client.

MODIFICATIONS AND RECOMMENDATIONS

Recommendations

Neuman's model is a conceptual model of a health-care system. It describes and seeks to explain man's interaction with the environment based upon his reactions to stress. It also seeks to describe and explain man's interaction with the health-care system, which is viewed as levels of prevention.

Primarily the model can be strengthened through research to establish it as a theoretical framework with a scientifically acceptable, predictive base for nursing practice in an interdisciplinary setting. The model can be strengthened by a clearer schematic and a parsimonious discussion of the interaction of the parts of the model. The nurse's role in the system needs to be clarified and the methods of intervention at the three levels of prevention need to be identified. Notions of the role relationships of health-care providers also needs to be clarified.

Proposed Modifications

Neuman's model has been modified to reflect the individual's interaction with the health-care system. This step is reflective of the future direction of the health-care system, toward the consumer's becoming the regulator of the interaction.

Figure 1 indicates the unidirectional movement of the client through the system. The arrows appearing at midpoints in the drawing indicate points of reentry into the system of interaction. The symbols in the drawing are defined as follows: The square blocks represent information points. The triangles represent points at which decisions are made based upon the information given. The small circles indicate the nature of the decision, Y = yes, N = no. The ellipse indicates the termination point in the system. The following comments describing the schematic are numbered to coincide with the numbers in the drawing in an attempt to clarify the meaning of the figure.

Figure 1 indicates that man is in continual interaction with the environment (1). The interaction with the environment may be positive and is perceived as positive (health state)(2). The individual is therefore in a state of equilibrium with the environment (3). However, the interaction with the environment may be negative (illness state)(4). If the individual does not perceive this interaction as negative (5), although in fact it is negative, there will be an attempt by the individual to adapt to the interaction (6), and maintain some semblance of equilibrium with the environment (7). If there is a failure to adapt to this negative interaction the eventual result is death (8). If the negative interaction (9) with the environment is perceived as negative (illness state) (10), the individual may enter the health care system for assessment. The health assessment is initiated by an appropriate member of the health care team and based on the assessment the client receives either primary, secon-

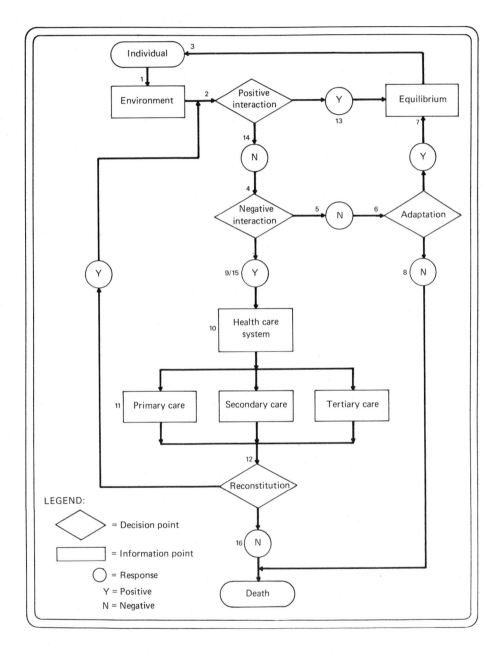

Figure 1 *Individual interaction with health-care systems.*

dary, or tertiary care (11). During the treatment period the client may begin to reconstitute (12). At the point of reconstitution, if the individual perceives a positive interaction with the environment (13), equilibrium is re-established. If the individual is reconstituted but perceives a negative interaction (14), the choice may be to reenter the health care system for further assessment (15). Finally, if reconstitution does not occur the individual expires (16).

The major premise of the schematic: the individual is the decision maker re: health/illness and entrance into the health care system. The individual's perceptions are the basis for decision making. Perception is influenced by the individual's values, beliefs, and attitudes. A positive or negative perception may occur at any point in the individual's environmental interactions regardless of the actual state of the client environment. It is the authors' opinion that such a depiction of the model establishes the consumers' role and responsibility in the system. If health care is a right, then the client must be given the opportunity to interact with the system, and he must accept this responsibility regardless of the consequences.

The nurses' role in the Neuman model has been identified as that of advocate for the client during his interaction with the health-care system. Kosik (1972) describes an advocate as a person who gives support, intercedes for the client in the system, sees that system expectations of the client are known to the client, identifies the client's rights, and sees that the system provides for the client's needs. This definition may imply that the nurse is the source of direct care or seeks appropriate direct-care providers through referral. Essentially it seems that Neuman concurs with the advocacy role when she points out that the nurse is concerned with all of the environmental variables affecting the individual and further indicates that the nurse can intervene at any level of prevention.

In conclusion it is recognized that further study needs to be done to clarify nursing's position in the health-care system. The Neuman model provides the necessary framework for an interdisciplinary approach to total health care for all clients. The time for this study is now, because of the growing debate over a totally regulated health-care system versus a more competitive system. The outcome of the debate will lead to an evolution of all health-care provider roles. The role of the nurse in the future, therefore, can be a dominate one. At this time as never before the nursing profession finds itself in a position to assume leadership in the unification of all health-care professions through the interdisciplinary approach to health-care delivery.

REFERENCES

Archer SE, Fleshman R: Community Health Nursing. Massachusetts, Duxbury Press, 1975

Baider L: Evaluation of the role of primary nurse in an oncology department. Ment Health Soc I: 110–117, 1974

Berrien TK: General and Social Systems. New Brunswick, Rutgers University, 1968

Bertalanffy L: General Systems Theory. New York, Braziller, 1968

Craven R: Primary health care practice in a nursing home. Am J Nurs 1985–90, 1976

Fagan J, Shepard J (eds): Gestalt Therapy Now: Theory, Techniques, Applications. Palo Alto, Science and Behavior Books, 1970

Kosik SH: Patient advocacy or fighting the system. In Spradley B (ed): Contemporary Community Nursing. Boston, Little, Brown, 1975

Laros J: Deriving outcome criteria from a conceptual model. Nurs Outlook 25:5:333, 1977

Logsdon, A. Why primary nursing? Nurs Clin North Am 8:2:283–291, 1973

Marram G, Schlegel M, Bevis E: Primary Nursing. St. Louis, Mosby, 1974

Neuman B: The Betty Neuman health-care systems model: a total person approach to patient problems. In Riehl JP, Roy C (eds): Conceptual Models for Nursing Practice. New York, Appleton, 1974

Pinkerton A: Use of the Neuman model in a home health-care agency. In Riehl JP, Roy C (eds): Conceptual Models for Nursing Practice. New York, Appleton, 1974

Reilly J: Why a conceptual framework. Nurs Outlook 23:9:566,

Selye H: The Stress of Life. New York, McGraw-Hill, 1976

Venable J: The Neuman health-care systems model: an analysis. In Riehl JP, Roy C (eds): Conceptual Models for Nursing Practice. New York, Appleton, 1974

Brenda Beitler
Barbara Tkachuck
Donna Aamodt

The Neuman Model Applied to Mental Health, Community Health, and Medical-Surgical Nursing

As nursing theory develops with an increasing emphasis on wellness, new frameworks for nursing education are essential. The department of nursing in our private, liberal-arts college provides a generic baccalaureate program. A major curriculum change made necessary a more wellness-oriented conceptual framework. The Neuman model was selected as a curriculum guide.

After the Neuman model was chosen, Neuman conducted a workshop on campus, clarifying the model for nursing faculty. Since the workshop, adaptations of the model to this particular setting were made with Dr. Neuman's permission. The total person approach, for instance, includes focus on the spiritual component of man.

Synopsis of two lesson plans, a patient interview, and plan of care utilizing the Neuman model follow. The assessment/intervention tool was used as a basis for these plans.

LESSON PLAN FOR PERSONALITY DISORDERS

In a unit on personality disorders, the lesson plan included the objectives and content. The latter encompassed the definition and categorization of personality disorders. In addition, because the curriculum base was the Neuman model, the lesson plan emphasized the following: stressors and primary, secondary, and tertiary prevention. These specific points are included in Table 1.

LESSON PLAN FOR WORKING WITH LOW-INCOME FAMILIES

To enable utilization of the Neuman model in the presentation of a lecture on low-income families for a class in community-health nursing, the following

TABLE 1. Stressors and Primary, Secondary, and Tertiary Prevention for Lesson Plan on Personality Disorders

Stressors	Denies anxiety	Broken relationships	Denies need for help	Adept at manipulation	Utilizes rationalization
Primary Prevention	Promote acceptance of frustration as part of life.	Promote trusting family relationships.	Establish trusting relationship with client.	Educate parents as to importance of consistent limits.	Establish open relationship with client. Support good parental role models.
Secondary Prevention	Provide activities for release of hostility.	Role model for authentic relationships.	Accept client.	Set reasonable but firm limits.	Role model for authentic relationships.
Tertiary Prevention	Involve client in activities for release of hostility.	Involve client in support systems.	Be supportive of client's support systems.	Positively reinforce previous successes, which did not utilize manipulation.	Be supportive of client's support systems.

aspects are presented in an outline form: the stressors inherent in the poverty culture, the intrapersonal, interpersonal, and extrapersonal factors that contribute to the problems of the low-income client, and the primary, secondary, and tertiary forms of prevention that nursing may utilize when working with low-income families.

I. Define poverty
   A. Acute and chronic
   B. Stereotypes of poverty
II. Identify stressors of low-income families, such as inadequate education, inadequate nutrition, inadequate medical care, crime, violence, substandard or overcrowded housing, and early marriage.
III. Health problems resulting from inability to cope with stressors
   A. Physical
   B. Mental
IV. Identify the intrapersonal, interpersonal and extrapersonal factors contributing to the problems of a low-income client.
   A. Intrapersonal factors
      1. Physical abilities and handicaps
      2. Mental and emotional abilities and handicaps
      3. Psychocultural: What values, attitudes and coping mechanisms are utilized?
   B. Interpersonal factors: What role does the client have within the family? With peers? With health professionals?
   C. Extrapersonal factors: community resources
      1. Availability
      2. Accessibility
      3. Adequacy
V. Primary, secondary, and tertiary prevention to utilize in working with low-income families
   A. Primary—The aim when working with low-income families would be to strengthen their defense against stressors as it may not be possible to decrease or eliminate the stressor.
   B. Secondary—When physical or mental health has been threatened, intervention must take place through proper referral.
   C. Tertiary—Stage of rehabilitation and reeducation involves health professionals, who help to prevent further disabilities, to attain optimum potential and to maintain stability.

THE ASSESSMENT/INTERVIEW TOOL

The assessment/intervention tool was used as a guide for interviewing a medical-surgical client in the acute-care setting. The intervention plan was developed based on the interview. Interventions and goals focused on secondary and tertiary prevention; primary goals were to be reestablished according to outcomes of tertiary prevention.

Definition Of Terms In The Model

Primary prevention—interventions initiated before or after an encounter with a stressor: includes decreasing the possibility of encounter with stressors and strengthening the flexible line of defense in the presence of stressors

Secondary prevention—interventions initiated after encounter with a stressor; includes early case finding and treatment of symptoms following a reaction to a stressor

Tertiary prevention—interventions generally initiated after treatment; focuses on readaptation, reeducation to prevent future occurrences, and maintenance of stability

Brief Admission Summary

Mr. Jones (pseudonym), age 41, married, father of three (ages 21, 19, 17), was readmitted on 12/22/78 for nausea and vomiting believed to be the result of tissue reaction (swelling) from recent radiation therapy. On November 29 surgery had revealed an unresectable 5 cm mass adherent to the portal vein, invasion of the transverse colon, multiple hard lymph nodes along the common duct and hepatic vessels, and a diffusely firm head of the pancreas. A gastrojejunostomy and side-to-side cholocolostomy were performed.

Patient Interview and Plan of Care

I. Stressors
  A. What do you consider your major problem, stress area, or areas of concern?
    1. Patient's perception
      a. "Getting stomach to accept food normally so radiation treatments can be resumed"
      b. "Cancer of the pancreas"
      c. "Stomach spasms—they really grab and squeeze my stomach"
    2. Care giver's perception
      a. Pre-holiday admission with nausea and vomiting as the result of edema from radiation treatments for adenocarcinoma of the pancreas. Client stated, "My family was a little upset that I had to come to the hospital just before Christmas" (Dec. 22).
      b. Inability to retain normal diet, maintained hyperalimentation.
      c. Denial of seriousness of illness. Said he had experienced similar

problems when, in reality, this current problem is different. Adenocarcinoma was not confirmed until after November surgery. Previous lesions causing obstruction of bile duct were benign. He knows his diagnosis.

B. How do present circumstances differ from your usual pattern of living?
1. Patient's perception
a. "I have to be in bed most of the time existing on IV's" (hyperalimentation).
b. "I haven't been able to go to work since Thanksgiving."
2. Care giver's perception
a. Normally able to eat and retain food, go to work, function as husband and father.
b. Now dependant on parenteral feedings.

C. Have you ever experienced a similar problem? If so, what was that problem and how did you handle it? Were you successful? (past coping)
1. Patient's perception
a. "Yes, I had an obstruction in June—they had to bypass my bile duct. I got better and went back to work."
b. "In July I had a lumbar laminectomy. I got better and went back to work after that."
c. "At Thanksgiving I had an obstruction of my duodenum. They did surgery and took it out. I went home for two weeks then started vomiting and came here. I have swelling of the anastomosis."
2. Care-giver's perception: No. Cancer of head of pancreas at MI stage diagnosed in November. Previous problems were resolved by surgery and he returned to work.

D. What do you anticipate for yourself in the future as a consequence of your present situation?
1. Patient's perception: "I'll start treatments again as soon as I can take food normally—I have had a full liquid diet starting yesterday and so far its all right."
2. Care-giver's perception: Current medical treatment is maintaining his normal body fluids, electrolytes, and nutrition (he has gained 10 pounds); the edema of the anastomosis is diminishing so that he is currently tolerating a full liquid diet. He should be able to return home in a few days and resume radiation and chemotherapy treatments.

E. What are you doing and what can you do to help yourself?
1. Patient's perception: "I can do most things for myself; I walk around the halls several times a day. I just have the nurses help me with my back; I can't reach it. They watch this IV, too."
2. Care-giver's perception: Maintain an optimal physical condition

through exercise, nutrition to tolerance. Build a support system—spiritual, psychosocial, family.
F. What do you expect care givers, family, friends, or others to do for you?
  1. Patient's perception
    a. "Not much, I can do most things myself. The nurses do help wash my back, watch the IV, and bring injections for pain.
    b. "My boss has told the fellows who work with me to stay away. He came to see me every day when I was in before. My wife comes every day. She got this rug for me to work on. She works on it when she is here, too. It is so big."
  2. Care giver's perception: This client is used to being independent. I do not see him "expecting" any more from care givers and others on whom he must rely as he is unable to meet his own needs. Currently he is doing almost everything for himself.

Summary of impressions (note any discrepancies or distortions between the patient's perception and that of the care giver related to the situation).

  I. Intrapersonal Factors
    A. Physical
      1. Abnormal function of digestive tract
      2. Unable to do total physical care because of subclavian and IVAC
    B. Psychosociocultural
      1. Feels he has no needs—denial stage of illness
      2. Has confidence in treatments offered. "My stomach must accept food so I can get on with the treatments."
      3. Has hope at this time.
    C. Developmental
      1. Has ego integrity.
      2. Denies concern about current situation.
      3. His job is secure; his boss will wait for him to recover.
  II. Interpersonal Factors
    A. Resources and relationship of family, friends, or care givers that either influence or could influence I
      1. Physical
        a. Needs assistance with bath and balance of fluid and electrolyte intake.
        b. Clinitest for glucose metabolism.
        c. Medications for control of nausea and pain
        d. Some control of environment because of low WBC from treatments
      2. Psychosociocultural: Current needs met by medical and nursing personnel, family, boss, friends and co-workers. As stages of acceptance of condition progress, he will need a strong support

system through the stages of his illness to help him maintain his independence as long as possible, to answer his questions, and to be available when he has needs.

3. Developmental: Greatest need will be to reaffirm his values of life, philosophical, religious, and social.

III. Extrapersonal Factors

A. Resources and relationship of community facilities, finances, employment, or other areas which either influence or could influence I and II.

1. Physical: Needs are cared for at present.
2. Psychosociocultural
   a. He has job security in spite of illness.
   b. Physicians are informing him of his illness.
   c. He has insurance.
   d. He has a supportive family, boss and co-workers.

IV. Formulation of the problem and rank-order of needs.

A. Admission problem
   1. Nausea and vomiting
   2. Pain
   3. Low WBC
   4. Hospitalization

B. Needs
   1. Nursing interventions
      a. Oral hygiene
      b. Pleasant room—neat and free of odors
      c. Implement medical plan
         (1) Medications for nausea
         (2) N G tube
         (3) Laboratory tests
         (4) Parenteral fluids and nutrition
         (5) Progressive diet post N/V
      d. Medication and procedures for reduction and control of pain
      e. Protection from infection
         (1) Control visitors
         (2) Avoid care by ill personnel
      f. Maintain maximum physical exercise to toleration
      g. Provide diversion
      h. Permit socializing as possible

Intervention Plan To Support Stated Goals

I. Primary Prevention
   A. Goal
      1. Reduce risk factors.

    2. Promote optimum health.

    3. Strengthen trusting relationships with family and friends.

  B. Intervention

    1. Avoid foods and environmental factors which could irritate condition.

    2. Physical and mental activities to tolerance.

    3. Continue family and social relationships as possible.

  C. Outcome

    1. Maintain line of defense.

    2. Reduce stressors.

  D. Comments

II. Secondary Prevention

  A. Goal

    1. Relieve N/V and pain.

    2. Prevent infection.

    3. Maintain physical strength and fitness.

    4. Identify client's goals.

    5. Build support system.

  B. Intervention:

    1. Oral hygiene, pleasant room, medications and treatments.

    2. Good handwashing, careful techniques, appropriate contacts.

    3. Encourage self-care, ambulation, bed exercises. Diversion.

    4. Discuss client's situation, *listen,* guide client to realistic analysis. Suggest appropriate support systems, i.e., pastor, family, friends.

    5. Be available to assist client in utilizing above suggestions.

  C. Outcome:

    1. Nausea relieved, food beginning to pass through

    2. No apparent infection, temperature normal

    3. Ambulates, does self-care, performs exercises.

    4. Client not yet ready to face seriousness of illness. Family and friends supporting.

    5. Staff listening, supporting.

  D. Comments:

    1. Normal line of defense in process of reestablishment.

    2. Lines of resistance building.

III. Tertiary Prevention

  A. Goal

    1. Maintain nutrition.

    2. Maintain support system.

    3. Keep pain at minimum, increase tolerance.

  B. Intervention

    1. Teach client how to maintain adequate nutrition.

    2. Encourage as normal a life as possible.

    3. Teach ways to reduce pain, i.e., diversion.

C. Outcome
1. Stabilization of body weight
2. Short-term goals for life-focused daily activities
3. Activities focused away from pain, i.e., to significant others.
D. Comments:
1. A line of defense reestablished.
2. Line of resistance strengthened.

SUMMARY

Application of the Neuman model was expedited by the adjunctive assessment/intervention tool. This adaptability promoted faculty acceptance of the model. Since application of the model in the content areas of psychiatric/mental health, community health, and medical-surgical nursing was accomplished, it is believed that the model is also adaptable to other content areas in nursing education.

15

The Roy Adaptation Model

The Roy Adaptation Model can be viewed primarily as a systems model though it also contains interactionist levels of analysis. The person as patient is viewed as having parts or elements linked together in such a way that force on the linkages can be increased or decreased. Increased force, or tension, comes from strains within the system or from the environment that impinges on the system. The system of the person and his interaction with the environment are thus the units of analysis of nursing assessment, while manipulation of parts of the system or the environment is the mode of nursing intervention. The person has four subsystems: physiologic needs, self-concept, role function, and interdependence. The self-concept and role function subsystems are seen as developing in an interactionist framework. Thus the interaction process is one of the elements to be assessed within the system. Likewise, one of the nurse's primary tools in manipulating elements of the system or the environment is her own or others' interaction with the patient. Within a systems model, therefore, interactionist concepts are relevant. They can be used in the explication of the Roy Adaptation Model.

The Roy model had its beginning in 1964 when the author was challenged to develop a conceptual model for nursing in a seminar with Dorothy E. Johnson, at the University of California, Los Angeles. The adaptation concept, presented in a psychology class, had impressed the author as an appropriate conceptual framework for nursing. The work on adaptation by the physiologic psychologist, Harry Helson, was added to the beginning concept and the model's present form began to take shape. In subsequent years the model was developed as a framework for nursing practice, research, and education. In 1968 work began on operationalizing the model in the baccalaureate nursing curriculum at Mount Saint Mary's College in Los Angeles. The first class of students to study with the model began their nursing major in the spring of 1970 and were graduated in June, 1972. Use of the model in nursing practice led to further clarification and refinement. In the summer of 1971 a pilot research study was conducted and in 1976–77 a survey research study was done that led to some tentative confirmations of the model. Thus the Roy model has been more fully developed and operationalized than some other models in spite of its relatively recent origin.

BASIC ASSUMPTIONS OF THE ROY ADAPTATION MODEL

An assumption is a statement accepted as true without proof. All models of nursing have certain underlying basic assumptions. Assumptions may be explicitly stated or they may be implied within the discussion of the model. The assumptions behind the Roy adaptation model are based on the model's approach to the concept of the person and to the process of adaptation. These assumptions are outlined and discussed in the following section.

Assumption 1 *The person is a bio-psycho-social being.*
This assumption states that the nature of the person includes a biologic component, such as his anatomy and physiology. At the same time, the person consists of psychologic and social components. Furthermore, the behavior of the individual is related to the behavior of others on a group level. Hence, methods of analysis of the person must come from the biologic, psychologic, and social sciences, and the person as a unified whole must be viewed from these perspectives.

Assumption 2 *The person is in constant interaction with a changing environment.*
Daily experience supports this assumption. One need only cite the vicissitudes of the weather, or of traffic conditions, as examples. The person confronts constant physical, social, and psychologic changes in his environment and is continually interacting with these.

Assumption 3 *To cope with a changing world, the person uses both innate and acquired mechanisms, which are biologic, psychologic, and social in origin.*
At times learned or acquired mechanisms are used to cope with the changing world. For example, on a cool day one might wear a sweater, then remove it as the temperature warmed. Other mechanisms are innate. An example is the natural reaction of thirst in response to water loss through perspiration. Reiner (1968) discusses the chemical control systems of the organism as an adaptive device.

Assumption 4 *Health and illness are one inevitable dimension of the person's life.*

This assumption states that each person is subject to the laws of health and illness. This dimension is therefore one aspect of the total life experience. The familiar greeting, "How are you?" attests to the validity of this assumption.

Assumption 5 *To respond positively to environmental changes, the person must adapt.*

Levine (1969) states that "a truly integrating system within the organism must be one that responds to environmental change." She describes this process as adaptation. Thus a changing environment demands a positive response which, hopefully, is adaptive.

Assumption 6 *The person's adaptation is a function of the stimulus he is exposed to and his adaptation level.*

The person's adaptation level is determined by the combined effect of three classes of stimuli: (1) focal stimuli, or stimuli immediately confronting the person, (2) contextual stimuli, or all other stimuli present, and (3) residual stimuli, such as beliefs, attitudes, or traits, which have an indeterminate effect on the present situation.

This assumption relies on the work of Helson (1964), whose systematic approach to behavior is assumed to be valid. Helson states that adaptation results from the response to a stimulus that stands in relation to the adaptation level. The strength of the confronting stimulus, the contextual or environmental stimuli, and other residual, or nonspecific stimuli go together to form an adaptation level. Thus, for example, the temperature outside, the humidity, and a person's previous experience with extreme temperatures all influence his adaptation to changing temperatures.

Assumption 7 *The person's adaptation level is such that it comprises a zone indicating the range of stimulation that will lead to a positive response.*

If the stimulus is within the zone the person responds positively. However, if the stimulus is outside the zone, the person cannot make a positive response.

This assumption, again based on Helson's theory, is illustrated in Figure 1. As noted in the example of assumption 6, adaptation to environmental temperature depends on the temperature outside, the humidity, and a person's previous experience with extreme temperatures. Thus a person raised in southern California has a narrow range of adaptability to extreme temperatures while someone raised in a high desert in New Mexico might have a much wider range of adaptability. If both persons were exposed to the same high temperatures with the same humidity, the New Mexican might respond

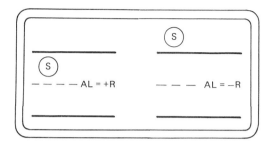

Figure 1 *Process of adaptation*

positively, or adapt, while the Californian would respond negatively, or fail to adapt.

Assumption 8 *The person is conceptualized as having four modes of adaptation: physiologic needs, self-concept, role function, interdependence relations.*

Roy defines a mode as a way or method of doing or acting. Thus a mode of adaptation is a way of adapting. Further, Roy assumes that the person has various ways of adapting. Based on an initial survey of 500 samples of patient behavior, Roy (1971) has tentatively identified four ways in which the person adapts in health and illness.

First, the person adapts according to his physiologic needs. The previous examples about adaptation to temperature changes illustrate this phenomenon.

Second, the person's self-concept is determined by his interactions with others. As outside stimuli affect him, the person adapts according to his self-concept. For example, when I switch from teaching to administration, my concept of myself adjusts; I may no longer think of myself as a mild, unperturbed individual, but rather as someone who can respond quickly and even vehemently.

Third, role function is the performance of duties based on given positions within society. The way one performs these duties is constantly responsive to outside stimulation. For example, the mother of a family constantly adapts her mothering activity to the changing developmental needs of her children.

Finally, in his relations with others, the person adapts according to a system of interdependence. This system involves his ways of seeking help, attention, and affection. Changes both within himself and outside cause changes in this subsystem. As an example, when a person is separated from a loved one, his mode of obtaining attention and affection is changed.

These eight assumptions about the person and his process of adapting are basic to the Roy adaptation model of nursing.

ELEMENTS OF THE MODEL

Values

The elements of a practice-oriented model were outlined in Chapter 1. These imply values and include goal, patiency, source of difficulty, and intervention. To begin with, Dickoff et al., say that a model must specify values that indicate that its goal is desirable of attainment. Like assumptions, the worth of values is not proved but is believed to be true.

The Roy adaptation model implies four basic values which, taken together, point to the desirability of the model's goal content. The goal of the model will be discussed later. The basic values behind the goal can be summarized as follows:

1. Nursing's concern with the person as a total being in the areas of health and illness is a socially significant activity.
2. The nursing goal of supporting and promoting patient adaptation is important for patient welfare.
3. Promoting the process of adaptation is assumed to conserve patient energy; thus nursing makes an important contribution to the overall goal of the health team by making energy available for the healing process.
4. Nursing is unique because it focuses on the patient as a person adapting to those stimuli present as a result of his position on the health-illness continuum.

These values are not proven within the model, but are assumed to be truths that make the overall goal of nursing worthwhile.

Goal of Action

Perhaps the most important distinguishing characteristic of a specific nursing model is the way the specific model describes the goal of nursing activity. The Roy adaptation model describes the goal of nursing as the person's adaptation in the four adaptive modes.

All nursing activity will be aimed at promoting the person's adaptation in his physiologic needs, his self-concept, his role function, and his relations of interdependence during health and illness. The criterion for judging when the goal has been reached is generally any positive response made by the recipient to the stimuli present that frees energy for responses to other stimuli. This criterion must be applied to each specific instance of nursing intervention for which a specific goal of adaptation has been set. For example, the patient may be confronted with the general stimulus of illness, and one necessary mode of adaptation is role function. The relevant literature reveals particular behavior cues indicating when there has been positive assumption of the sick role (e.g., Martin and Prange, 1962). When the patient is no longer fixated on the restrictions imposed on him but is able to take these in stride and to free his energies for other things, then adaptation regarding the sick role has occurred.

Patiency

A practice-oriented model must clearly describe who or what is the recipient of the activity. According to the Roy adaptation model, the patiency of nursing is described as the person as an adaptive system receiving stimuli from the environment which are inside and outside his zone of adaptation.

The person as a bio-psycho-social being in constant interaction with his changing environment has been discussed in conjunction with the assumptions of this model. Also, the process of adaptation and the person's four modes for adapting have been explored. At this time it should be pointed out that the recipient of nursing is the person in the dimension of his life related to health and illness. Thus the patient may be ill, or may be potentially ill and require preventive services. Also he may be adapting positively or not. If the patient is adapting, the nursing goal is to maintain that response. For example, when a public health nurse makes a postpartum visit and finds a new mother adapting positively to her changing role, she aims to maintain this positive response. The person adapting in health and illness is the patiency of nursing care.

Source of Difficulty

The source of difficulty, the next element of the model, is described as the originating point of deviations from the desired state or condition. The current view of this deviation is implied in Figure 2. A need is a requirement in the individual that stimulates a response to maintain integrity. As internal and external environments change, the level of satiety for any need changes. When satiety changes, then a deficit or excess is created. This deficit or excess triggers off the appropriate adaptive mode. Within the modes are coping mechanisms whose activity is aimed at integrity. The manifestations of this activity are the adaptive or ineffective behaviors. The source of difficulty, then, is coping activity that is inadequate to maintain integrity in the face of a need deficit or excess.

Intervention

Intervention, as described earlier, includes both focus and mode. The intervention focus is the kind of problems found when deviations from the desired

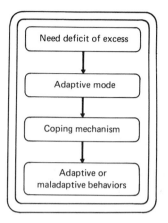

Figure 2 *Source of difficulty*

state occur. It describes the kinds of disturbances in the patiency that are to be prevented or treated. Roy has identified some commonly occurring adaptation problems in each of the adaptive modes. These can be thought of as a failure of coping mechanisms when excesses or deficits are present in the modes. Those currently identified are listed below.

A. Basic Physiologic Needs
   1. Exercise and rest
      Immobility
      Hyperactivity
      Fatigue and insomnia
   2. Nutrition
      Malnutrition
      Nausea and vomiting
   3. Elimination
      Retention and hyperexcretion
      Constipation and diarrhea
      Incontinence
   4. Fluid and electrolytes
      Dehydration
      Edema
      Electrolyte imbalance
   5. Oxygen
      Oxygen deficit
      Oxygen excess

6. Circulation
   Shock
   Overload
7. Regulation
   a. Temperature
      Fever
      Hypothermia
   b. Senses
      Sensory deprivation
      Sensory overload (pain)
   c. Endocrine system
      Endocrine imbalance
B. Self-Concept
   1. Physical self
      Loss, e.g., depression following mastectomy
   2. Personal self
      a. Moral-ethical-guilt, e.g., child with rheumatic fever blames illness on disobeying his mother
      b. Self consistency-anxiety, e.g., patient pacing the floor the night before surgery
      c. Self-ideal and expectancy-powerlessness, e.g., teenager in traction unable to try out for varsity
   3. Interpersonal self
      a. Social disengagement, e.g., elderly woman refuses to communicate with staff
      b. Aggression, e.g., cardiac patient yells at nurse
   C. Role Mastery
      Role failure—perceived inability to perform behaviors related to role, e.g., amputee: former truck driver concerned about supporting family
      Role conflict—perceived expectations of others regarding role behavior differs from own expectations, e.g., wife with threatened abortion whose husband expects sexual relations
D. Interdependence
   Alienation, rejection, aggression, rivalry, competitiveness, hostility, loneliness, disengagement, dominance, exhibition

The intervention mode is the major means of preventing or treating the problems identified in the intervention focus. It is the action that can be used to change the course of events toward the desired end product. In this model, it is what the nurse can do to promote patient adaptation. According to the Roy adaptation model, the nurse acts as an external regulatory force to modify stimuli affecting adaptation. Her mode of intervention is to increase, decrease, or maintain stimulation. This mode of intervention takes place within the nursing process, a problem-solving approach to diagnosing patient problems and to planning, carrying out, and evaluating patient care.

Roy has developed a two-level assessment process. The first level includes the identification of patient behaviors in each of the adaptive modes and the recognition of the person's position on a health-illness continuum. This assessment can be carried out rapidly and utilizes both objective data and subjective reports from the patient. The nurse may read on the chart that the postoperative patient refused his breakfast tray and she may also hear the patient state that he is not hungry. For any behavior that the nurse is concerned about, either for purposes of reinforcement or modification, she begins a second level of assessment. In this she looks for the focal, contextual, and residual factors influencing the behavior. For example, the nurse may question the patient further about his statement that he is not hungry. She may learn that the immediate cause for the patient refusing the tray is that he is afraid of gas pains. But she may also learn that the patient dislikes to eat in bed, a contextual factor. In addition the patient lacks knowledge about return of peristalsis and about the effects of nutrition on healing. Finally, the diet may not be as well seasoned as the patient prefers. These conditions all would enter into a nursing assessment for possible intervention.

Based on the information from her assessment the nurse makes a diagnosis. This is either a summary label that connotes the nature of the problem (for example, one of the adaptation problems) or a statement of the relationship between the behavior and the impinging stimuli. Thus in our example the diagnosis might read, "Refused breakfast tray related to fear of gas pains."

At present, the Roy adaptation model is not sufficiently developed to include a typology of nursing interventions. Generally interventions are devised by the selection of influencing factors that can be manipulated. If possible, the focal stimulus is manipulated first, since it is the primary cause of the behavior. If this stimulus cannot be manipulated, as, for example, when the focal stimulus is a necessary but painful treatment, then the appropriate contextual or residual stimuli are manipulated. An example is the support given during treatment. In the situation we have been discussing the nurse might try to help the patient resolve his fear of gas pains by exploring this fear, and the basis for it, with the patient. The intervention focus thus is adaptation problems and the mode is the changing of stimuli through the process of assessment, diagnosis, planning, effecting, and evaluating nursing care.

SUMMARY

The Roy adaptation model has been developed as a nursing model and can thus be more easily analyzed according to the characteristics of models. However, this brief explanation of the model already points to the need for continuing development of many of its aspects. Some assumptions about the model should be validated, for example, the assumption that the person has four modes of adaptation. Assumed values, particularly the value concerning the uniqueness of nursing, need to be made more explicit, and perhaps should also be supported. The model's goal, patiency, source of difficulty, and intervention in terms of focus and mode are all replete with possibilities for further clarification. A particularly fruitful field for study is the patient's use of adaptive mechanisms and the nurse's support of these in each of the adaptive modes.

REFERENCES

Helson H: Adaptation Level Theory. New York, Harper & Row, 1964

Martin HW, Prange A: The stages of illness—psychological approach. Nurs Outlook 10:30:168, 1962

Reiner JM: The Organism as an Adaptive Control System. Englewood Cliffs, NJ, Prentice-Hall, 1968

Roy C: Adaptation: a conceptual framework for nursing. Nurs Outlook 18:3:42, 1970

Roy C: Adaptation: a basis for nursing practice. Nurs Outlook 19:4:254, 1971

Roy C: Adaptation: implications for curriculum change. Nurs Outlook 21:3:163, 1973

Suzan L. Starr

16

Adaptation Applied to the Dying Client

In caring for the dying client, the nurse must focus her attention on stimuli, internal and external, in the client's environment that directly effect the client's experience of dying with dignity. In order to identify and manipulate these stimuli, the nurse must examine adaptive behaviors, stimuli, and nursing interventions relative to the terminally ill client.

PHYSIOLOGIC MODE

Adaptive physical behaviors are verbal and nonverbal expressions of freedom from pain and physical discomfort.

Stimuli effecting physical adaptation are pain medications that alleviate pain and allow the client to have a "clear mind," restful nights, good appetite, absence of nausea and vomiting, respiratory rales, productive cough, dyspnea, decubitus ulcers, fecal impactions, flatus, toothaches, footdrop, and physical odors.

Nursing interventions are directed to the overall goal of the client's freedom from pain and the maintenance of his physical comfort. For pain management, the nurse will assess the site, duration, pattern, and precipitating factors of pain, administer pain medications as ordered, and assess their effects, for instance, on relief, respiration, or alertness. The nurse must be knowledgeable of medications that promote physical comfort and freedom from pain. Bromptom's mixture, methadone, morphine, tylenol, and aspirin are pain medications effective in controlling pain and allowing the client to have a clear mind in order that he might feel in control of his environment (Prilook, 1977). Back rubs, positioning, and distraction also are effective interventions for relieving pain or increasing the effect of pain medication.

To prevent sleep disruption, the nurse will administer sleeping medication at the hour of sleep and spend time, prior to sleep, talking to the client to alleviate his or her fears and anxieties of falling asleep and not ever waking up again. The administration of Valium, 5 to 10 mg per physician's orders, is effective in promoting a restful night (Prilook, 1977, Saunders, 1976).

To support a client's good appetite, the nurse will encourage the client's family to bring in foods from home. To alleviate nausea and vomiting, the nurse will administer, per physician's orders, Compazine, 5 to 10 mg, p.o. or I.M. (Huff, 1975).

To alleviate respiratory rales, productive coughing, and dyspnea, the nurse will assist the client in coughing and deep breathing, administer suctioning, oxygen, and atropine, 0.4 mg, per physician's orders. Atropine given every eight hours within 48 hours preceding death drys the secretions in the respiratory tract and quiets the "death rattle" (Paige, 1977).

The nurse will turn, position, and apply body lotion over bony prominences every two hours to prevent decubitus ulcers. The nurse will administer, as ordered, laxatives daily to prevent constipation and fecal impactions due to immobility and the administration of narcotics for pain. The nurse will assist in mouth care every shift to prevent toothache due to poor oral hygiene. The nurse will actively/passively perform range of motion exercises with the client, position the client every two hours, and use a footboard, as needed, to prevent footdrop. The nurse will assist in bathing the client daily to prevent physical odors and to maintain the integrity of the skin. The use of room deodorizers and the sprinkling of spirits of peppermint on bed linen are effective nursing interventions in alleviating lingering odors (Paige, 1977).

SELF-CONCEPT MODE

Adaptive self-concept behaviors of the dying client are the conviction that the self has control over the environment, and expressions of self-worth and value.

Stimuli affecting adaptation of the self-concept are physical comfort and freedom from pain, the client's concept of death, and his or her spiritual needs.

Nursing interventions are intended to promote physical comfort and freedom from pain, to explore the concept of death by the nurse's listening and responding to behaviors that express a need to discuss the client's dying, and to assess spiritual needs by questions to the client on how he or she perceives God in relation to his or her illness. The nurse can offer to read scriptures from the Bible and to pray with the client.

ROLE MODE

Adaptive behaviors of the client in the "death role" include freely discussing dying with cooperative others, i.e., family, physicians, nurses, and friends, and actively making social arrangements for his or her death.

Stimuli effecting "death role" adaptation are active cooperation, participation, and availability of cooperative others and the setting of realistic goals during the dying process both by the client and by cooperative others.

Nursing interventions are to assist the client and cooperative others in setting realistic goals, to encourage the client to participate in decision making regarding these goals, and to assist the client and cooperative others in making social arrangements for the client's death when appropriate.

INTERDEPENDENCE MODE

Adaptive interdependent behaviors of the dying client include the client's acceptance of his or her impending loss of significant other and support systems and discussion of this loss with them.

Stimuli effecting these behaviors are the significant others' and support systems' understanding of the emotional stages the dying client may experience, their coping with the client's impending death, the availability of significant others and support systems, the continuity and consistency of care, and the commitment of the care givers.

Nursing interventions include meeting with the dying client's family and helping them to understand the emotional stages their loved one is experiencing, and assisting the family in coping by spending time with them and allowing them to ventilate their feelings about their impending loss. The nurse should encourage the family to become involved in the client's daily care, explain to family members of semicomatose clients that hearing remains so that families may express feelings to the client in final meaningful words (Paige, 1977), extend visiting hours around the clock, and allow *all* family members and pets to visit the dying client. The nursing staff must provide continuity of care and be committed to care for the dying. This builds trust in the nurse-client relationship, increases the dying client's sense of security, and decreases his fear of abandonment.

SUMMARY

This presentation of the adaptive behaviors of the dying client has defined the elements of an adaptive death as (1) a physical self that is free of pain and discomfort; (2) a self-concept that includes a sense of control over the environment, which is expressed by behaviors of self-worth and value; (3) the ability of the client to accept his role of dying, and the exhibition of this acceptance by his freely discussing his dying with cooperative others and his making social arrangements for his death; and (4) the client's acceptance of his impending loss of significant other and support systems, as evidenced by his discussing the loss with them. I have also presented stimuli that affect adaptive dying and nursing interventions that manipulate these stimuli to promote death with dignity.

REFERENCES

Huff B (ed): Physicians' Desk Reference. Oradell, New Jersey, Litton, 1975, p. 1374.

Paige RL: When the patient is dying. Hospice care for the adult. Am J Nurs 77:1813, 1977

Prilook ME: Roundtable. Dying and death. Easing the final hours or days. Patient Care, part 5, vol. 11, (June 15, 1977), p. 121.

Saunders C: Care of the dying: mental distress in the dying. Nurs Times 30:1174, 1976

Mary Schmitz

17

The Roy Adaptation Model: Application in a Community Setting

When the setting for practice is the client's home rather than the hospital, it is necessary to modify the use of the adaptation nursing process. Within the parameters of the adaptation model, the recipient of care, the goals and mode of intervention, and the contextual stimuli are redefined for the home environment.

The individual whose need precipitates contact with the health-care system is not the sole recipient of care in the home. The concept of client is expanded to include not only the individual with an identified need, but the "family of care" as well. In this context, "family" may refer to the available biological family, the primary-care giver, or significant others. During a home visit, the nurse not only intervenes with an individual but assesses the availability, adequacy, and needs of those who constitute the family of care. This broadened definition of the client is necessitated by the goals of home care.

Unlike hospital personnel, the home-care nurse is not available to the client 24 hours a day. The hombound individual must be able to function alone or aided by the family of care with only occasional interventions by the nurse. As the frequency of the nurse's input is diminished, the goal of client independence predominates. The kardex of every home-care client is replete with goals aimed toward the individual's and family's ability to verbalize and demonstrate independence in care.

In any community health setting, primary and secondary prevention are fundamental goals. As an individual moves out of the acute phase of an illness and toward the positive pole of the health-illness continuum, his energies are freed to respond to goals of disease prevention and health promotion. The man convalescing after an MI may be quite receptive to a discussion of stress management, nutritional awareness, and physical fitness. High-level wellness is a goal congruent with adaptation nursing. Man adapting in health and illness is the recipient of nursing care. (Roy, 1970).

The nurse's manner of intervention with the client is also modified by the home setting. While in the hospital, the client is a temporary participant in the health professional's territory. The hospital nurse's intervention by "doing for" the client is appropriate if the person is not able to manage his care independently. In contrast, the home is the territory of the client, and the visiting nurse becomes a guest in this environment. She is likely to experience the client as more assertive, more creative, or possibly less compliant with a care regimen when he is in his more familiar setting. Instead of a doer, the nurse necessarily becomes a collaborator, a teacher, a supporter of adaptive behaviors. The client assumes greater responsibility for the outcomes of care in the home.

In the home setting, the variables influencing care differ in their predictability and complexity. Quite often the client's primary concern does not emanate directly or exclusively from the disease process, disability or health situation precipitating the home visit. The client's primary concerns may relate to the transition from hospital to home care, a change in role relationships within the family due to the presence in the home of a dependent member, and occupational, financial, or other adaptation problems.

One 68-year-old woman was discharged from the hospital following surgery for formation of a colostomy due to cancer of the rectum. The nurse went to her home expecting to deal with problems of elimination, nutrition, and altered self-image. During the home visit the client identified her sole concern as confusion about where in the bathroom she should hang the bag of water during the irrigation procedure. The community nurse has to be especially astute in assessing and assisting with client priorities. It is these variables, in addition to those theoretically related to the health-illness situation, which so decidedly influence the outcomes of home care.

Community Case Study

The Roy Adaptation Model was used in the following case study for assessment and intervention with a family referred for home nursing care. The L family included 23-year-old Ms. L, her six-year-old son, five-year-old twin daughters and a 2-month-old son. This black family lived in a modestly furnished two-bedroom apartment in the projects. The youngest son's father lived nearby. The referral for home nursing was initiated by a private physician after he received numerous phone calls from Ms. L requesting information about the care of her youngest son. The referral stated that the mother was anxious, slow to learn, and needed teaching.

A birth history of the infant, JL, was obtained from the community hospital. JL was born six weeks prematurely by Cesarean section to a severely pre-eclampsic mother. Interuterine growth retardation was suspected. JL weighed 3 pounds 8 ounces at birth and was discharged 18 days later weighing 5 pounds 2 ounces. Ms. L returned home 13 days prior to her son's discharge following an uncomplicated post-surgical convalescence.

At six weeks of age, JL was rehospitalized for repair of bilateral incarcerated inguinal hernias. At that time he weighed 7 pounds 4 ounces and was 19.5 inches in length. JL was discharged afebrile on 125mg of Polycillin every six hours. Ten days after discharge he developed gastroenteritis and was started on Parapectalin for diarrhea. During the next four days, Ms. L contacted the child's doctor six times to inquire about different aspects of child care. A home-care referral was initiated for maternal teaching and continued physical assessment of the infant.

Behavioral Assessment
The home-care nurse made four visits over a period of two weeks. The care plan was established on the basis of an assessment of each family member and the family as a unit. However, the major findings related to JL and his mother.

Physiological Mode
Nutrition. JL was taking 4 ounces of formula every two to three hours, from a bottle which held only 4 ounces. Prior to the onset of gastroenteritis, JL was eating strained foods, including chicken, fruits, and cereals, and taking up to 2 ounces of sweetened water each day. Ms. L reported that JL used to be a good eater but was increasingly fussy the last few days. He ate less of the strained foods but seemed to want more formula. JL weighed 8 pounds 12 ounces. He had good skin turgor and muscle tone and looked small for his age. His abdomen was soft and not extended.

Elimination. After each feeding, JL had a small amount of liquid to soft green stool. Ms. L was unsure of the distinction between diarrhea and normal stools. She asked numerous questions about this. She related that JL had two days of liquid stools prior to hospitalization for repair of the inguinal hernias. JL voided clear urine in sufficient amounts. Ms. L administered the Polycillin and Parapectalin as directed. JL's diarrhea was a significant problem for the infant and a concern for his mother.

Fluid and Electrolytes. Two days prior to the initial home visit, the physician had ordered Pedialyte, an oral electrolyte solution, to be started with the discontinuance of usual foods and liquids. Ms. L was not able to get transportation to the store to purchase this solution and did not understand exactly how to give it.

Oxygen and Circulation. JL's respiratory rate was 44 without retractions. His lungs were clear to auscultation. He had no evidence of cynosis.

Skin Integrity. JL's bilateral inguinal incisional sites were healing without infection or discharge. Milia were present on his forehead and an umbilical hernia was observed. JL had a mild diaper rash which Ms. L. had not tried to treat. JL's circumcision was clean and healed.

Exercise and Rest. JL slept soundly during the day, up to three hours at a time. However, he was more restless at night.

Regulation. The moro, grasp, sucking, rooting, and tonic neck reflexes were present. JL was able to visually follow a large colorful object when it was passed in front of him. JL's rectal temperature was 99.8 F. Immunizations were current for all the children except JL. Ms. L understood that his schedule was interrupted by the hospitalization and episode of diarrhea. JL's testes were descended.

Maladaptive behaviors in this mode included JL's liquid to soft stools after each feeding and Ms. L's failure to purchase and administer the Pedialyte. Ms. L was unable to distinguish between diarrhea and normal infant stools. This behavior was related to responses identified in other modes. Adaptive behaviors in the physiological mode were JL's healing surgical sites and Ms. L's involvement and concern for the infant's care when she understood the regimen.

Self-Concept Mode

There is an intimate relation between the parent's conception of the child and the self-concept of the parent.

Children are believed to be seen by their parents as extensions of themselves; they idealize the child not only as they perceive themselves but also as they would like to be perceived. An unstable self-concept on the part of one or both parents can be further threatened by a child who is imperfect (Tudor, 1973).

Physical Self. Ms. L described herself as heavier than she would like to be. During the home visits, however, she was more focused on her son's status than her own. Ms. L described JL as small for his age and incapable of controlling his stools like healthy infants.

Personal Self. JL's physical problems precipitated threats to Ms. L's personal self and to her perception of JL. Ms. L heard the word "retarded" used in the hospital in reference to JL. She stated that she wasn't exactly sure what the doctor meant by that and asked the visiting nurse if she thought the child was slow. Ms. L's primary concern was that JL had not begun to laugh. She had been told by a neighbor that other children laughed by this age. The nurse assessed that Ms. L was experiencing anxiety due to the conflict between her desire for a normal child and any sign of slowed development in her son. Ms. L perceived the nurse's visits as a threat to her personal adequacy. Because she had not been informed by the doctor of the referral to home care, Ms. L interpreted that the nurse had to visit because she was doing something wrong.

Interpersonal Self. It was difficult for the nurse to assess the relationship between Ms. L and the infant's father. The hospital chart included entries indicating that he was a frequent visitor both times the child was hospitalized. Ms. L made only vague statements about this man and averted her eyes from the nurse when speaking about him.

Ms. L displayed ambivalent behaviors toward health-care personnel. She referred to the nurses and doctors in the hospital as "those people." Although Ms. L had called her private physician frequently about JL's care, she perceived him as "too busy to really explain things to me." Ms. L's response to the visiting nurse varied from active communication with questions, clarifying statements, and smiles to withdrawal behaviors such as long periods of silence and nonresponsiveness to questions.

Role Function Mode

Both the instrumental and expressive components of role function require a recipient, a response, resources and cooperation. JL was Ms. L's recipient in the performance of her maternal role. A cooperative system existed in the L family with the participation of the other children, Ms. L's mother, and possibly JL's father in the care of the infant. The nurse identified deficits in both the resources and response requirements for Ms. L's maternal role. Ms. L was limited in her knowledge of normal growth and development and normal elimination patterns for infants. She expected JL to be laughing at an age when infants usually do not do so, and she perceived his normal stools as diarrhea. Because of this resource deficit, Ms. L thought that JL was not responding to her like a normal infant—an expressive requirement.

Contextually, Ms. L was influenced by the availability of child-care information from her mother, a neighbor, and the health-care provider. Although Ms. L had three other children, it had been five years since the last birth. She frequently sought details related to

TABLE 1. Nursing Assessment of Infant's Physiological Behaviors and Related Stimuli

Behaviors	Stimuli		
	Focal	Contextual	Residual
1. Liquid to soft stools after every meal. 2. Increased indication of desire for liquids.	Hyperperistalsis due to bacterial/chemical irritation of intestinal mucosa.	1. Mother giving strained foods 2×/day, plus formula. 2. Mother does not understand importance of Pedialyte. 3. Mother had not purchased Pedialyte. 4. Mother does not understand how to administer Pedialyte. 5. Mother unable to distinguish diarrhea from normal stools. 6. Polycillin 125 mg q 6 hours PO QID ac given by mother. 7. Parepectalin 2.5 cc q 6 hours PO given by mother. 8. Last hospitalization of J.L. preceded by 2 days of diarrhea.	Cultural perception of meaning of elimination problems.

maternal role performance. JL's normalcy was closely tied to her adequacy as a mother. Any indication that JL was slow in development could theoretically be perceived as an indication of Ms. L's failures in mothering.

Interdependence Mode

The established organization and interaction within a family unit can be upset by the introduction of a new child into the family unit. In addition, family members usually have few role models or traditions to guide them in coping with an infant who deviates from the norm of wellness. In adjusting to a new child who is frequently ill, the family may experience a temporary disorganization and confusion of their interdependence patterns.

Help Seeking. Ms. L was able to seek help from her daughters, her mother, a neighbor, and the physician. During the home visits, Ms. L asked her daughters to help with JL's care by getting her a washcloth and bottle from another room. Ms. L occasionally asked her mother to babysit while she went shopping. She called the physician frequently to report new symptoms or changes in J.L.'s status.

Affection Seeking. Ms. L was able to seek affection and give it to her infant. She held JL close to her, patted his back, and hugged him gently. J.L. responded by cuddling in his mother's arms. No physical contact was observed between Ms. L and the other children.

Initiative Taking. Ms. L was capable of taking initiative in most tasks of mothering. However, she did not buy the Pedialyte when it was ordered by the doctor because she did not consider it urgent.

The L family demonstrated a balance of both dependent and independent behaviors in most of their interactions. When JL's physical needs increased, the family showed greater dependency needs. An example of this was Ms. L's numerous phone calls to the physician. "There is evidence . . . that objectively trivial medical problems also can prove to be a real threat for the postpartum mother" (Carey, 1977).

Nursing Diagnosis

Behaviors observed in the L family were grouped into those caused by the same focal stimulus and prioritized for intervention. Focal, contextual, and residual stimuli were identified for each group of behaviors (Tables 1,3,5).

The primary adaptation problems of the infant, the mother, and the family as a unit were identified by nursing diagnoses. The liquid

TABLE 2. Nursing Care Plan for Mother of Infant with Diarrhea

Nursing Diagnosis	Goal	Intervention	Evaluation	Modification

Disruption of intestional elimination pattern.	1. Maintenance of fluid and electrolyte balance.
	  a. Mother will purchase Pedialyte.
	  b. Mother will give meds and Pedialyte as directed.
	  c. Diarrhea will cease.
		1. Explain importance of solution, how it will help infant.
		2. Explore resources to facilitate prompt purchase of solution.
		3. Contact MD to verify directions for use.
		4. Write directions in clear terms for mother.
			1. By the second visit mother had purchased Pedialyte.
			2. She had stopped strained foods and was giving meds and Pedialyte according to written directions.
			3. According to her description of stools, diarrhea had ceased but she was not convinced.
				1. Reinforce adopted behavior.
				2. See goal 2.

2. Mother will be able to distinguish diarrhea from normal stools.
   a. Mother will verbalize J.L.'s usual stool when taking formula and Pedialyte, and when strained foods are added.
   b. Mother will identify three normal stools.

3. Mother will:
   a. Verbalize home tx of diarrhea.
   b. Verbalize indicators of need to notify MD.
   c. Decrease calls to MD.

5. Explain relation between type of intake and stool.
6. Explain wide variety of color, consistency and general appearance of bowel movements in healthy babies.
7. Practice with mother the identification of normal stools.
8. Reinforce correct judgment with praise.
9. Give mother handout on diarrhea and review.
10. Compare handout descriptions with J.L.'s status.
11. Reinforce correct judgment re: notification of MD with praise.

4. Mother able to identify J.L.'s normal stools related to type of intake.
5. Mother able to identify several normal stools. Stated she felt better about knowing the difference now.
6. Mother able to verbalize home tx both with Rx meds and without.
7. Still unsure if she can know when to call MD.
8. Mother had not called MD, she reported progress to him on regular visit.
9. Review and reinforce.

TABLE 3. Nursing Assessment of Mother-Child Social Behavior and Related Stimuli

Behaviors	Stimuli		
	Focal	Contextual	Residual
1. Mother thinks J.L. should be laughing at this age and he doesn't.	IUGR infant with health crisis.	1. J.L. is recipient of maternal role performance.	1. Unvalidated relationship with J.L.'s father.
2. Mother questions nurse, "Is he slow?"		2. Other children available to assist with care.	2. Previous experience with health-care providers.
3. Mother asked nurse, "Did you come because I was doing something wrong?"		3. Mother lives nearby and is available to assist with care.	3. Ethnic differences between black family and caucasian visiting nurse.
4. Mother provided basic care for J.L.		4. Ms. L. has little knowledge of normal growth and development.	4. Cultural prescriptions for maternal role functions.
5. Mother focused on needs of J.L.		5. Neighbor, mother, MD available for input re: appropriate role behavior.	
6. Mother described J.L. as small for his age.		6. Five years since last birth.	
7. Mother stated that the baby was called retarded in the hospital.			
8. Mother called physician frequently.			

TABLE 4. Nursing Care Plan for the Anxious Mother

Nursing Diagnosis	Goal	Intervention	Evaluation	Modification
Anxiety—self-concept mode with maternal role conflict.	1. Ms. L. will continue to demonstrate adaptive instrumental behaviors.	1. Reinforce need for family involvement in care. 2. Support adaptive behaviors of appropriate feeding, bathing, providing for rest.	1. Adaptive instrumental behaviors continued.	
	2. Ms. L. will verbalize appropriate behavior for 2-month-old compared to J.L.'s.	3. Give and review list of appropriate behaviors. 4. Explain variance in developmental abilities. 5. Ask Ms. L. to identify which behaviors J.L. is now able to do.	2. Ms. L. appreciated the list but on subsequent visits was again confused.	1. Review more slowly; demonstrate behavior with J.L.
	3. Ms. L. will verbalize feelings about J.L.'s development with nurse.	6. On each visit spend time listening to Ms. L.'s perception of J.L.'s changes.	3. Ms. L. was hesitant to discuss feelings with nurse.	2. Encourage verbalization with significant other.
	4. Ms. L. will verbalize ways in which she can stimulate J.L.	7. Give and review list of age-appropriate stimulants.	4. Ms. L. responded well to this. She was excited to recount that she had bought a bright red plastic key chain for J.L.	
	5. Ms. L. will verbalize satisfaction with herself as a good mother.	8. Praise realistic indicators of adequate mothering skill. 9. Ask Ms. L. to identify ways in which she cared for J.L. during the week.	5. Awkward beginning of verbalization. Ms. L. hesitant to say she's a good mother. This change in perception would result from a more long-term relation with client.	

TABLE 5. Nursing Assessment of Mother with 2-Month-Old Child and Related Stimuli

| | | Stimuli | |
Behaviors	Focal	Contextual	Residual
1. Ms. L. asks children to assist with care. 2. Ms. L. seeks her mother's assistance and advice. 3. Ms. L. seeks neighbor's advice about behaviors of 2-month-old infant. 4. Ms. L. gives affection to J.L., which he responds to. 5. Ms. L. calls physician frequently.	Entry of infant into family constellation. Increased physical needs of infant.	1. Availability of family members and neighbors to assist with care. 2. Ms. L.'s initiative-taking ability. 3. Family's growing trust of RN. 4. Reinforced behaviors are likely to be repeated. 5. Insufficient knowledge re: child care. 6. Last hospitalization of J.L. was preceded by 2 days of diarrhea. 7. Mother's last childbirth was 5 years ago.	1. Interdependence patterns of family prior to birth of J.L. 2. Availability of J.L.'s father as a resource.

TABLE 6. Long-Term Nursing Care Plan for Mother's Adaptive Behavior

Nursing Diagnosis	Goal	Intervention	Evaluation	Modification
Adaptive interdependent relationships.	1. Adaptive interdependent behaviors will continue.	1. Acknowledge perception of interaction pattern.	1. On two occasions, Ms. L. thanked her daughters for helpful behaviors. Ms. L. continued to provide care for children. Unable to observe interaction of other family members.	This must be considered a long-term goal. Thorough evaluation of goal attainment inadequate on four visits.
Increased dependency.	2. Family resources will be sufficient for adequate child care. a. Ms. L. will verbalize proper food, elimination pattern, rest, exercise and stimulation for 2-month-old. b. Ms. L. will verbalize indicators of need to notify physician.	2. Elicit Ms. L.'s concern re: child care. 3. Review handout on foods, elimination, rest, exercise and stimulation needs of 2-month-old. 4. Reinforce knowledge each visit. 5. Review and reinforce indicators of need to notify physician.	2. Ms. L. altered dietary intake of J.L. She verbalized correct knowledge re: child care but was not sure she could distinguish when to call physician.	More than four visits needed to meet this goal.

to soft stools after every feeding indicated the infant's physiological problem: disruption of the normal elimination pattern. Ms. L was concerned about the discrepancy between her conception of the ideal child and mother and her perception of the behaviors of JL and herself. She sought information from others, which resulted in conflicting prescriptions for her role. Ms. L's nursing diagnosis was self-concept mode anxiety with maternal role conflict. The family as a unit demonstrated adaptive interdependent relationships, with increased dependence behaviors in response to JL's changing physiological needs.

Goals for each group of behaviors were established. Interventions, evaluations of goal attainment and modification of goals are listed in Tables 2, 4, and 6.

Summary
The Roy Adaptation Model was used in this case study to assess and intervene with a family receiving home nursing care. The client, goals, interventions and influencing variables were defined specifically for the home environment. The infant, JL, along with his mother, siblings, and grandmother composed the client constellation. Goals and interventions were designed to provide sufficient resources for the family to function independently. The most predominant client priority was for information and reassurance about JL's developmental adequacy. Although limited by the number of allocated visits, the nurse was able to assess needs, prioritize, set goals, and intervene efficiently and effectively by application of this adaptation nursing model.

REFERENCES

Carey W: Psychological sequelae of early infancy health crisis. Clin Pediatr 8:8:259, 1969.

Roy C: Adaptation: A Conceptual Framework for Nursing. Nurs Outlook 18:3:42, 1970.

Tudor M: Family habitation: a child with a birth defect. In Hymovich D and Barnard M (eds): Family Health Care. New York, McGraw-Hill, 1973.

Dorothy E. Johnson

18

The Behavioral System Model for Nursing

The behavioral system model for nursing has been developed from a philosophical perspective, supported by a rich, sound, and rapidly expanding body of empirical and theoretical knowledge. Philosophically, starting with nursing's traditional concern for the person who is ill, nursing's specific contribution to patient welfare has come to be as the fostering of efficient and effective behavioral functioning in the patient to prevent illness, and during and following illness. The goal of nursing is to assist a person (1) whose behavior is commensurate with social demands, (2) who is able to modify his behavior in ways that support biologic imperatives, (3) who is able to benefit to the fullest extent during illness from the physician's knowledge and skill, and (4) whose behavior does not give evidence of unnecessary trauma as a consequence of illness. Thus we see nursing offering a service that is complementary to that of medicine and other health professions, but which makes its own distinctive contribution to the health and well-being of people.

With this focus on efficient and effective behavioral functioning, it has been useful to accept a theoretical view of the patient as a behavioral system in much the same way physicians have accepted a theoretical view of the patient as a biologic system. Such acceptance is made possible by the relatively recent development and rapid expansion of a literature contributing to our understanding of man as a behavioral system. It is an interdisciplinary literature developed by behavioral and biologic scientists, animal and human ethologists. Scientists in these disciplines have focused on the behavior of the individual as a whole—on what he does, why, and on the consequences of that behavior—not on why or how he has changed over time in an intraorganismic sense. They study the output of intraorganismic structures and processes as they are coordinated and articulated, and as they respond to changes in sensory stimulation. More specifically, they focus on social behavior, that is, behavior that takes into account the actual or implied presence of other social beings, and especially on those forms of it that have been shown to have major adaptive significance.

At this point, research and theoretical attention have been directed primarily toward specific response systems within the total complex of the whole behavioral system; an empirical literature supporting the notion of the behavioral system as a whole* is largely yet to be developed. This is not unlike the case of the growth of knowledge about the biologic system, in which knowledge of the parts preceded knowledge of the whole. Fortunately, there is also developing concurrently a body of knowledge about systems in general and the laws that govern the operation of all systems, on which we can rely in a tentative way until further knowledge of the behavioral system is developed (Buckley, 1968).

Let us first consider the ideas and assumptions critical to understanding the nature and operation of the whole system. According to Rapport (1968), "A system is a whole that functions as a whole by virtue of the interdependence of its parts." Therefore, by the use of the construct "system" in reference to behavior, we assume there is "organization, interaction, interdependency, and integration of the parts and elements" (Chin, 1961) of behavior that go to make up the system. The interrelated parts are called, under certain conditions, subsystems; the subsystems of behavior will be discussed more fully later.

We assume also that a system "tends to achieve a balance among the various forces operating within and upon it" (Chin, 1961), and that man strives continually to maintain a behavioral system balance and steady states by more or less automatic adjustments and adaptations to the "natural" forces impinging upon him. At the same time we recognize that man also actively seeks new experiences that may disturb his balance, at least temporarily, and that may require small or large behavioral modifications to reestablish balance.

We assume further that a behavioral system, which both requires and results in some degree of regularity and constancy in behavior, is essential to man; that is to say, it is functionally significant in that it serves a useful purpose both in social life and for the individual. Finally, we assume that behavioral system balance reflects adjustments and adaptations that are successful in some way and to some degree. This will be true even though the observed behavior may not always match the cultural norms for acceptable or healthy behavior.

It seems likely that for most individuals most of the time the behavioral

---

*It should be noted here that the conception of man as a behavioral system, or the idea that man's specific response patterns form an organized and integrated whole is original with me, so far as I know. There are indications in the literature that others support the idea, however.

system is at a level of balance that is functionally efficient and effective. There appears to be built into the system sufficient flexibility to take acount of the usual fluctuations in the impinging forces and enough stress tolerance for the system to adjust to many common, but extreme, fluctuations. Most individuals probably experience at one or more times during their lives a psychologic crisis or a physical illness grave enough to disturb the system balance and to require external assistance. Nursing is (or could be) the force that supplies assistance both at the time of occurrence and at other times to prevent such occurrences.

The discussion to this point has referred to the laws that govern the operation of all systems and has indicated that a behavioral system must operate according to these same laws. Compare, for example, the biologic system, which is also made up of parts, or subsystems, with the organization, interaction, and interdependency of those parts. They too tend to achieve a balance and this balance is essential to effective system functioning. Finally, we know that the level of balance achieved by the biologic system is not always optimal, and all too frequently not even ''healthy.''

Specifically then, all the patterned, repetitive, and purposeful ways of behaving that characterize each man's life are considered to comprise his behavioral system. These ways of behaving form an organized and integrated functional unit that determines and limits the interaction between the person and his environment and establishes the relationship of the person to the objects, events, and situations in his environment. Such behavior is orderly, purposeful, and predictable; that is, it is functionally efficient and effective, most of the time, and it is sufficiently stable and recurrent to be amenable to description and explanation.

The behavioral system has many tasks or missions to perform in maintaining its own integrity and in managing the system's relationship to its environment; thus the parts of the system evolve, or subsystems develop, each to carry out its own specialized tasks for the system as a whole. A biologic system, too, has many tasks to perform and so its subsystems have evolved. The more complex and highly organized the system, the more parts or subsystems evolve to manage the increasing variety of tasks to be performed.

Each subsystem of the behavioral system is formed of a set of behavioral responses, responsive tendencies, or action systems that seem to share a common drive or goal. Organized around drives (or some type of motivational structure) these responses are developed and modified over time through maturation, experience, and learning. They are determined developmentally and are continuously governed by a multitude of physical, biologic, psychologic, and social factors operating in a complex and interlocking fashion. These responses are reasonably stable, though modifiable, and regularly recurrent, and their action pattern is observable.

Consider, for example, the proximity-seeking or contact-seeking behavior so clearly seen in young children: the visual seeking and following, the turning and later the creeping toward the caretaker, the following, the reaching out (Ainsworth, 1964). Under usual conditions, these behaviors stimulate the caretaker's reinforcing responses of regarding, smiling, talking to, and picking up (Robson, 1967). Patterned behavior of this kind is triggered by genetic propensities and shaped by maturation, experiences with the caretaker, and the general learning conditions. It serves some function for the individual. Here, proximity-seeking behavior fulfills in the broadest sense the function of survival for the young infant and more specially for all individuals the function of intimacy or inclusion (Ainsworth, 1972). This is called attachment or affiliative behavior.

The subsystems are linked and open, as is true in all systems, and a disturbance in one subsystem is likely to have an effect on others. Just as cardio-respiratory dysfunction may affect urinary function, so too is the behavioral system one may find aggressive responses precipitated by dysfunctional attachment behaviors; or, if dependency behaviors are not met with care-giving behaviors, attachment behaviors may be increased.

Although each subsystem has a specialized task or function, the system as a whole depends upon an integrated performance. This is sometimes a source of difficulty for the person. A good example can be traced to the present-day changing conditions for women in our society. Many women, particularly young women, today find themselves not infrequently with two conflicting drives operating simultaneously: the achievement and the sexual drives. This creates for the behavioral system at best tension, and at worst erratic and disorganized behavior.

Each subsystem has structure as well as function and can be described and analyzed along these axes. There are at least four structural elements in each subsystem. Although only one of these elements, the actual behavior of the individual, can be observed, the behavior is instigated or inhibited and shaped by other structural elements whose nature can be inferred. First, from the form the behavior takes and the consequences it achieves can be inferred what *drive* has been stimulated or what *goal* is being sought. The drive or goal of each subsystem is the same for all people when stated in general terms, but there are variations among individuals in the specific objects or events that are drive-fulfilling, in the value placed on goal attainment, and in drive strength. To illustrate, it can be inferred from the courting behavior of individuals that sexual gratification or procreation is being sought, although the person (object) toward whom the behavior is directed may be the same or the opposite sex. Further, this drive is stronger in some individuals than others; the goal is less valued by some than by others, and all of these (goal, object, strength, and significance) can and do change over time.

Secondly, the individual's *set* in each subsystem must also be inferred from observation. By set is meant the person's predisposition to act, with reference to the goal, in certain ways rather than in other ways. This concept takes into account the fact that within the range or scope of behaviors that might be possible for the individual, given a particular goal, the action alternatives of the individual are not only comparatively few and highly selective but also hierarchically arranged. In essence, through maturation, experience, and learning, the individual comes to develop and use preferred ways of behaving under particular circumstances and with selected individuals. Although more difficult to describe and analyze in the concrete case, through history, test, and structured observations, it is possible and diagnostically and therapeutically useful to determine, for example, whether the young child tends to call for help from one person or many, from adults or peers; whether he asks directly or indirectly for assistance; and how he varies his approach from those who are familiar to those who are strangers.

The third structural element in each subsystem is the totality of the behavioral repertoire available to the individual for the achievement of a particular goal. This constitutes his choices, or the scope of action alternatives from which he can choose. We rarely use all the action alternatives in our behavioral repertoires, and those observed tend to be the most preferred ones. Individuals frequently have others, however, on which they can fall back if under different or unusual circumstances the preferred ones do not work. Throughout life, people continuously acquire new action choices or modify old ones, although the rate of acquisition tends to decrease with increasing age, being highest at birth and lowest with old age. It should be noted, however, that people vary markedly at any given age level in the number and complexity of the action alternatives available to them, and no doubt many individuals operate at a less than optimal behavioral level because their choices are limited. Recognition of this fact is quite evident in current nursing practice in the techniques (for example, teaching, role modeling, counseling) used to help people find new or "better" ways of behaving. These techniques in effect contribute to an enlargement of choices. Finally, it must also be noted that larger behavioral repertoires characterize more adaptable individuals.

The fourth structural unit, which we can observe directly, is the person's behavior. Here our concern is the efficiency and effectiveness of the behavior in goal attainment. Is the behavior succeeding or failing to achieve the consequences sought? Are more skillful motor, expressive, or social skills needed? Are the choices appropriate? Is the sequence of action purposeful and orderly; does it demonstrate economy mf action; is the action socially and biologically appropriate? These and other questions of a similar nature are necessary for an analysis of system functioning. And for the analysis to be sound, the behavior observed must be described and organized into functional units when possible, for example, attention or approval seeking behaviors, requests for assistance, proximity seeking, courting.

In addition to the structural units just described, each of the subsystems and the system as a whole has a function. Some of the functions have already been alluded to in an illustrative way in the description of the structure. The full list of the subsystems with their functions will be presented later as each is discussed individually. Before this, a few other comments about the subsystems as a group are pertinent.

Each of the subsystems, and the system as a whole, has certain functional requirements that must be met through the individual's own efforts, or through outside assistance, for each to grow, develop, and remain viable. The biologic system and all other living systems have the same requirements: Each must be *protected* from noxious influences with which the system cannot cope, *nurtured* through the input of appropriate supplies from the environment, and *stimulated* for use to enhance growth and prevent stagnation. To illustrate, the attachment subsystem of the behavioral system of the young infant must be protected from prolonged separations from the main caretaker, nurtured by receiving appropriate responses to his signals to the caretaker, and stimulated by experiences that allow new, more highly developed responses and signals to be shaped as he is developmentally ready.

Finally, it should be noted that the subsystems and the system as a whole tend to be self-maintaining and self-perpetuating so long as conditions in the internal and external environment of the system remain orderly and predictable, the conditions and resources necessary to their functional requirements are met, and the interrelationships among the subsystems are harmonious. If these conditions are not met, malfunction becomes apparent in behavior that is in part disorganized, erratic, and dysfunctional. Illness or other sudden internal or external environmental change is most frequently responsible for such malfunctions.

A number of subsystems have been identified. Those included here are found cross-culturally and for the most part across a broad range of the phylogenetic scale. This latter connection would support the idea that these response systems, or at least the primary releasers for them, are genetically programmed. The great variability in human responses also points to the significance of social and cultural factors in their development. The ultimate group of response systems to be identified in the behavioral system will undoubtedly change as research reveals new systems or indicates changes in the structure, functions, or behavior pattern groupings in the original set.

One of the first response systems to emerge developmentally, and probably the most critical one for it forms the basis for all social organization, is the *attachment* or *affiliative* subsystem. At its most general level, it serves the function of (survival) security, while more empirically it has the consequence of social inclusion, intimacy, and the formation and maintenance of a strong social bond. The literature on attachment behavior, particularly in the infant and young child and the mother-child dyad is a rich and growing one.

Descriptions and explanations of *dependency* behavior (Heathers, 1955,

Gerwitz, 1972; Rosenthal, 1967) have been found in the literature for some time, but the term served as a kind of umbrella concept that included attachment. With the isolation of attachment behavior and its functions, dependence behavior appears to have more limited and more precise functions. In the broadest sense, it is succoring behavior that calls for a response of nurturance. More specifically, it is behavior that has as its consequence approval, attention or recognition, and physical assistance. Developmentally, dependency behavior in the socially optimum case evolves from almost total dependence on others to a greater degree of dependence on self, with a certain amount of interdependence essential to the survival of social groups.

Because of our previous association of the *ingestive* and *eliminative* subsystems with the biologic system, it is important to make clear at the outset that these response systems have to do with when, how, what, how much, and under what conditions we eat, and when, how, and under what conditions we eliminate (Walike, 1969; Mead, 1953; Sears, et al., 1954). Ingestive behavior can thus be ssen to serve the broad function of appetitive satisfaction in its own right. This may be, and all too often is, at odds with the biologic requirements for food and fluids. What, how, how much, et cetera, we eat are all governed by social and psychologic considerations far more potent in affluent societies than food per se. The function of the behavioral eliminative subsystem is more difficult to differentiate from that of the biologic subsystem, yet clearly all humans must learn expected modes of behavior in the excretion of wastes, and these behaviors often take precedence over or strongly influence purely biologic eliminative acts.

The *sexual* subsystem also has strong biologic system connotations, though we are more likely to recognize that biologic factors play only one role in the sexual behavior expected and learned in any given culture (Kagan, 1964; Resnik, 1972). With its dual functions of procreation and gratification, the response system originates with the development of a gender role identity and covers the broad range of those behaviors dependent upon one's biologic sex, including but not limited to courting and mating.

The postulated function of the *aggressive* subsystem is self- (and thus societal) protection and preservation. This follows the line of thinking of Lorenz (1966) and other ethologists (Feshbach, 1970) rather than that of the behavioral reinforcement school who think that aggressive behavior is not only learned but has as its primary intent the injury of others. It should be noted, however, that even in animal societies, the imperatives of collective life demand that limits be placed on modes of self-protective behavior and that there be protection and respect for the person and property of all.

Development of the *achievement* system probably is first manifested by exploratory behavior and attempts to manipulate the environment. Its function is mastery or control of some aspect of the self or environment as measured against some standard of excellence. The significance of intellectual achievement behavior has long been recognized, but other areas in which achievement behavior has been described are physical, creative, mechanical, and social skills (Atkinson, Feather, 1966; Crandal, 1963). Still other areas may emerge with further research; tentatively included now are care-taking skills, encompassing physical care of children, spouses, home, et cetera.*

In summary, then, the behavioral system has seven subsystems, each carrying out a specialized task for the system as a whole. The system operates at some level of efficiency and effectiveness in its internal affairs and external relationships so long as it is able to maintain overall balance and dynamic stability. Nursing problems arise because there are disturbances in the structure or function of the subsystems or the system, or because the level of behavioral functioning is at less than a desired or optimal level. To the extent that any problem that might arise can be anticipated and appropriate methodologies are available, preventive nursing action is also in order. The goal of nursing action in each case is to restore, maintain, or attain behavioral system balance and stability at the highest possible level for the individual.

Nursing is thus seen as an external regulatory force which acts to preserve the organization and integration of the patient's behavior at an optimal level under those conditions in which the behavior constitutes a threat to physical or social health, or in which illness is found. This force operates through the imposition of external regulatory or control mechanisms, through attempts to change structural units in desirable directions, or through the fulfillment of the functional requirements of the subsystems.

Adoption of this model for practice carries with it direct responsibilities in education. The user will need a thorough grounding in the underlying natural and social sciences. Emphasis should be placed in particular on the genetic, neurologic, and endocrine bases of behavior; psychologic and social mechanisms for the regulation and control of behavior; social learning theories; and motivational structures and processes. The next level of instruction is devoted in large measure to nursing's basic science—the study of man as a behavioral system, that is, study of the system as a whole and each of the subsystems. Also appropriate at this level of instruction, although not a part of nursing's basic science, is the study of pathophysiology of the biologic system, of medicine's clinical science, and of the health system as a whole. The last level of basic instruction would emphasize nursing's clinical science, the study of behavioral system problems in man, which would include the relevant diagnostic and treatment rationales and methdologies. It must be noted that at this level, selection of course content is difficult because the needed years of patient and painstaking investigation are still to come, and the knowl-

*Differences will be noted in this listing of the subsystems and their functions from that of Grubbs in this volume, and those writing elsewhere. The presentation here is the original one and the one to which I continue to subscribe.

edge base tends to be disorganized and more intuitive and speculative than scientific.

The research path for the investigator committed to this model is two-directional. Those more interested in nursing's basic science will tend to join those basic scientists already engaged in studies of the several subsystems in the behavioral system or will attempt to learn more about the operation of the system as a whole. Those more interested in immediate results for practice will tend to focus on the identification, clarification, or explanation of behavioral system problems, or will direct their attention toward diagnostic or treatment rationales or methodologies. Clearly, knowledge in both areas is needed, and the need for knowledge of behavioral system problems is urgent.

By any of three criteria brought to bear, the behavioral system model for nursing seems defensible and promising. It has already proved its utility in providing clear direction for practice, education, and research. Insofar as it has been tried in practice, the resulting nursing decisions and actions have generally been judged acceptable and satisfactory by patients, families, nursing staff, and physicians. More important, the resulting actions have been thought to make a significant difference in the lives of the persons involved—an important test for professional actions. It has been and continues to be used as a basis for development of curricula. It has generated many questions for research. Clearly the knowledge base for the model is incomplete, both empirically and theoretically; knowledge about behavioral systems is in its infancy. Its further development is open to and dependent upon the creative efforts of all those attracted to it, practitioners, educators, and researchers.

REFERENCES

Ainsworth M: Patterns of attachment behavior shown by the infant in interaction with mother. Merrill-Palmer Quart 10:1:51–58, 1964

Ainsworth M: Attachment and dependency: a comparison. In J Gewirtz (ed): Attachment and Dependency. Englewood Cliffs, NJ, Prentice-Hall, 1972

Atkinson JW, Feather NT: A Theory of Achievement Maturation. New York, Wiley, 1966

Buckley W (ed): Modern Systems Research for the Behavioral Scientist. Chicago, Aldine, 1968

Chin R: The utility of system models and developmental models for practitioners. In Benne K, Bennis W, and Chin R (eds): The Planning of Change. New York, Holt, 1961

Crandal V: Achievement. In Stevenson HW (ed): Child Psychology. Chicago, University of Chicago Press, 1963

Feshbach S: Aggression. In Mussen P (ed): Carmichael's Manual of Child Psychology, 3rd ed, vol. 2. New York, Wiley, 1970

Gerwirtz J (ed): Attachment and Dependency. Englewood Cliffs, Prentice-Hall, 1972

Heathers G: Acquiring dependence and independence: a theoretical orientation: J Genet Psychol 87:277–291, 1955

Kagan J: Acquisition and significance of sex typing and sex role identity. In Hoffman, Hoffman (eds): Review of Child Development Research. New York, Russell Sage Foundation, 1964

Lorenz K: On Aggression. New York, Harcourt, 1966

Mead M: Cultural Patterns and Technical Change. World Federation for Mental Health, UNESCO, 1953

Rapoport, A: Foreword to Modern Systems Research for the Behavioral Scientist. Buckley W (ed): Chicago, Aldine, 1968

Resnik HLP: Sexual Behaviors. Boston, Little, Brown, 1972

Robson KS: Patterns and determinants of maternal attachment. J Pediat 77:976–985, 1967

Rosenthal M: The generalization of dependency from mother to a stranger. J Child Psychol Psychiatry 8:177–183, 1967

Sears R, Maccoby E, and Levin H: Patterns of Child Rearing. White Plains, Row, Peterson, 1954

Walike B, Jordan, HA, and Stellar E: Studies of eating behavior. Nurs Res 18:108–113, 1969

Judy Grubbs

19

An Interpretation of the Johnson Behavioral System Model for Nursing Practice

There are many frameworks within which to view man. This paper will present a view of man based on a systems theory, whereby man is seen as a collection of behavioral subsystems that interrelate to form a whole person or behavioral system.* To operationalize this model, assumptions about nursing will be presented first, followed by an analysis of the specific components of the theory. The purpose of this paper is to present a clear and logical view of the model, so that its value as a systematic guide to nursing practice will seem both feasible and prudent.

BELIEFS AND ASSUMPTIONS ABOUT NURSING

The assumptions as presented by Johnson (1968) are given in Table 1. The narrative which follows will present an elaboration of the assumptions based on the present writer's interpretation.

The intent of these statements is to demonstrate that nursing does provide a distinctive service to society that can be differentiated from the other health professions. The predominant focus of nursing is on the person who is ill, or threatened with an illness, while the primary focus of medicine is on pathologic changes. The concern of the nurse is to assist the patient to cope when the stress, or the threat, of illness exists. Questions nurses might raise would relate to how this illness is perceived by the patient, how it has changed his usual behavior, and how it has changed, or threatens to change, his

---

*This model was conceived and developed by Dorothy Johnson, professor of nursing at the University of California at Los Angeles. The author wishes to express her gratitude to Ms. Johnson for her inspiration. This paper is, however, the author's interpretation of the model.

TABLE 1. Beliefs About Nursing and Its Practice

1. Nursing is concerned first with the person who is ill rather than his disease.
2. Achievement by nurses of the mission expressed in this model would be congruent with society's expectations and would provide a socially valued service.
3. Nursing will continue to assist medicine in the fulfillment of medicine's mission both because of the intrinsic value of that mission and because doing so will facilitate the fulfillment of nursing's mission. As medical technology places increased demands upon nursing, it will be essential to set limits based on rational criteria.
4. These two missions—medicine's and nursing's—are in an important sense complementary.
5. Nursing's role in coordination must be limited to nursing services and possibly in some settings to patient care. Specifically excluded is coordination of patient care services at any level.

life-style or self-concept. It is assumed that this role of the nurse is congruent with society's expectations of nursing and that nursing's contribution to health care is a socially valued service. Nursing and medicine are seen as complementary roles that are inextricably intertwined.

Given such a responsibility, nurses cannot be involved in the coordination of patient care to the extent that they are now, but they must concentrate on coordinating the nursing care for individual patients. This commitment means that in many institutions tasks with which nurses are now involved must be delegated to other personnel, so that nurses can optimally fulfill their nursing obligations to the patients. The question now is what are the aspects of care for which nursing can be held accountable? To help clarify this, Table 2 summarizes the model's assumptions about the value system and goals that direct the nurse's focus (Johnson, 1968). The discussion that follows elaborates on these assumptions.

How can one respond to the frequent question, what is a nurse and what does she do? What does it mean to state that the nurse is responsible for the person with an illness? To begin, one might say that the nurse is an external regulator. Although she actually regulates the environment within which the patient functions, she also uses resources in that environment to assist the patient to regulate his own adaptation to the situation.

Regulating the environment encompasses the caring and nurturing tasks with which nurses are most commonly associated. The nurse determines what the patient is accustomed to and attempts to match, within the limits of the illness, the present setting to his usual patterns. She scrutinizes the environment with an eye toward monitoring either too little or too much stimulation. She provides the patient with the equipment and the stimulation to manage his personal hygiene and the activities of daily living, given the restrictions that may have been imposed by illness or institutionalization. She protects the patient from unnecessary or overwhelming threats or deficits from his immediate environment. Her goals are the patient's comfort, the appropriate use of his energy to adapt to the illness, and the maintenance of his developmental level of functioning.

Using herself as a primary resource, the nurse mobilizes all other resources in the situation to stimulate and nurture the person to the point of optimum functioning within the given psychologic and biologic limits. Prevention of problems involves the nurse in instructing the patient or preparing him for impending experiences. Intervention for existing problems calls forth such goals as resocializing the patient and members of his family to take on desired and appropriate roles, managing the affective responses accompanying the stress of illness, and mobilizing coping abilities for actual or potential stresses. The end result is the modification of the patient's behavioral patterns to meet the demands of the unmodifiable elements in his life. Hopefully this will bring him closer to realizing a satisfying personal and social life. These are the goals of the model and the responsibilities of the nurse.

Although the goals of the model seem appropriate and perhaps somewhat optimistic, what are their limitations? How does the nurse avoid modifying a patient's behavior to create congruency with her own value system? Clearly the lower limit of acceptable behavior that a nurse cannot support is behavior so deviant that it tends to exceed society's limits. Or it is behavior that threatens the survival of the individual either biologically or socially.

TABLE 2. Assumptions About the Value System to Guide the Scope of the Nurse's Role

A. The Lower Limits of Acceptable Behavioral-System Balance and Stability
  1. There is a wide range of behavior tolerated by this society (or any other) and only the middle section of the continuum can be said to represent cultural norms.
  2. So long as the behavior at either extreme does not threaten the survival of society, it is tolerated by society.
  3. The outer limits of tolerated behavior are therefore set for the professions by society; in fact, the limits of tolerated behavior set by the professions, including nursing, tend to be narrower in many areas than those set by society.
  4. In essence, then, nursing does not purposefully support (maintain), certainly over a prolonged period or in the absence of other counteractive measures, behavior so deviant that it is intolerant to society or constitutes a threat to the survival of the individual (socially or biologically) and ultimately of society.

B. Desired Behavioral-System Balance and Stability
  1. Just as medicine has the obligation to seek the highest possible level of biologic functioning and overall stability, so too nursing has the obligation to seek the highest possible level of behavioral functioning. Both are limited by current knowledge and the value judgments of society.
  2. There are no established and universally accepted standards for behavior that represent a "better" or "higher" level in any absolute way.
  3. Nursing can contribute, through research, to further understanding of the significance and consequences of certain behaviors. Nursing can also use, but judiciously, the knowledge available. In no case, however, can the individual nurse afford to impose upon the patient her judgments as to what is desirable.

However, caution must be taken to judge the patient's behavior in light of his specific social environment and his biologic and psychologic capacities. Obviously, operating exclusively either consciously or unconsciously on the basis of one's own biases and value system is unacceptable for professional nurses.

What then are the upper limits of nursing's responsibilities? Within the boundaries of available knowledge of man's behavior and within the values of the particular society, nurses strive to achieve the highest possible level of behavioral functioning for all individuals. However, after the determination of the potential a person is able to attain, the means to attain it, and the consequences of a lower level of functioning, the patient is the final judge of his behavioral goals. This decision is every person's right and must be respected.

Within this model, therefore, the nurse can define problems of individual behavioral instability and group instability. However, she must take into account the biologic, psychologic, and sociocultural factors as these regulate behaviors. And she must retain the belief that the individual ultimately holds the key to his own destiny.

BASIC CONCEPTS OF THE JOHNSON NURSING MODEL

Systems Theory

The recent popularity of systems theory perhaps attests to its usefulness in understanding complex situations. Analyzing a system merely implies the theoretical cessation of its process in order to remove an imaginary section for closer scrutiny. It is assumed that any section is more or less representative of the whole. Since the basic concepts of systems theory have been discussed earlier in this book, this writer will simply list for clarification and review the definitions that will be used in the remainder of this paper.

Definitions of Terms

Boundary—the point which differentiates what is inside from what is outside the system; the point at which the system has little control over, or impact on, outcomes.

Function—the consequences or purposes of a particular action in relation to the whole system.

  Manifest function—the apparent or primary outcome of an action.

  Latent function—the unintended result of a behavior, which is less observable, unconscious, or of secondary value.

Functional requirements—the input in the form of protection, nurturance, and stimulation that the system must receive from the environment in order to survive and develop; also termed *sustenal imperatives.*

Homeostasis—the actual process of maintaining stability.

Instability—that situation which occurs when there is an overcompensation by the system to deal with a strain, also when extra energy output is used to respond to a stressor with the result that the energy source needed to maintain stability is depleted. The resultant stress state is demonstrated by one or more of the following behaviors:

  Disorderly behaviors—those behaviors that are not organized and methodical, or that do not build sequentially toward a purpose.

  Purposeless behaviors—those behaviors that have no rational pattern or goal.

  Unpredictable behaviors—those behaviors that are at variance from that which is usually repeated under similar circumstances.

Stability—the situation that exists when a system is able to maintain a certain level of behavior within an acceptable range; synonyms are *balance* and *steady state.*

Stressor—any stimulus within or outside the system that results in *stress* or instability.

Structure—those parts of the system that make up the whole.

System—a whole which functions as a whole by virtue of the organized interdependent interaction of its parts (Rapoport, 1968).

Subsystem—a minisystem with its own particular goal and function that can be maintained as long as its relationship to the other subsystems or the environment is not disturbed.

Tension—that state in which the system adjusts to demands for changes or adjusts to actual disruptions; tension is essential for the system to grow and change over time.

Variables—factors outside the system that influence behavior within the system, but which the system has little power to change.

The resultant image of a system encompasses a whole that includes efficient interdependent parts defined by a boundary. The whole is highly dependent upon the outside environment and may be disrupted by deficits or excesses from without. A stress on any part of the system affects the interdependent parts and disrupts functioning of the whole. Such disruptions may be observed as dysfunctional behavior with a resultant concentration of energy to handle the stress. Success of the system is dependent upon its ability to adjust to a continuously changing environment, and to change. The success of a nurse using this model of nursing depends upon her ability to alter her conceptualization of man from the traditional view of being only a physiologic system to the view of man as a behavioral system.

Assumptions About Man and His Behavior

Man can be viewed as many different types of systems depending upon the focus and purpose of the viewer. If man is viewed as a health-care system rather than a physiologic system, an entirely different image can be conceptualized. To look at a person and be able to "see" a collection of behavioral subsystems with the familiar psychologic, sociocultural, and physiologic factors operating outside them is a necessary prerequisite to using this model. Over time many of these factors do become an integral part of each subsystem, so aspects of these variables may act as external influences while other aspects act within the system to influence behavior. For most students this shift of thinking involves discarding old ways of conceptualizing the individual. One must consciously strive to "see" the behavioral subsystems and their boundaries.

Behavior

Basic to the model is the concept of behavior. But what is behavior and how does it develop? Table 3 summarizes the points about behavior that will be discussed in the following paragraphs (Johnson, 1968). *Behavior* is defined as those observable features and actions that a person displays in response to external or internal stimuli. Behavior is primarily concerned with social behavior. The focus is on how one interacts with other people. A *behavioral system*, then, is the organized, interrelated complex of subsystems each with behavioral patterns that determine and limit how the person interacts with his environment. Behavioral patterns develop over time and are influenced by such outside variables as physical, biologic and social factors.

TABLE 3. Assumptions About Man and Behavior

1. Behavior is determined by multiple complex interactions of physical, biologic, and social factors.
2. The behavior of an individual at any given point is the product of the net aggregate of consequences of these factors over time and at that point.
3. Man strives continuously to bring into balance the forces operating within and upon him and through adjustment and adaptation to maintain order and stability in his behavior.
4. Man also actively seeks new experiences (and exposure to new forces) that require adjustment and adaptation.
5. The observed regularities and constancies in human behavior are functionally significant for the individual and for social living, serving such purposes as, for example, economy of energy, efficiency of action, and facilitation of social interaction.
6. When these regularities and constancies are disturbed, the integrity of the person is threatened and the functions served by such order are not adequately fulfilled.

Stability

The model assumes that man constantly strives to bring into balance forces operating within and upon him in order to maintain stability. Behavioral balance is a dynamic state of interaction between the individual and his environment that allows for a range of behaviors and also adapts to a range of input without resulting in disruption. Through the processes of adjustment and adaptation the individual changes or grows to meet external demands and constraints. The development of patterns of behavior or habits helps him to maintain a constant relationship with his environment. Patterns assure economy of energy, efficiency of action, and facilitation of social interaction. The goals of the system are thus met and living becomes as predictable and orderly as is possible. The concepts pertaining to stability are included in Table 4 (Johnson, 1968).

Inherent in a systems theory are assumptions about mechanisms whose purpose is to maintain stability. The primary concepts involved are input, output, and regulating and control mechanisms. The latter two concepts will be discussed in detail later in the paper. *Input* is any type of stimulus or material taken from the environment. *Output* is the observable release of energy or materials into the environment. Output not only rids the body of waste, but may also be used as a feeler to gather information about how successfully the individual is functioning. Through the sensory input modes, the individual judges the effectiveness of his verbal or nonverbal output by the reactions of his environment. Adjustments are made to alter further input or output according to the evaluation. This feedback mechanism is analogous to

---

TABLE 4. Assumptions About Behavioral-System Balance

A. Behavioral-System Balance or Stability
1. Demonstrated by behavior which is purposeful, orderly, predictable.
2. Achieved and maintained at a variety of different levels (when judged on the basis of optimal, desirable, or possible) over time and within a particular time segment.
3. Stabilized, for varying periods of time, at levels that represent adaptation and adjustment (to changing conditions) which are successful for the individual in some way and to some degree.
4. Self-maintained and self-perpetuated so long as the functional requirements of the subsystems are adequately met and fluctuations in environmental conditions are within the system's current capacity to adjust.
5. A necessary condition for an output of behavior that is efficient and effective for the individual.

B. Consequences of Behavioral-System Balance
1. A minimum expenditure of energy is required.
2. Continued biologic and social survival are insured, i.e., the behavior does not violate essential biologic imperatives and is commensurate with the demands of social life.
3. Some degree of personal satisfaction accrues.

the physiologic feedback mechanisms that monitor and control physiologic states. Messages received through the behavioral feedback mechanisms guide the quality and quantity of the individual's activities and responses. Actual consequences of behaviors are thus constantly evaluated in terms of those desired.

Change Of Behavior

Since the environment is not always predictable and orderly, the system has to develop strategies for coping with change. According to the model, three situations would motivate an individual to modify his behavior. Table 5 summarizes the three states associated with behavioral change.

The first situation exists when a basic drive is not adequately satisfied. The response to this state might be an increase in the drive and, thus, an increase in the behavior directed toward satisfying that drive. Another response might be to change the direction of the drive, in other words, to direct the energy toward achievement of a goal different from the original. The second situation leading to impetus for change is a lack of fulfillment of a subsystem's functional requirements. Without sufficient stimulation, protection, or nurturance, the subsystem will be impelled to make adjustments to seek new sources of fulfillment or to alter its functional requirements. The last source of impetus for change is the result of fluctuations in environmental conditions that exceed the system's capacity to adjust. Instances of illness or hospitalization are the stressful situations of this type that nurses are perhaps most familiar with in their practice.

Instability

When a person is unable to act within the range of his usual behavioral patterns, or when the environmental pressures call for behaviors with which he is not prepared to respond, the behavioral system may become unstable. If the individual can alter his behavior to fit the situation, the instability is temporary. However, other situations may be beyond the person's ability to cope without outside assistance. For example, illness may be a stressful constraint on usual behavior. Another example would be a crisis state. This is a situation in which the individual has no effective adaptive responses. Instability results when stress exceeds the individual's coping abilities.

TABLE 5. Assumptions About Change in the Behavioral System

Change in the Structure and Dynamics of the Behavioral Subsystems and/or the Whole System is Associated with:

1. Inadequate drive satisfaction
2. Inadequate fulfillment of the functional requirements of the subsystems
3. Fluctuations in environmental conditions that exceed the system's capacity to adjust

---

In behavioral system theory instability is described as behaviors that are not efficient and effective enough to meet the goals of the subsystems. Thus, instability is indicated by behaviors that require so much energy that other subsystems are unable to function efficiently, and behaviors that threaten the individual's biologic or social survival. Since these unstable behaviors can be observed, patients who require nursing care to help them regain stability can be identified and described.

Behavioral Discrepancies

Behavioral instability may be observed either as physiologic changes or as behavioral changes. The physiologic cues that indicate imbalance are changes in pulse and respiration, for example. Prolonged stress may be evidenced by those physiologic changes described by Selye as the stress syndrome.

Beyond the physiologic cues, nurses might also identify actual changes in overt behavior indicative of instability. These changes comprise categories that will be called behavioral discrepancies—disorderly, unpredictable, and purposeless.

Disorderly behavior might be displayed either as regression or as the failure to carry out usual routines. *Purposeless behavior* may manifest as repetitious actions with no apparent goal, or with a goal that does not benefit. *Unpredictable behaviors* are those which differ from what one would expect. The baseline of expectations may be established by comparing the patient's present behavior with his past behavioral patterns, with common patterns observed in other patients, or with response patterns described in the literature. Unpredictable behaviors might also appear as alteration in the varieties of activities usually undertaken, or as accentuated, perhaps inappropriate, use of one type of behavior. If instability does in fact exist, an individual will be unable to suppress the resultant behavioral discomfort. Either physiologic or behavioral cues will be manifest. Patients in need of nursing assistance will therefore be obvious to the astute observer.

Summary

With systems theory as a framework, man is seen as a dynamic whole responding to an ever-changing environment. That environment is both internal and external. Through learned patterns of habitual responses man can adjust to daily stresses and strains. His ability to modify behavior patterns maintains the growth and development of new adaptive responses. At times the stressors impinging upon this system are beyond its ability to cope without assistance. If this instability arises when the stressor is related to health or illness, nursing's assistance may be beneficial in helping the patient to achieve his previous level of stability.

BASIC ELEMENTS OF THE MODEL

Subsystems

Having discussed the assumptions underlying the model and reviewed the concepts of systems theory as they apply to human behavior, it is necessary to consider the behavioral subsystems that are the core of this model. The assumptions upon which this section is based can be found in Table 6 (Johnson, 1968).

The whole behavioral system of man is composed of eight subsystems: affiliative, achievement, aggressive, dependency, eliminative, ingestive, restorative, sexual (Figure 1). Each subsystem has its own structure and function. The structure of each is comprised of a goal based on a basic drive, a set, choices, and the ultimate action or behavior (Figure 2). Each of these four factors contributes to the observable activity of a person in any given situation.

Goals

The goal of a subsystem is defined as the ultimate consequence of behaviors in it. The basis for the goal is a universal drive whose existence can be supported by available scientific research. With drives as the impetus for the behavior, goals can be identified, and are also considered universal. The goals of each of the subsystems are as follows:

Achievement subsystem—to master or control oneself or one's environment; to achieve mastery and control.

TABLE 6.   Assumptions About Man's Behavioral Subsystems

The Recurring, Patterned Behavior Characteristic of the Individual is a Function of the Operation of a Behavioral System in which:

1. Drives serve as focal points around which, over time, originally random and purposeless behaviors are differentiated and organized to achieve specific goals.
2. This process of goal-directed behavioral differentiation and organization is furthered by the concurrent development within the organizational structure of each grouping of such differentiated behaviors as a tendency (or predisposition) to act in specific selected ways (set), and a repertoire of alternative behaviors (choice).
3. The specialized parts or subsystems of the behavioral system that are so formed, each with its *structure of goal, set, choice,* and *actions,* and each with observable functional consequences, are linked and open, and the structure, function, and operation of each affects each of the others.
4. These interactive and interdependent subsystems tend to achieve and maintain a balanced relationship within each subsystem and between the subsystems through the operation of control and regulatory mechanisms (including feedback), which monitor the system under a variable standard of operation.

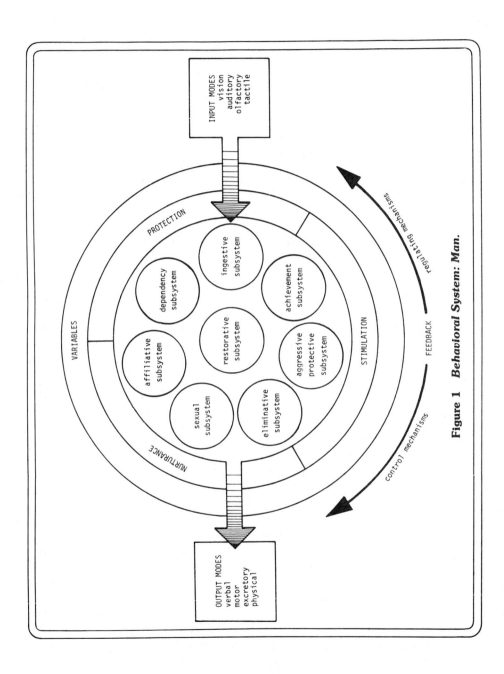

Figure 1 *Behavioral System: Man.*

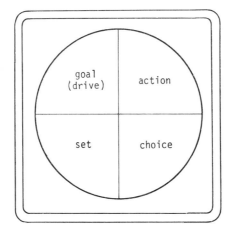

Figure 2 *Structure of each subsystem.*

Affiliative subsystem—to relate or belong to something or someone other than oneself; to achieve intimacy and inclusion.

Aggressive/Protective subsystem—to protect self or others from real or imagined threatening objects, persons, or ideas; to achieve self-protection and self-assertion.

Dependency subsystem—to maintain environmental resources needed for obtaining help, assistance, attention, permission, reassurance, and security; to gain trust and reliance.

Eliminative subsystem—to expel biologic wastes; to externalize the internal biologic environment.

Ingestive subsystem—to take in needed resources from the environment to maintain the integrity of the organism or to achieve a state of pleasure; to internalize the external environment.

Restorative subsystem—to relieve fatigue and/or achieve a state of equilibrium by reestablishing or replenishing the energy distribution among the other subsystems; to redistribute energy.

Sexual subsystem—to procreate, to gratify or attract, to fulfill expectations associated with one's sex; to care for others and be cared about by them.

Each subsystem has its own input and output mechanisms so that communication, for example, may serve a purpose for all the subsystems. The taking in of information would not be classified as ingestive behavior. The question to ask to analyze the taking in of information would be to what end is the information being used. Thus one can determine which subsystem is receiving input. The conceptual problem to avoid is the equation of input and output with the eliminative and ingestive subsystems. The latter two are more specific to bodily secretions and appetitive pleasures.

For each subsystem there are several functions that serve to achieve the goal. Functional behaviors would be those activities executed to meet the goal of the subsystem. Each subsystem has analytic or conceptual goals, which were previously stated, but each subsystem also has actual or concrete goals set by the individual that ultimately meet the conceptual goals if his choices are effective. The functional behaviors vary with each individual depending to some degree upon the concrete goals he chooses to reach the conceptual goal of the subsystem. The concrete goals an individual chooses are influenced by the person's age, sex, motives, cultural values, social norms, self-concept, and rewards from others. Activities engaged in are determined by the individual goals set. To clarify the functions that subsystem behaviors might serve, some examples will be given.

Within the achievement subsystem, some functions that achievement-directed behaviors might serve are to gain control over one's body, to establish one's position in a group, to set both long- and short-term goals. Within the affiliative subsystem, behaviors might be directed toward sharing objects or feelings, relating to nonhuman objects, becoming intimate with another person, establishing maternal attachments to a child, or accepting loss of loved objects or persons. To summarize then, each subsystem has an ultimate conceptual goal that must be met. Several types of activities are functional for meeting that goal, which are directed toward concrete goals. These concrete goals can usually only be inferred by observing the consequences of the behavior in each subsystem.

Action

The action is defined as the observable behavior of an individual. The actual action is restricted by the individual's size and abilities. Behavior can be loosely interpreted to include physical changes as well as excretory and motor outputs. Thus a change in the condition of the skin, and crying, both might be considered as actions. Actions are any observable responses to stimuli. Action can be analyzed by the consideration of individual movements or entire behavioral sequences, depending upon the type of data required.

Choice

Choice refers to the alternate behaviors the individual sees himself as being able to use in any given situation. Another person, such as the nurse, may see many other choices that an individual may use to accomplish a goal. Thus, many interventions often involve letting the person know what choices are actually available to him. This type of choice expansion is usually called problem solving. The selection of a behavior and the range of choices considered feasible are dependent upon one's past experiences, the way the present situation is perceived, energy levels available, learning, external restraints or pressures, and age. As one develops, one learns what choices are viable alternatives in a given situation.

Set

A set may be defined as a tendency or predisoposition to act in a certain way in a given situation. Once developed, sets are relatively stable and resistant to change. Set formation is malleable to such influences as societal norms, status in the society or group, the family life-style, perception and cognitive abilities, and accrued knowledge. One's set is limited by motor and language skills.

Sets can be divided into two types: the *preparatory* set and the *perseverative* set. Preparatory set describes what one attends to or focuses on in a situation. For example, during an emergency situation, a child may focus on the painful injections he is given, while an adult focuses on the cause of the illness. This perception will determine the subsequent nursing interventions. The perserverative set refers to the habits one maintains. The term "perseverative" is derived from the infinitive "to persevere" which implies persistence. The flexibility or rigidity of the set varies with each individual. Many colloquial phrases, such as rigid, compulsive, adaptable, and unstructured, are used to describe an individual's usual set. In short, the set plays a major role not only in the choices a person considers, but in his ultimate behavior. Hence one's set also influences his selection of goals. For each subsystem there is a general set, and for any given situation there is a more specific set.

Summary

Man as a behavioral system is viewed as having eight subsystems, which are interrelated and interdependent. Each subsystem has its own structure, which is composed of an overall goal (drive), action, choices, and set. Each subsystem has functions, which serve to meet the goal. Over time, originally random and purposeless behaviors are differentiated and organized to achieve specific functions. Individuality of behaviors is assured by the development of sets. An individual also learns a repertoire of behaviors for use in any given situation and, thus, has alternate choices. An individual can be differentiated in any given moment by the strength of his drive, the direction or goal of the drive, his set in the situation, his usual choices, and the observable action. This type of systems analysis can be applied to any of the eight subsystems for the understanding of a nursing problem.

Input to the subsystems is through the sensory modes; output is seen as verbal, motor, or physical exchanges with the environment. The feedback system that monitors the input and output is composed of regulating and control mechanisms. While highly organized as a system, the human organism is dependent upon the outside environment. In order to grow and survive, the system's functional requirements of protection, nurturance, and stimulations must be met. Also, variables beyond the system boundary affect behavior within each subsystem. It may be helpful next to examine what the environment must supply and what influence it exerts on the survival and growth of the human behavioral system.

SUSTENAL IMPERATIVES OR FUNCTIONAL REQUIREMENTS

In order for the eight subsystems to develop and maintain stability, each must have a constant supply of functional requirements. The environment must supply the sustenal imperatives of protection, nurturance, and stimulation; these are the necessary prerequisites to maintaining healthy behavior. The analogy familiar to many nurses would be the "needs concept." For example, one might meet the patient's need to sleep by protecting him from disturbing stimuli. Thus, as mentioned earlier, the nurse becomes an external regulator of the environment, which in turn has the capacity to influence the patient's responses. The nurse meets the patient's basic needs or maintains his supply of functional requirements so that he can adapt to stresses. Any person in the patient's environment may meet these requirements, but for this discussion the supplier will be referred to as the nurse, and the recipient or patient, as a behavioral system. However, all humans require sufficient supplies from the environment all the time. Only when illness poses a threat does the nurse become a source of functional requirements.

Protection
Protection includes (1) safeguarding the patient from noxious stimuli, (2) defending the patient from unnecessary threats, and (3) coping with a threat in the patient's behalf. Any of these three methods ultimately serve to help the behavioral system maintain stability in the face of actual or potential threats. Often nurses need only identify the patient's present adaptive response and determine whether it is the most effective. If the patient's coping is not adequate or if the threat is severe, the nurse might choose one of the three methods to assist him. A judgment of ineffective coping would be based on the criteria of the patient's biologic or social integrity. Coping that threatens either of these factors would have to be modified.

An illustration of each of the three types of protection may be helpful. The first method is well known to nurses. It consists of measures to prevent damage from actual threats to the person either physically, psychologically, or socially. For example, to prevent physical damage, the nurse turns the patient frequently. The second method, decreasing any potential or unnecessary threats, increases a person's control in a situation so that he will not experience feelings of total helplessness. For example, preoperative teaching pre-pares a person for a stressful event and thus protects him from unnecessary fears. The consequence is that the person's own ability to handle the threat is enhanced. The third method is used when the patient is unable to handle a threat by himself. The nurse often intercedes to monitor and control stressful stimuli until such time as the patient can protect himself. Nurses working in pediatrics, geriatrics, and intensive care units frequently use these protective measures. Another example of this type of protective intervention is patient advocacy in a bureaucratic system.

In summary, when patients are most vulnerable, labile, or helpless, pro-tective interventions serve to supplement inadequate responses until such time as the person develops more efficient responses, if that is possible. In any case, the withdrawal of protection must be based on a realistic appraisal of the person's capacities and abilities to defend himself on his own.

Nurturance

Nurturance is the second sustenal imperative. As the word implies, one nur-tures or supports the patient's adequate adaptive behaviors. Akin to a paren-tal role, nurturance includes the following:

1. The provision of necessary nourishment and training to help an indi-vidual incorporate and cope with new environmental stimuli
2. The provision of conditions that support the progressive growth and development of behaviors
3. The encouragement of effective behaviors
4. The discouragement of ineffective behaviors

Nurturance supports successful adaptation to new stimuli, which may arise normally in the course of development or may stem from an illness. As new behavioral repertoires are being developed, limits must be set on disrup-tive behaviors while encouragement is given for independent exploration of new behaviors. Crisis intervention perhaps best exemplifies the first type. It is an attempt to help the patient develop new coping mechanisms in the face of a situation he is unable to handle without a great deal of anxiety.

Nurturance also implies the maximum utilization of all available re-sources. Resources include anything from a formalized agency to a significant other to a balanced diet. Much of health education is directed toward inform-ing the individual of how best to utilize those resources available to him. Without appropriate and sufficient resources neither growth nor development will progress.

The last two methods of nurturing are often used simultaneously. Praise and reward would encourage behavior, while punishment or ignoring would discourage a behavior. The principles of reinforcement theory best exemplify use of stimuli either to increase or decrease a behavior. The nurse attempts to shape a behavior that is adaptive.

In summary, when the behavioral system exhibits the capacity to make its own choices in a new situation, it requires the support or nurturance from its environment to develop the necessary ability to manage the new or changed stimuli. The new behavior may then have to be encouraged, while the old ones are discouraged, until the final behavior becomes stabilized. Ultimately, the individual may become his own best source of reward or punishment.

Stimulation

Stimulation, the last sustenal imperative, implies stimuli that arouse action. While nurturance influences the quality of behaviors, stimulation affects the quantity of behaviors. As research in sensory stimulation and deprivation accumulates, it becomes clear that without appropriate stimulation behavior does not develop and, in fact, deteriorates. Adequate and meaningful stimulation is necessary to maintain behavioral stability.

Stimulation includes:

1. Provision of stimuli that bring forth a new behavior
2. Provision of stimuli that increase an actual behavior
3. Provision of opportunities that allow for appropriate behaviors to increase
4. Provision of stimuli to increase the motivation for a particular behavior

Keeping in mind that quantity is to be influenced, the first of these types of stimulation attempts to draw out a behavior that does not at the time exist. The behavior desired may have been lost through regression or, as frequently happens with a child, the behavior may be entirely new. An example would be the stimulation a nurse provides a deaf child in teaching him sign language. The second type of stimulation identifies a behavior that occurs, but only infrequently. Rewarding the behavior when it does occur tends to increase its occurrence. The learning in these two situations may involve either the development of a completely new behavior or the use of a previously acquired behavior in a new situation.

The third type of stimulation requires use of a previously acquired behavior in a different situation. The intervention is intended to provide an opportunity for the appropriate behavior to occur. Frequently, a patient's misperceptions of what the hospital staff expects of him will result in regressed or dependent behaviors. When the nurse clarifies expectations and sets the scene for more appropriate behaviors, a patient will often comply with the desired change. This method necessitates manipulation of cues, expectations, and perhaps actual opportunities for the occurrence of a behavior.

The last type of stimulation brings in the concept of motivation. Rather than use the more direct approaches discussed above, the nurse must attempt to increase the patient's motivation to respond in a certain manner. Examples of stimuli she may use are a reward system, a significant other, or mobilization of unconscious motives. A direct motivation of a behavior such as the insertion of a catheter to increase coughing would be an intervention. In either case, the nurse is manipulating the patient to bring forth a behavior she decides is beneficial.

In summary, stimulation is used to increase a desired behavior. A decision must be made by the nurse about what is desirable. Based on societal expectations and existing capacities of the patient, a nurse has the obligation to try to stimulate a patient to function at his optimum potential. However, since it is the patient who in the end holds the key to his destiny, stimulation may have to cease before that optimum is reached.

Supply of Sustenal Imperatives

All of the eight subsystems need a certain amount of each of the three functional requirements discussed above. While the source of these requirements at birth is almost entirely external, the individual later learns either to supply himself or to seek efficiently the sources of supply. Thus the types of functional requirements and the amount needed vary with each stage on the health-illness continuum and with each stage of life. The nurse must judiciously assess the patient in terms of the amounts needed and the present sources available. Restrictions imposed by the setting or illness on the usual patterns of meeting the requirements must also be taken into account. Next the priorities of needs among the eight subsystems should be estimated based on the patient's age and state of illness. With this type of analysis completed the nurse then decides on the type and amount of stimuli to be supplied to each subsystem. Adequate intake is illustrated by stability and optimum functioning in every subsystem.

REGULATING AND CONTROL MECHANISMS

To monitor and coordinate the interrelationships between the eight subsystems, regulating and control mechanisms exist to guide and limit behavior. Complete behavioral chaos would result if these mechanisms were either nonexistent or inadequately developed. For the human system to operate effectively, there must exist internal guidelines. Although theoretical distinctions can be made between the two mechanisms, for purposes of clarity the two will be considered as one mechanism. The regulating and control mechanisms serve to establish a desired level of performance and then attempt to control the performance of the subsystem at that desired level. Few biologic control mechanisms have been clearly delineated and almost none have been adequately described relating to control of behavior, so this area is at best speculative.

Regulating and control mechanisms are methods the individual uses to evaluate and decide on a desirable behavior. Upon this evaluation he then adjusts his actual behavior to match the desired behavior as closely as possible. The result is efficiency. Learning is the mode through which behavioral patterns and ways of maintaining efficient behavior are incorporated. Skills or habits are developed that regulate behavior for the most efficient use of energy.

In addition, each person has methods of adjusting behavior to adjust to changing conditions. These methods are also the control and regulating mechanisms. Internalized values, beliefs, rules, self-concept, and cognitive level are types of these mechanisms. As Toffler (1970) illustrates in his book *Future Shock,* man must learn how to cope with change now more than perhaps at any other time in history. Man must develop concepts and values that will help him to maintain his emotional and intellectual equilibrium while being constantly bombarded with changing and often unpredictable stimuli. In order to achieve independence from the environment each person learns and adopts rules to guide his behavior so that it is consistent despite changing situations. One's value system, for example, directs behavior in social situations. One's self-concept dictates other aspects of social behavior. Control and regulating mechanisms are learned and are usually fully internalized during adolescence.

There are three major types of mechanisms: biophysiologic, psychologic, and sociocultural. *Biophysiologic mechanisms,* such as the autonomic nervous system responses, are not subject to conscious control. One learns what stimuli are threatening and responds involuntarily with a "fight or flight" response. *Psychologic mechanisms,* include one's self-concept and commonly used defense mechanisms. One witnesses the growth of mechanisms in the development of a child's social behavior; he learns through the socialization process the difference between right and wrong and then internalizes these guidelines.

Lastly, *sociocultural mechanisms* are learned through the socialization and enculturation process. Enculturation involves the learning of patterns of behavior consistent with successful functioning in society. Thus the child incorporates the language, belief systems, and value systems of his environment. Socialization entails learning behaviors consistent with the individual's social position. The child learns the behaviors expected of him based on such parameters as his age, sex, race, and socioeconomic group. A person who does not follow the expected guidelines may be termed deviant depending upon the society's tolerance for a range of behaviors within its generally acceptable boundaries.

Thus sociocultural mechanisms are internalized guides that give direction to behaviors and limit them within a learned acceptable range. Childhood is the time when the individual is groomed for later roles in life; it is a time when the child learns to want to do that which societal and familial expectations anticipate of him.

These concepts introduce a positive view of human behavior. If a nurse considers that at any given time the patient makes the best choice he can based on his learning and values, she is less likely to become critical if she deems the behavior unacceptable. The patient may not have known any other way to react. The questions to be raised do not concern how the patient could possibly have done what he did but what he did do, and the choices he sees for himself. The inquiry focuses on the patient's values, philosophy, and culture. These insights help the nurse to understand why the patient exhibits a particular behavior. Only then can the nurse decide whether or not the behavior is discrepant, from both the individual's and society's standards. Given the situation and the patient's past experiences, his behavior at any moment is, after all, conceived by him to be his best choice.

Variables

The term "variable" encompasses all those factors outside the boundary of the behavioral system that have the capacity to alter or change behavior within the system. The term "variables" is synonymous with the concept of environment. Variables are the supply source from which the individual draws sustenal imperatives. Variables may be internalized over time as regulating or control mechanisms so that they are no longer outside the system only. Since control mechanisms are internalized, they can often be inferred only by an examination of past or present variables. The quality and quantity of variables greatly influence behavior. For example, the pathologic variable of diabetes influences an individual's choice of behaviors in many subsystems.

Nine categories of variables have been defined by the author. The depth of consideration of each category as it affects behavior is directly proportional to the individual nurse's understanding and knowledge in that particular area. The categories are as follows:

1. Biologic—those factors encompassing the givens; those capacities a human is born with or those capacities based on maturation and growth; related to biologic capacities that are dependent on anatomic and physiologic functioning.
2. Developmental—those abilities modified by experience; acquired skills realized through biologic growth and organization of behaviors; a process beginning at an undifferentiated state and progressing to a more highly organized one.

3. Cultural—factors affecting attitudes, beliefs, and behaviors that are learned through education, discipline, and training.
4. Ecologic (environmental)—those stimuli available to the sensory intake modes; environmental stimuli influencing the mutual relationship between a person and his environment; would include the immediate environment such as a hospital and also the environment of a person's upbringing.
5. Familial—those persons of common ancestry or those living in the same household.
6. Pathologic—anatomic and physiologic deviations from the norm; abnormal tissue changes.
7. Psychologic—factors relating to the unconscious or internal psychic processes; would include chronic or acute reaction states or cognitive functioning.
8. Sociologic—expectations and behaviors related to one's role based on rank, status, or position in society; one's relation to society's institutions.
9. Level of wellness—responses in relation to position on the health-illness continuum.

Behavior in each subsystem is intimately related to each particular variable. As mentioned earlier, some of these factors remain outside the behavioral system while others are incorporated over time into the structure of each subsystem to influence goals set, choices made, and set toward situations. For example, each category of variable could be associated with particular types of affiliative behavior. We expect a two-year-old to socialize differently from a ninety-two-year-old. For a complete analysis of a subsystem, the nurse must have information about the possible effects of any or all of the variables. To define the total system, one must examine the behaviors and the variables as they give information about the source of sustenal imperatives, and infer the regulating and control mechanisms present.

Summary

Despite the apparent complexity of the elements of the model, man as a total system encompasses only the individual's behavior and his environment. From his environment he receives his sustenal needs and is molded through the internalization of concepts. Also his immediate responses are dependent upon stimuli impinging on him from the environment. The basic concepts are probably familiar to most nurses; only the terminology and categorization may be new. The total behavioral system as described in all its complexity is, in the end, the total person familiar to us all.

THE MODEL AS A GUIDE FOR THE
NURSING PROCESS

Successful incorporation of the model into professional nursing is predicated on the nursing process itself. The nursing process is composed of four essential stages—assessment, diagnosis, intervention, and evaluation. Systematic use of the model in each successive stage will dictate patient-care goals. An oversight or omission in any of the stages will often lead to decisions based on intuition rather than thoughtful, scientifically based patient-care choices. Use of the model successfully to guide the nursing process will assist the nurse to perform interventions that will assure, as much as possible, that the patient's course along the health-illness continuum is predictable and progressive.

Assessment

An individual becomes a patient when his behavioral system is threatened with the loss of order and predictability through illness (Johnson, 1968). The assessment stage establishes as accurately as possible a picture of the patient as he is at the time, and as he has been. Many different sources may be used to create this picture, e.g., information from the patient and his family, from other health-team members, and from the chart. The nurse will be looking for changes in the patient and for his effectiveness in adapting to the new stimuli in the patient role.

There are two levels of assessment. An initial general, but thorough, examination of the patient's behavior and the significant variables helps the nurse to determine if a nursing problem exists. If there is an actual or predicted problem, a second level of assessment is initiated. During this stage, the nurse closely analyzes the unstable subsystem and determines which variables she may be able to manipulate.

First-Level Assessment

The objective here is to determine the actual or perceived threat, and the abilities of the patient to adapt to the threat without resultant instability. Existence of behavioral discrepancies, as described earlier, would also be determined. An attempt would be made to validate the usual behaviors in each subsystem to establish a baseline of behaviors for comparison.

Observing the environment, the nurse collects information on the source and sufficiency of the sustenal imperatives for each subsystem. The present milieu is carefully scrutinized for restrictions imposed by the patient's illness, situation, or his setting.

Change attracts attention the most. Changes of behavioral patterns or changes in any of the variables become readily apparent. The changes may be benign. Often, however, change is painful, and patients may indicate a need for assistance to adapt successfully. Lack of change in a situation requiring a new way of acting might be a less obvious source of difficulty.

A sample outline for a first-level assessment tool is included in the appendix to this chapter. Appropriate questions and observations are developed to coincide with the patient's age group, illness state, and setting. Information is collected systematically for each variable and subsystem, producing a total picture. An alternate and equally effective tool is one based on the examination of major areas of activity in the patient's life. For example, questions relevant to each subsystem could be asked with the focus on such activities as work, social interaction, or play. With a child, rather than ask questions, the nurse might observe play behavior and derive data pertinent to many subsystems in that manner.

From the first-level assessment, the nurse will know if instability exists or is predicted. When such is related to illness, behavioral instability becomes a nursing problem.

Second-Level Assessment

If instability does exist or is predicted, a second more in-depth diagnostic assessment is required. The first-level assessment highlights those behavioral subsystems in which the actions are not functional for meeting the goal of the subsystem. Each subsystem suspected must be analyzed in terms of structure and function. Besides pinpointing the problem, the nurse will also collect information that may be useful to her in the intervention stage.

The following guide may be used to analyze problematic behavior within any subsystem.

Observable behavior (action)—describe the verbal and nonverbal behavior, when it occurs and what stimuli instigate or terminate it.

Function of the behavior (manifest and latent)—what are the intended and unintended consequences of the behavior, for what subsystem is the behavior functional, what is the effect of this behavior on the other subsystems?

Set: Preparatory—what is attended to or focused on by the individual in the situation, what need is he aware of, can he communicate this need or concern?

Set: Perseveratory—what is the usual or preferred behavior?

Choice—does the individual use or know of alternative behaviors for the situation, what other choices are realistically available, is the behavioral choice appropriate, how does the individual perceive the appropriateness, are actual and perceived restrictions of choice the same?

Drive (direction and strength)—how often does the behavior occur, what factors either inhibit or increase the desired actual behavior?

Sustenal imperatives—what is the source of nurturance, protection, and stimulation for the actual and the desired behavior, is the source consistent and sufficient?

Variables—what internal or external factors beyond the person's control are positively or negatively affecting the behavior, is a variable causing or influencing the behavior, can it be manipulated?

Regulating and control mechanisms—what physiologic, sociologic, cultural, or psychologic mechanisms might be operating, as inferred from the variables or from the behavioral patterns observed?

From her analysis of the collected data, a synthesis of pertinent facts will emerge and assist the nurse to determine her diagnoses. The analysis will also indicate the type of intervention that might be most successful for the patient. It is recommended that a nursing history that categorically summarizes the assessment and the problems identified be written and included in the chart. The analogy is the physician's written history and data from the physical exam. Communication of this sort is a necessary step on the road to clarifying the nurse's area of concern and expertise, and makes explicit those areas for which she may be held accountable.

Diagnosis

Having assessed the patient, the nurse proceeds to the nursing diagnosis. "Diagnosis" essentially means to make a decision. What does the nurse decide are the underlying dynamics of the patient's problematic behaviors in a situation? Her dilemma, like the physician's, is how to differentiate healthy signs and symptoms from abnormal ones. Once the dysfunctional behaviors have been identified, clustering them and analyzing their interrelatedness is a key to accurate diagnosing. Validating with the patient is another method that can be used.

Identification and validation of the problem leads to the nursing diagnosis. The nursing diagnosis is a description of that behavior which is at variance with the desired state or that which does not meet the goal of the system. The behavior illustrates existing or anticipated instability in the system and requires some type of nursing intervention to maintain or regain stability. The diagnosis dictates treatment and provides a basis for evaluation of patient outcomes.

This model differentiates four diagnostic classifications. Disorders originating within any one subsystem are manifested either by (1) *insufficiency* which exists when a particular subsystem is not functioning or developed to its fullest capacity due to inadequacy of functional requirements, or (2) *discrepancy*—a behavior that does not meet the intended goal. The incongruity usually lies between the action and the goal of the subsystem, although the set and choice may be strongly influencing the ineffective action.

Disorders manifested within more than one subsystem are either

(1) *incompatibility*—the goals or behaviors of two subsystems in the same situation conflict with each other to the detriment of the individual—or (2) *dominance*—the behavior in one subsystem is used more than any other subsystem regardless of the situation or to the detriment of the other subsystems.

Under each of these categories for each subsystem, specific nursing problems or subcategories can be listed. For example, grief is a manifestation of an insufficiency in the affiliative subsystem; the etiology would be the loss of a source of sustenal imperatives represented by the loss of someone or something significant to the person. By classifying the problem, clues are offered for intervention tactics. There is first a need, however, to further differentiate and individualize the problem using the second-level assessment discussed earlier. Once this is done, the decision must be made whether the etiology of the instability is internal or external and whether the patient is an active or passive participant in the etiology.

An ill person is in a state of stress. There are two types of stress states: structural and functional. *Structural stress* is that which occurs within the subsystems. Structural stress involves internal control mechanisms and reflects inconsistencies between the goal, set, choice, or action. *Functional stress,* on the other hand, most often arises from the environment. Overload or insufficiency of any of the sustenal imperatives results in functional disorders. With the strain of environmental changes or restrictions, the usual supply of any of these requirements may no longer be sufficient.

For diagnostic purposes, it is helpful to determine whether the stress is the result of a functional or structural cause. For example within the achievement subsystem, the internal structural stress might be deliberate avoidance of achievement situations. On the other hand, an external functional stress might be the lack of achievement opportunities. With the former, the problem is the difference between the goal of the subsystem to master and control and the behavior that is not meeting the goal; the patient is an active participant by choosing not to achieve. In the latter situation, the patient is essentially a passive victim of his environmental situation. With the probable source of stress identified, the intervention course becomes clearer.

The statement of the diagnosis identifies the nursing problem, the diagnostic classification, and whether the problem is functional or structural. A sample diagnosis might be: maternal deprivation, insufficiency of the affiliative subsystem, functional. This diagnosis describes the phenomena both categorically and individually.

Interventions

When a behavioral system is threatened by illness, a person becomes a patient because his internal demands exceed his capacity to adjust. The result is behavioral disequilibrium. The overall objective of any nursing intervention is to establish regularities in the patient's behavior so that the goal of each subsystem will be fulfilled. When this state is achieved, it can be observed as the economic use of energy, efficient actions, and social interaction, coupled with some degree of personal satisfaction.

For each patient, more specific objectives must be established based on the nursing diagnosis. After the objectives are set, the method of intervention and the anticipated behavioral outcomes can be established. To decide on a method of intervention the nurse first clarifies what her focus of action will be and what mode or general approach she will use.

The focus will be on either a structural part of a subsystem or the supply of sustenal imperatives. If the problem has a structural stressor, the nurse will focus on either the goal, set, choice, or action of the subsystem. If the problem is functional, the nurse would focus on the source and sufficiency of the functional requirements since functional problems originate from an environmental excess or deficiency.

The mode is the general method used to change behavior. Again, if the problem is structural, the nurse may direct her activities toward such consequences as broadening the choices, altering the set, changing the action, strengthening the dirve, or altering the goal. Her choices in structural problems are to manipulate the structural units or to impose temporary controls and thus regulate the interaction of the subsystems. If the problem is functional, the nurse chooses a mode that will supply the functional requirements. She may either supply a sustenal imperative herself or mobilize other resources to meet the demand.

There are four categorical choices available to the nurse to carry out the mode of intervention: restrict, defend, inhibit, facilitate.

Restrict—the imposition of limits or external controls on behavior; supplements immature or ineffective control and regulating mechanisms.

Defend—supplies protection by preventing damage from exposure to unnecessary stressors or coping with threats in the patient's behalf.

Inhibit—supplies nurturance by suppressing ineffective responses.

Facilitate—supplies nurturance and stimulation to expedite the incorporation of new demands and to increase the use, or opportunity to use, a behavior.

A statement of an intervention would include the focus and the mode, both categorically and specifically. For example, given the diagnosis "fear of injections, dominance of aggressive/protective subsystem, with structural stress between goal and action," the intervention would include the following: focus—choice and action in the aggressive/protective subsystems; mode—stimulate to broaden choice with resultant change in action. The focus, the categorical choice, and the mode are stated in that order. Having established this groundwork, the nurse then decides what technique to use to stimulate a new behavior. To follow with the previous example, she may decide to use needle play as a technique. For each of the categorical choices, one could list techniques appropriate to that intervention mode.

The intervention techniques themselves are familiar to most nurses; the novelty here stems from our analysis of the categorization of methods and the explicit identification of means and goals. Herein lies the secret to the successful application of this model to practice. Consistency and logic are preserved, and these will lead to interventions which assure the patient's progressive and purposeful adaptation.

Evaluation

Identification of means and goals is mandatory to evaluation of patient outcome and professional competence. To evaluate, one first must predict expected outcomes. This helps to assure as purposeful and predictable a course as is possible given one's skills and the limitations of current knowledge. To evaluate effectively the nurse sets both long-term and short-term goals and behavioral objectives that will indicate the progress made toward achieving those goals.

The first step in evaluating is to set the long-term goal. What is the ultimate desired result of the nursing intervention? These goals are usually broad and apply to many patients in a similar situation. An example from a pediatric setting would be the successful incorporation of the hospitalization experience without extreme regression or detrimental effect on development. With the long-term goal identified, the nurse proceeds to consider which short-term goals would prepare the way and lead up to the achievement of the overall goal.

Short-term goals are more individualized and are derived from the diagnosis. At this point the nurse examines her intervention methods and attempts to find evaluative criteria that will indicate the successfulness of the intervention techniques. What will be accomplished if the techniques are effective? Consistency would be maintained if the short-term goals were stated in terms of the change in any of the subsystems or variables. For example, two short-term goals might be maintenance of affiliative bonds between mother and child and increased involvement of the family, particularly the father and siblings. These two examples illustrate the attempt to tie in the affiliative subsystem and the familial variable. Given these still rather broad short-term goals, the nurse asks what specific behaviors would indicate that these goals have in fact been achieved. What specific outcomes might be expected?

Expected outcomes are expressed as behavioral objectives. As the term implies, objectives are observable and accessible behaviors or patient responses that one might expect to see following a nursing intervention. The current observable behaviors of a patient are used as a baseline from which to derive expectations of reasonable and realistic behavioral changes, given the time limitations and the patient's capacity for change. The objectives are based upon the predicted behavioral change that is expected if the goal is achieved. These objectives are established from the nurse's knowledge collected during her assessment of a patient's particular patterns of response. Her knowledge of expected behaviors of patients in similar situations, derived from her experience and the nursing literature, is also used to guide her in deciding upon expected outcomes.

Time limits within which the nurse expects to see the predicted change are also based on her knowledge and experience. A single, observable, realistic expectation is set within a probable time limit. For example, a short-term goal may be to establish maternal attachment, with a behavioral objective stating that the mother will hold the infant close to her body within three days. Upon completion of the act or at the end of three days, the nurse either sets a new objective or reevaluates the effectiveness of her intervention. In either case, a new behavioral objective would be established.

The nurse might set objectives one at a time, or in the beginning set a progression of objectives which ultimately lead to the desired behavior. Step-by-step behavioral objectives serve as a guide for staff and patient to follow progress and monitor regressions. Flow sheets facilitate the systematic monitoring of changes. A flow sheet for the previously mentioned example of the mother of a premature infant would begin with her present behavior and predict increments of change until attachment, or discharge, occurs. Thus the flow sheet might appear as shown in Table 7. Careless evaluation is worse than no evaluation as it salves the wound without healing. The validity and reliability of criterion measures must be continually examined. Validity is enhanced if the measures are derived from theories and knowledge of human behavior. Standardized instruments or measurements augment the use of behavioral objectives to follow progress. Moreover, use of two different types of measures strengthens the reliability of the evaluative process.

Using the model consistently through all the steps in the nursing process necessitates pulling out salient findings and categorizing them on a nursing-process work sheet. Table 8 offers a guide to analyzing a nursing problem.

TABLE 7. Sample Flow Sheet

Activity:	Mon	Tues	Wed	Thurs	Fri
Touches infant with fingertips	X	X			
Asks to hold infant		X	X		
Holds to her breast with arms			X	X	X
Takes infant out without asking					X

TABLE 8. Nursing-Process Work Sheet

	Assessment				Diagnosis		
Behaviors	Structural Unit	F or D	Variables	I or C	Nursing Problem	Diagnostic Classification	Functional or Structural Stress
Subsystem: (list significant behaviors)							

TABLE 9. Sample Diagnostic Analysis

Behavior	Structural Unit	F or D	Variables	I or C	Nursing Problem	Category	F of S[4]
Subsystem Affiliative 1. cries when mother leaves	action	F	Develop. 25 months old	C	Separation anxiety	Dominance Agg/Prot Subsystem	Functional perceived loss of protection
			Family— 2-month-old sibling	I			
Dependency 1. clings to mother	action	F	Patho. receives shots q4h	I			
Ingestive 1. Refuses to eat	action	D	Health-Ill. never hospitalized before	I			

System

Goal		Method	
Focus	*Mode*	*Category*	*Technique*
Source of sustenal imperatives to alter set of fear of separation and pain	Supply protection	Defend	Rooming-in by mother Decrease number of staff with child Mother to stay with child during injections

Evaluation

Behavioral Goals

Long-Term	*Short-Term*	*Behavioral Objectives*	*Time Limit*
Successful incorporation of experience without residual instabilities	1. Maintain mother-child relationship 2. Stabilize all subsystems	1. continue to prefer mother, e.g., crying when she leaves	Until discharge
		2. decrease crying with staff	3 days
		3. eat usual solid foods	3 days
		4. cry, but not fight shots	3 days

State if representative of goal, set, choice, action.
F for functional behavior; D for dysfunctional behavior.
I for influencing; C for causing behavior.
To assure consideration of all pertinent variables, one may label variables such as developmental or pathologic.
Write F or S, then state stress.

TABLE 9.—*Continued*

Intervention				Evaluation		
System Goal		Method		Behavioral Goals		Time Limit
Focus	*Mode*	*Category*	*Technique*	*Long-Term*	*Short-Term*	*Behavioral Objectives*

Table 9 presents a sample analysis of a problem. Use of such a guide assures the systematic approach to decisions on patient care. Data from this form can then be transferred to the nursing-care plan in terms that all professionals will understand. The benefit to the patient is that he receives consistent care based on the fact that a single nurse has carefully collected all the data available and set up a rational guide for his treatment. And also, the nurse has communicated this guide to the other nursing personnel so that all interactions will be purposeful and directed toward the same goals.

SUMMARY

Ultimately, patient goals are considered in terms of the functional consequences for the person as a behavioral system. These outcomes of minimal expenditure of energy, congruency with biologic and social survival, and existence of some degree of personal satisfaction have already been discussed. The dilemma returns to the question of how. How one can tell when these outcomes have been accomplished, given the infinite variability of human responses, has yet to be determined.

Summarization might best be accomplished by reviewing what the nurse intends to achieve using this model of nursing. What are her goals as congruent with the model and how might she evaluate her success in using the model? Outcomes are often seen in terms of the consequences for the patient. The intended consequences are behavioral stability, adjustment to the situation, and adaptation to stressors. Absence of behavioral discrepancies and use of effective coping mechanisms would indicate these outcomes. Behavior would be purposeful, predictable, and orderly (Table 10).

TABLE 10.   **Summary of Behavioral Subsystems**

Subsystems	Behaviors*		Variables†	
	Subjective	Objective	Influencing	Causing
Affiliative				
Achievement				
Aggressive/Protective				
Dependency				
Eliminative				
Ingestive				
Restorative				
Sexual				

*Behavioral discrepancy, marked "D"
†Manipulatable variable, marked "M"
Patient profile—narrative description of patient and situation

Unintended consequences exist but are more difficult to identify. Questions to be asked might involve such issues as possible increased dependency of the patient, or imposition of expectations on the patient that are congruent with the nurse's life-style but not the patient's. Increasing one's thoughtful and rational approaches to patients, while decreasing thoughtless intuitive measures, may guarantee fewer unintended outcomes.

Consequences might also be viewed from the perspective of behavior that has changed. With this in mind, one would consider the altered level of behavioral equilibrium, previous level of functioning compared to the present, or evidence of added choices and altered set to increase the repertoire of behaviors available to the patient.

In addition to benefiting the patient, evaluation of patient progress upon termination of service also benefits the nurse. It provides her a critical examination of her nursing practice. Did she successfully incorporate the model into her practice? Was there a successful blend of past knowledge and theories with the behavioral systems model? Areas to scrutinize would include the accuracy of the assessment tools, accuracy of the diagnosis, and effectiveness of the interventions. Was there consistency of approach and were changes noted and responded to appropriately? How successful was the communication with, and cooperation of, other persons involved with the care? Was there consistent awareness of self as a variable, and of the unintended outcomes? What might be derived from this case that might indicate need for improvement or study of nursing-care problems and techniques? The latter might involve the review of a range of cases from time to time to seek out significant constellations of cues and success or failure of treatments which would lead to more accurate description of the etiology and course of nursing problems. The model provides the framework for categorizing all aspects of the nursing process so that the science of nursing, the personal satisfaction of the nurse, and ultimately the welfare of the patient will improve.

REFERENCES

Johnson Dorothy: UCLA School of Nursing, class notes and handouts 1968 and 1972

Johnson Dorothy: "One Conceptual Model of Nursing," unpublished paper presented April 25, 1968 at Vanderbilt Univ, Nashville, Tenn.

Rapoport A: Foreword to Buckley W (ed): Modern Systems Research for the Behavioral Scientist. Chicago, Aldine, 1968

Toffler A: Future Shock. New York, Random House, 1970

Nursing Assessment Tool Using Johnson Model

Basic information: name, age, sex, date, and place of examination. Source of information. Present situation: patient's perception of reason for seeking help, any current crisis, changes or stresses in patient's life.

Medical history (pathologic variable): present illness, pertinent past history, present medical regime (medications, treatments, diet, and/or activity restrictions), prognosis and future medical plans (biologic variable), restrictions of functioning due to maturation or genetic defects, any anomalies, visual or hearing defects, immunization status.

Health-illness response: what patient or parents have been told, reactions to past illnesses or hospitalizations, compliance with medical regime, adaptation to present situation, interaction with medical and nursing staff.

Psychologic status (psychologic variable): cognitive state and level of perception, estimate of presence of anxiety, fears, grief or other unconscious factors, changes such as moves, divorces, deaths in last year, usual reaction to stress or change.

Family history (familial variable): family structure and state of health of persons now living in the patient's dwelling, involvement of members with the patient, patient role in the family, interaction patterns and problems, main person responsible for care of the patient, problems caused because of the illness.

Cultural variable: religion, identification with cultural or ethnic group, apparent childrearing techniques, language and/or communication modes, value system particularly regarding health (home remedies, beliefs about cause of illness, etc.), present vs. future orientation to planning, cultural regulators of behavior (expressions of "right" vs. "wrong," "good" vs. "bad," etc.).

Social history (sociologic variable): status in terms of educational level, socioeconomic group, occupation, roles patient has such as student or employee, usual source of medical care, financial situation, accessibility to medical services (transportation, insurance), relation to any other social agencies.

Environmental history (ecologic variable): living situation (adequacy of location, neighborhood, stimulation deprivations or excesses), hazards to health or development (play areas, infestations, poisons or drugs, etc.). For an inpatient evaluate also in terms of the hospital situation (type of room, position in room, noise level, light source, temperature, roommate).

Developmental history: current level of functioning in relation to age (motor, language, peer interaction, cognitive skills). For a child secure information on the developmental milestones (sitting, standing, walking, etc.).

REVIEW OF BEHAVIOR SUBSYSTEMS

Achievement

1. Skill and control of body (speech, motor, bowel, and bladder)
2. Accomplishments appropriate for age and sociocultural position (occupation, progress in school)
3. Interpersonal control—drive to be dominant vs. passive; takes leader or follower role; competitiveness
4. Drive to control own life and actions—evidence of powerlessness or assertiveness
5. Expects rewards from others or is self-rewarded for accomplishments
6. Desire to learn or master situations
7. Able to set and work toward appropriate goals; presence of short- or long-term goals; ability to delay pleasure to achieve another goal
8. Development of identity and self-concept
9. Ability to care for own activities of daily living
10. Methods of externalizing internal thoughts (able to express self, talks freely, writes or draws, nonverbal behaviors)
11. Ability to perceive environment as influenced by level of consciousness, intelligence, awareness of time and place, confusion or disorientation, memory and recall skills
12. Intake of information or knowledge; aware of lack of knowledge

Affiliative:

1. Relationship to persons with whom patient is intimate
2. Interpersonal skills—sharing, reaction to strangers, approach vs. avoidance of social interactions
3. Access to sources to meet group inclusion needs (family, residence, work, clubs, church)
4. General manner of relating (friendly, shy, hostile)
5. Awareness of others' reactions or feelings
6. Influence of significant others on behavior and beliefs

Aggressive/Protective:

1. Commonly used defense mechanisms
2. Overt aggressive actions to self or others (accidental, instrumental, or hostile)
3. Verbal aggression, such as demandingness, silence, vulgarity, criticism, hostility
4. Protection against perceived threats to identity and self-concept (confident, cooperative vs. fearful, lying, sensitive to criticism, withdrawal when approached)
5. Reactions to real or imagined threats, which may be objects, persons, or ideas, that the nurse should try to identify if possible
6. Reactions to frustration and failure
7. Protection of property or perceived territory; availability ot one's own territorial space
8. Behaviors externalizing internal feelings (holds things in, easily angered, projects feelings on others, scapegoats, denies, expression of positive and negative feelings appropriate to occurrence of event

Dependency:

1. Able to identify to another person one's own psychologic, physiologic, sociocultural needs and desires and thus receives appropriate responses
2. Strength of drive and behaviors to secure sympathy, pity, attention
3. Reactions to demands to be independent (refusal, self-confidence)
4. Reactions to dependency (accepts or seeks help when needed, reluctant to act without permission, resists dependency)
5. Security needs (seeks reassurance and/or explanation, self-deprecating comments, needs encouragement to act)

6. Trust vs. suspicious behaviors, especially in those upon whom person is dependent (parent, doctor); physiologically related

Eliminative:

1. Daily habits and patterns related to urination, defecation, and menstruation if appropriate
2. Modesty, control of functions
3. Presence of excessive externalization of physiologic wastes (diaphoresis, vomiting, drainage, fever, increased exhalation)

Ingestive:

1. Habits and preferences regarding food and drink, appetite
2. Normality of inspiration and need for oxygen
3. Intake modes intact (vision, hearing, tactile, taste, smell, kinesthetic); presence of overload or deprivation of environmental stimuli
4. Administration of medication or treatments
5. Intake of nonfunctional materials for pleasure (smoking, drinking, drugs)

Restorative:

1. Rest and sleep patterns; conditions necessary to induce sleep
2. Daily hygiene habits
3. Methods used to relax (recreation)
4. Methods used to reduce feelings of tension
5. Level of physical activity (range of motion, restrictions real or imagined); exercise
6. Responses (psychologic and physiologic) to pathologic stressors; preventive health habits (immunization status, regular dental and medical check-ups, etc.)
7. Appropriate use of energy for situation and potential of patient (restless, relaxed, drowsy, fidgety); supportive measures needed to prevent or cure pathologic condition; presence of stimuli preventing restorative behavior (pain, noise, anxiety, medications)

Sexual:

1. Physical sexual development
2. Behaviors indicating sexual identification (clothing, interest areas, play, peer selection)

3. Significant sexual related behaviors (VD, pregnancy, abortions, mastur-
   bation, intercourse)
4. Grooming concern and habits
5. Sexually aggressive behavior
6. Activities associated with sexual roles (parent role, husband-wife roles,
   male-female roles)
7. Cares about and is also able to care for significant others

Bonnie Holaday

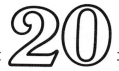

Implementing the Johnson Model for Nursing Practice

The use of a theoretical framework or a conceptual model of nursing practice represents the use of scientific knowledge and methods to study a patient. The focus of this article is to demonstrate how this knowledge and these methods may be applied to an individual patient. This article will discuss operationalizing the model and the nursing process: assessment, nursing diagnosis, intervention, and evaluation. Because clinical concepts are most clearly understood by reference to clinical data, clinical case material will be used throughout this article.

Once a nurse has selected a conceptual model for use in her practice, her next step is to operationalize the model. To accomplish this, one must define terms, define the function, goal, set, choice, and action of each subsystem, define the variables, and then design the assessment tool and the framework of the model that will guide the nurse through the nursing process.

The Johnson model is one model currently being tested in nursing practice and is the one used by this author. It is based on systems theory and contains eight subsystems, as discussed by Judy Grubbs in the previous article.

DEFINING THE TERMS

One practitioner may define the function of a subsystem somewhat differently than another practitioner, if it suits her needs and does not contradict systems theory. For example, I have defined the function of the eliminative subsystem as follows:

1. To express verbally and nonverbally one's feelings, beliefs, and emotions
2. To relieve feelings of tension

3. To expel waste products
4. To maintain physiologic equilibrium by excretion

The goal of the subsystem may also differ from one practitioner to another. I defined the goal of the eliminative subsystem to be that of externalizing the internal environment.

The set, choice, and action of each subsystem must be considered. In the eliminative subsystem the set may involve a person's attitudes and beliefs about (1) modesty and self-expression, (2) being a quiet or rowdy person, and (3) physiologic processes of defecation, urination, or vomiting, as well as past experence. The choice for this subsystem is simple; either retain it or expel it. Actions for this subsystem would include talking, perspiring, urinating, and defecating, to name a few. The process of determining what the set, choice, and action include must be done for each system.

Variables are those elements liable to influence or change behavior. The following list of variables may be used as a guide to areas of behavior that should be assessed: biologic, cultural, developmental, ecologic (environmental), familial (family history), pathologic, psychologic, sociologic (social history), and situational (health-illness response) (Grubbs, 1971).

THE ASSESSMENT TOOL

The purpose of the assessment is to study the behavior of the patient. The method of assessment should be derived from established theoretical principles. Although the Johnson model is a systems model, developmental theory, which is commonly used in working with children, can easily be a part of such a tool.

The task of the assessment process is to obtain samples of the patient's behavior as it occurs in a natural setting by observation, by interview, or by some type of test that requires the person to act or respond to something. In the process of assessment the nurse has two concerns: (1) As a practitioner, the nurse may find that the patient's behavior and physical condition require some clinical attention, and (2) as a scientific investigator the nurse is trying to describe general patterns of behavior. Since I function as a practitioner, the discussion presented will be from that frame of reference.

In assessment of all patients, the type of patient determines (1) which variables are most important and (2) which subsystems to concentrate upon. I work with chronically ill children and their parents. The types of questions in my assessment tool will be somewhat different from those of a nurse working with geriatric patients. First, with regard to variables, under the familial variable, both the nurse working with a geriatric patient and I would be interested in the family structure, the relationship and ages of the people living in the house, the patient's role in the family, the main person responsible for care of the patient, and problems that the illness has caused the family. Yet our questions about these would differ in that mine would take into consideration the needs of the child. Second, with regard to the subsystems, all the behaviors exhibited by the patient are classified under one of the eight subsystems. In my work with chronically ill children, ages 6 to 12 years, past experience and previous research (Jordan, 1962) revealed that the achievement, dependency, and affiliative subsystems should be carefully assessed.

In the assessment of children, a knowledge of facts and theories of human behavior is essential. The term "theories" needs to be emphasized because no one theory has been evolved that is complete enough to cover child development. Theories of development proposed by Piaget (1955, 1959, 1960) and Erikson (1950, 1964) were valuable to me in assessing the chronically ill child. I will illustrate their use in the following paragraphs.

Piaget's theory deals strictly with cognitive development and is one of the few theories that can be used at all levels of the nursing process. To illustrate, I used Piaget's theory in assessing the eliminative subsystem (in this example, the ability to express oneself verbally). I assessed the child's cognitive level so that I could effectively plan to teach the child the facts about his illness or surgery. A complete assessment would test states versus transformations, concreteness, transductive reasoning, conservation of number, and composition of classes.

Some of the Piagetian techniques I used to assess Nancy, a six-year-old who was scheduled for surgery, are presented below. The first is a test for centering and irreversibility (Figure 1). Two clay balls of equal size were shown to the child. She was asked: Are they the same size or does one have more clay in it than the other? Nancy answered that they were the same. Then, right before her eyes, one of the balls was rolled into the shape of a hot dog, and Nancy was asked the same question as before. A child in the preoperational subperiod will say that the longer object has more clay than the other.* Nancy answered that the "hot dog had more clay."

Piaget and Inhelder (1956) designed another test for checking egocentricity in the representation of objects, called the "three mountain problem" (Figure 2). Three cones or blocks are set on a table and a chair is placed on each side of the table. Nancy sat in one of the chairs and a doll was moved from chair 1 to chair 2 to chair 3. Nancy was asked to draw what the doll saw from each place. The preoperational child cannot do this, and neither could Nancy.

---

*A child in the preoperational stage, age two to seven years, has language, and objects and events begin to take on symbolic meaning. Thought is still based on simple characteristics of an object, and the concept is not separated from the concrete perceptual experience. The child in this stage does not have a mental representation of a series of actions.

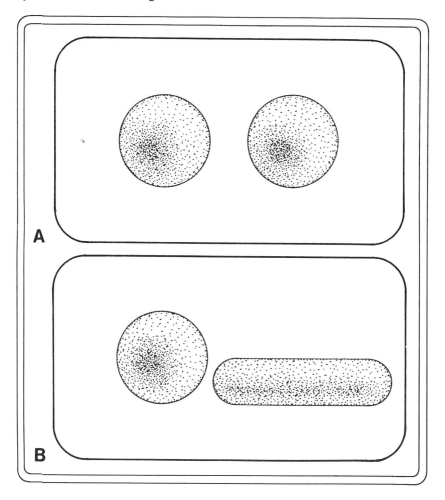

Figure 1 *Clay test.*

Once the assessment is complete the nurse can make a diagnosis and plan some appropriate interventions. Nancy's complete assessment revealed she was still in the preoperational stage of cognitive development. Thus, her preoperative teaching must involve more than just talking about her surgery. To enhance Nancy's understanding, my approach must involve her other senses, such as touching, hearing, and seeing. I must focus on who is involved and what will happen since Nancy does not seem to notice how something happens; she only attends to the end result. By using Piaget's theory to assess the situation and plan some interventions, the results are logical and more effective.

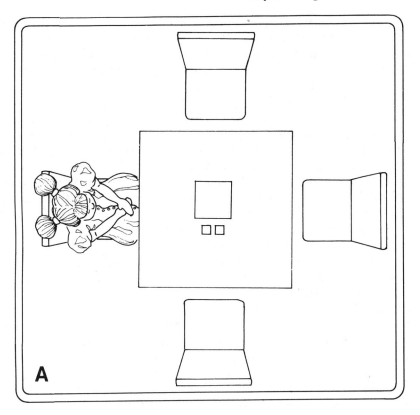

Figure 2   *Three-mountain problem.*

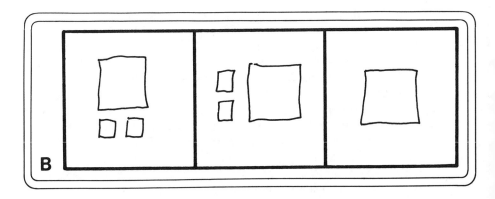

Figure 2.B.   *Figures the child should draw.*

Erikson's theory offers a set of opposites—pathology and health—each cast at one of the critical stages. These begin with the concept of basic trust versus mistrust (birth to 1 year), followed by autonomy versus shame and doubt (1 to 3 years), initiative versus guilt (3 to 5 years), industry versus inferiority (5 to 12 years), and identity versus role diffusion in the years through adolescence. I used this theory to evaluate behavior patterns in my assessment of chronically ill children. Did the child's behavior represent a deviation from normal according to Erikson? The following paragraphs summarize the information I obtained from my assessment tool regarding the affiliative and dependency subsystems. The informants are the mother and the patient, Paul. Paul is a 12-year-old boy with a diagnosis of (1) meingomyocele, (2) neurogenic bladder secondary to no. 1, and (3) chronic urinary tract infections. He was admitted to the hospital for an anterior YV plasty and wedge resection of the posterior bladder.

First, information was obtained from the mother about the affiliative subsystem. Paul lives at home with his parents and two older brothers, ages 19 and 17. He gets along well with his brothers, although they do not play much together now that they are older. The mother describes Paul as being the "middleman," who gets very upset when his brothers argue. Paul and his father enjoy watching football and basketball games on TV. The mother believes Paul will miss his dog and his brothers the most while he is in the hospital. As for the dependency subsystem, information revealed that the mother saw Paul as being "mild and shy." He likes to play with other children, but "he needs a little push." When asked how much attention Paul wanted, his mother responded "a lot, especially the past year." She explained that Paul had been having a lot of "bladder problems and infections, and so we have been helping him."

Second, responses from Paul were noted about the affiliative subsystem. When asked whom he would miss the most while he was in the hospital, Paul mentioned his mother. Paul said he enjoyed watching TV with his father and playing games like Clue and checkers. The question about interacting with his brothers brought a long silence; then he said, "Well we watch TV some, but they spend most of their time with their motorcycles." Paul admitted he spent most of his time with his mother. When asked what they did together he shrugged and said, "Watch TV and talk." I tried to discuss activities he enjoyed with his friends and found that he did not consider anyone at school or in his neighborhood to be a friend. I tried to discuss whether or not it was easy for him to meet people and make friends, but Paul would not answer. When I attempted to ask questions concerning the dependency subsystem, he refused to answer. However, he did admit he did not like being in the hospital because he lost a lot of freedom to do things.

With the knowledge I had from Erikson's theory, Paul's behavior was meaningful. It indicated that existence of disequilibrium in the dependency and affiliative subsystems. The disequilibrium present in these two subsystems caused several problems during Paul's hospitalization. One of these problems will be discussed later in the paper.

At the completion of the assessment, the nurse should be able to make an appraisal of the child's behavior. The assessment should point to present or potential deviations from normal, and should also identify the major variables causing the behavior. For example, after completing her assessment, the nurse states a diagnosis, such as insufficiency of the restorative subsystem; causative variable is the environment—noises and lights in the hall make it impossible for the patient to sleep.

As stated earlier, the purpose of an assessment is to study a patient's behavior to see if disequilibrium exists. If it does, then the nurse must determine the nature and extent of the disequilibrium in order to select an intervention. The nurse wants to define the problem so carefully that the intervention will appear obvious. A thorough assessment makes it easier to examine the potentialities of various interventions. This is why the first steps of operationalizing the model are so important.

INTERVENTIONS

The method of intervention is derived from the model, but may incorporate other theories. For example, Dave is a 15-year-old retarded boy who was diagnosed as having a discrepancy of the eliminative subsystem. Postoperatively, he refused to take oral fluids. The causative variables were biologic since Dave was retarded, and developmentally his language and cognitive skills were at age four years. A choice for intervention would be for the nurse to act as a temporary external control mechanism using the method of behavior modification. The goal of behavior modification is to change behavior through alteration of the environment (Bandura, 1969). The desired behavior is rewarded, and the undesirable behavior is ignored or punished. In this case Dave received a star for every glass of fluid he drank, and three stars earned him a piece of his favorite chocolate candy.

To make the entire process of intervention clear, I will illustrate use of the Johnson model in an actual case and discuss a problem which occurred during Paul's hospitalization using the Weed (1970) method of problem-oriented charting.

Problem 1 Little verbal communication with the nursing staff or myself.
Problem 2 Unable to keep accurate intake and output (secondary to 1).

A. Subjective data
   1. The nursing staff reports that Paul is not telling them how much he is drinking or when he needs a dressing change.

B. Objective data
1. Leaking large amounts of urine from around the suprapubic tube.
2. Urinary tract infection diagnosed on 5/26.
3. Wound infection diagnosed on 5/27.
4. Paul is 12 but still turns to his parents and asks them to answer questions for him. For example, when asked what he drank for breakfast, he answered, "You tell 'em Dad."

C. Variables
1. Developmental: Except at school, Paul has little verbal interaction with adults or peers. This is a causative variable and can be manipulated.
2. Familial: In the family, the child's pattern of interaction with his parents is that of child to adult, and never of adult to adult or adult to parent. This is a causative variable and can be manipulated.

D. Diagnosis
1. Incompatibility of eliminative subsystem (action and goal) and the affiliative subsystem which is probably secondary to an insufficiency of the affiliative subsystem (lack of social skills with peers and adults).

E. Plan
1. The intervention goal is to stimulate a change by broadening Paul's set and choice.

F. Methods
1. The intervention is geared towards helping Paul develop social skills with adults and peers. I will spend at least ½ hour to 1 hour a day talking with Paul. The conversation is to be structured to encourage adult-to-adult and adult-to-parent conversation (Berne, 1964).
2. To discuss Paul's responsibilities as a patient with him as far as informing the staff about fluid intake, pain, and need for dressing changes.
3. To secure a roommate for Paul, and provide opportunities for Paul to go to the activities room and to the weekly picnic.

G. Criteria to evaluate interventions
1. After three days of our meetings, Paul's eye contact with me will increase.
2. After three days of our meetings his verbal communication with me will increase.
3. By the end of five days, there will be an increase in Paul's verbal interaction with the nursing staff.

H. Evaluation
1. My observations confirmed that the first two objectives were met.
2. The outcome of the third objective was inhibited by the almost constant presence of one or both parents. Once the parents decreased the number of hours they visited there was an increase in Paul's interaction with the staff.

SUMMARY

Use of a model will increase the nurse's ability to give effective and scientifically based nursing care to patients. The assessment allows the nurse to describe objectively the patient's behavior, which serves to indicate the presence of any disequilibrium. A thorough assessment also provides data for planning an intervention in sufficient detail that the method to be used can be made clear to the patient, the parents, and the nursing staff.

This article was based on the assumption that the use by nurses of a conceptual model and its derived systematic assessment will represent a major improvement in the methods of providing nursing care. In the past, nursing care consisted almost exclusively of carrying out the orders of others. The emphasis in the future will almost certainly be on the use of a systematic method of assessment by nurses as a basis for planning and giving care.

Unfortunately, at present, the nurse's findings still do not play a significant part in deciding how the patient can be helped. As nurses continue to work with models, the validity of the models can be tested, and perhaps nursing will eventually occupy a more esteemed position in the medical hierarchy. For now, the overriding need in nursing is to develop a wide range of assessment techniques to obtain a fuller body of data on patients as individuals and as groups.

REFERENCES

Bandura A: Principles of Behavior Modification. New York, Holt, 1969

Berne E: Games People Play. New York, Grove Press, 1964

Erikson E: Childhood and Society. New York, Norton, 1950

Erikson E: Toys and Reasons. In Haworth M (ed): Child Psychotherapy: Practice and Theory. New York, Basic Books, 1964, pp 3–11

Grubbs J: Class material, Spring, 1971

Jordon T: Research on the handicapped child and the family. Merrill-Palmer Quarterly, vol. 8, 1962, pp 243–255

Piaget J: The Language and Thought of the Child. New York, World, 1955

Piaget J: Judgment and Reasoning in the Child. Paterson, NJ, Littlefield, 1959

Piaget J: The Child's Conception of the World. Paterson, NJ, Littlefield, 1960

Piaget J. Inhelder B: The Child's Conception of Space. London, Routledge and Kegan Paul, 1956

Weed L: Medical Records, Medical Education, and Patient Care. Chicago, Case Western Reserve U. Press, 1970

Beverley Small

21

Nursing Visually Impaired Children with Johnson's Model as a Conceptual Framework

An interest in assessing the needs of visually impaired children resulted in a research study that evaluated and compared the visually handicapped with normally sighted preschool children. The study compared the perceived body image and spatial awareness of these two groups in order to evaluate the role of vision in the development of object permanence and the relation of objects in space. These two concepts are necessary for the development of the child's body image and for his awareness of the body and objects in the space surrounding his body.

Two hypotheses were tested in the study. The first hypothesis stated that there would be no significant difference between the perceived body image of visually impaired and normally sighted preschool children. The second hypothesis stated that there would be no significant differences between the spatial awareness of visually impaired preschoolers and those who were normally sighted.

STUDY DESIGN

The Subjects

The testing of the hypotheses was undertaken with two groups of preschool children. One group, designated as group A, consisted of seven visually impaired preschool children. These children were selected by a purposive sampling technique from an agency offering educational services to visually impaired children. The population of visually impaired preschool children was limited. However, the sample chosen did include all children available for study that had some residual vision of functional use. By definition these children were not blind; that is, their vision included more than light perception. Each subject had a different degree functional vision due to the particular cause of his or her visual impairment. Two subjects were visually impaired because of optic nerve disease. The causes of visual impairment in the other five subjects were as follows: bilateral colobomas, retinitis pigmentosa, meningitis, microophthalmos, and one unknown. Each subject had been visually impaired since birth.

Group B, the control group, was composed of seven normally sighted preschool children. These children were chosen from a day-care center. This group was matched as closely as possible for age and sex to the visually impaired children. The parents of these children (Group B) reported that they had no indication that a visual problem existed with their children.

No child over 48 months was included in either group. The ages of all subjects ranged from 18 months to 46 months. Both sexes were represented in each of the groups.

The Instrument

Data for this study were collected by utilizing Scale I and Scale V of the six Uzgiris-Hunt Ordinal Scales of Psychological Development (Uzgiris and Hunt, 1976). The six scales identify behavioral actions of infants and are designed to assess the infant's progress in different areas of intellectual functioning. The level of cognition is established by observation of an infant's response to objects and toys presented at points along the continuum of intellectual development. These scales are not based on an intelligence quotient, nor do they parallel the chronologic age of the infant. The scales are ordinal, which implies a hierarchical relationship: What an infant is able to do at one level is based on his incorporating what he or she has accomplished at a lower level. These scales represent a sequence of development; that is, they are normative and are meant to be reported as stage equivalent not age equivalent. Scale I (Development of Visual Pursuit and Permanence of Objects) and Scale V (Construction of Object Relations in Space) were extracted and presented to each subject as a play activity in order to elicit a behavior response.

Methodology

During the administration of the two scales, each subject was supine on a flat surface, in an infant seat, sitting unaided, and/or propped in a sitting position. The positions of the subjects were determined by the directions for each item to be tested on each scale and with regard to the age of the subjects or limitations due to physical inabilities.

Scale I consisted of fifteen separate items for evaluation. The investigator began with item one regardless of the age of the subject and proceeded down the item list in chronologic order. Each item was presented at least two times in an attempt to achieve success with the item. When it was determined, after a predetermined specific number of trials, that the subject was unable to exhibit the expected behavior (perform the task presented), that section of the evaluation was terminated.

Each child in both groups was shown an object or toy that attracted his or her interest from a specified list of toys and objects. This toy or object attracted the subject's attention by either sight or sound. The object was hidden from the subjects in a variety of ways, for example, covering it with three nontransparent screens. The subject had to remove each of these three screens to find the toy/object. If the subject was successful with the task, then a higher level task was presented. In the latter case, the toy/object was placed in a small box as the subject observed the action. The box was then turned over under the screen, and the subject was shown the empty box. The subject was encouraged to find the toy/object which had been left under the screen.

Scale V was comprised of eleven items for evaluation. Again, each item was presented in chronological order with at least two trials to measure successful accomplishment. The subjects were presented with two different toys or objects that elicited an interest. The initial situations included, for example, the child's observing two objects alternately, or localizing an object by its sound. As the children progressed to more complex situations, the higher level responses involved their ability to build a tower of at least two objects and to acknowledge the absence of a familiar person by gesture or word. All of these concepts relate to the infant's development of an appreciation of spatial relationships between objects.

The behavioral responses of Group A and Group B on both Scale I and Scale V were compared using Fisher's exact probability test (Siegel, 1956). Age was summarized for each of the groups with computation of the mean, median, and range. Frequency counts were obtained on demographic data to include sex and race.

STUDY RESULTS

The null hypothesis, that there would be no significant difference between the perceived body image and the spatial awareness of the two groups, was rejected. The alternate hypothesis was accepted due to the overwhelming number of significant differences between the two groups on each scale utilized in the study.

Scale I, object permanence, parallels Piaget's theory of sensorimotor cognitive development. The role of vision was found to be significant in the development of this concept. Visual impairment hindered the ability of the subjects in Group A to master the tasks with items evaluated at higher levels.

Piaget's theory states that overt sensorimotor activity is the infant's only means of environmental awareness. This sensorimotor period of cognitive development begins at birth and constitutes approximately the first two years of life. This period is divided into six sub-stages (Appendix I). It is during this period that object permanence is established. A month-old infant exhibits sucking and kicking. If an object is brought into the infant's line of vision and removed, he does not search for it. As the infant's ontogeny advances, his senses become more refined, and by six months, substage three, he is able to reach for a rattle. He is beginning to grasp and manipulate objects. He can move a rattle hung over his head and repeat the action, but will not search for it if it falls from his line of vision.

During substage four, designated by Piaget as the coordination of the secondary schemes, the nine- to twelve-month-old infant begins to search for lost objects. If a toy is hidden by a cloth cover in two places, the infant will search in the first place. The subjects in Group A in this study were all beyond the age of one year. The average age was equal to 32.9 months and only 57 percent of Group A subjects were able to find an object that was covered by a screen.

Piaget theorizes that by the time the infant is nearing his second birthday, he is able to search for objects hidden by superimposed coverings and invisible displacement. To determine if the subject had mastered object permanence, the final item, 13, of Scale I was evaluated. In this test, three nontransparent screens were placed side by side in front of the subject. While the subject was watching, a small toy was then put into a box with one end open. Then the box was placed under one of the three screens and turned over to leave the toy hidden under the screen. The empty box was removed and shown to the subject. Not one subject from Group A could find the object following this invisible displacement. However, six subjects, which represented 85.7 percent of all the normally sighted subjects in Group B, were able to follow this invisible displacement of an object.

Scale V evaluated the behavioral responses of both groups in regard to the relation of objects in space. The visually impaired subjects, Group A, had not reached the level of development necessary to attain the more complex tasks on this scale. This level is reached at approximately 24 months of age when the infant is beginning to develop memory skills. His imagination and pretending abilities are evolving (Piaget and Inhelder, 1969). If a toy that has attracted an infant's attention is placed out of reach and he has a stick, he will attempt to retrieve the toy with the stick. Substage six is conceptualized as the invention of new ways and means as the infant begins to interiorize schemes. One subject in Group A was able to satisfactorily perform the final item evaluated. All but one of the normally sighted subjects was able to perform the highest level evaluated on this scale. This subject had not reached the age of 24 months when a positive response in this category would be expected.

It was concluded that because of a visual impairment (degeneration of the optic nerve, a tumor of the eye, or congenital cataracts, for example), not all visually impaired children will perceive their body image or spatial awareness in an identical way. The rate of the child's development of these concepts will vary. Two of the visually impaired subjects, close in age, reached the higher stages of sensorimotor cognitive development in regard to object permanence and the relation of objects in space. These subjects had developed the ability to integrate structures (items evaluated) at lower levels. These two subjects appeared to have more functional vision. Three questions could be posed. Did these subjects have experience or more instruction in following displacement of objects? Did they have continuous stimulation of their residual vision? Or did they possess a higher intelligence quotient?

Other physical handicapping conditions were not controlled for and therefore had a bearing on the ability of the child to perform all of the items evaluated on each scale of assessment. Due to the extreme heterogeneous nature of the sample of subjects evaluated, one cannot generalize, from the results, about a larger population of visually impaired preschool children.

One purpose of this study was to determine whether or not Scales I and V could be used in the assessment of learning and thought competencies of visually impaired children. These scales were developed and validated for use with normally sighted infants from birth to two years. The results of this study further validate the use of these scales for normally sighted preschool children. Also, Scales I and V do give identifying measures of the cognitive development of visually impaired preschool children and are useful as tools to record longitudinally the progress of the child's development.

IMPLICATIONS FOR NURSING

This study, submitted as partial fulfillment of the requirements for a master's degree, can be considered as a guide for pediatric nurses. It will give the nurse information for assessing the learning and thought processes (the cognitive development) of visually impaired preschool children as well as of normally sighted preschool children. The investigation adds to basic nursing knowledge of visual impairment and the concomitant effect this sensory deprivation has on a child's developing body image and his awareness of his body in space. This knowledge and its adaptation to the Johnson nursing model gives direction for nursing practice.

Johnson's nursing model, based on a systems theory, represents a conceptual framework, a model, for nursing practice. This model considers man as a human system, a behavioral organism, continuously in interaction with the environment. Man is a whole system divided into eight subsystems, or minisystems, each with its own goals or functions. Each subsystem is interrelated and interdependent. The particular goals (behaviors) and functions that serve to achieve the goals of each of the subsystems can be maintained if the human system is not subjected to excessive stress and change. The nurse, as an environmental regulator of the human system, is seen as intervening in the stress of illness and disability. Nursing interventions are protection, nurturance, and stimulation. These three areas are referred to as sustenal imperatives. It is in these three areas that the role of nurse can influence the development and maintenance of stability of human behavior (Grubbs, 1980).

Holaday (1980) combined the Johnson model and Piagetian theory to assess the cognitive development of a six-year-old, chronically ill child. Holaday looked at the eliminative subsystem of the Johnson model in regard to the child's ability to express himself verbally. Observations of play behavior, utilizing Piaget's tests for centering, irreversibility, and egocentricity in the representation of objects, revealed the level of the child's cognitive development. This was invaluable information for the nurse in preparing the child preoperatively for surgery (Holaday, 1980).

Familiarity with visual impairment and resultant handicaps, as well as with attitudes toward blindness, comprises two explicit parameters of nursing knowledge. A nurse demonstrates her knowledge of the control of ophthalmia neonatorum by the instillation of a 1 percent silver nitrate solution (or other equally effective agent) in the conjunctival sac of the infant at birth. The nurse in this instance is seen in the protective role in relation to the newborn.

As the visually impaired child grows, he must be considered and evaluated as a total person who is allowed through trial and error to encounter the challenges of life. This child needs to develop a feeling of self-permanence, which evolves from the development of a sense of the permanence of objects and the meaning of space. Both of these concepts are developed from the experiences of the child acting on the environment and adapting to the environment. As the child acts on the environment, he assimilates the action and its results, which become part of his inner organization. The child accommodates the environment, which has acted on him. The resultant balance between these two mechanisms represents a state of equilibrium (Piaget, 1973; Piaget and Inhelder 1969; Marlow, 1977; Stephens, 1972). This allows the child to differentiate self from others and leads to a satisfactory self-concept, autonomy, and independence.

An important aspect in the assessment of the total child is an understanding of his intellectual level in the context of Piaget's theory of sensorimotor cognitive development. This assessment of the child's cognitive development is necessary to establish goals for nursing intervention. Uzgiris-Hunt Ordinal Scales of Psychological Development can be of value to nurses in determining behavioral responses during play activities (Uzgiris and Hunt, 1976). These responses will indicate the child's development of a sense of the permanence of objects. By determining the level (the sensorimotor stage) of a child's thinking process, the nurse can apply what the child is able to do in real life situations. Important criteria to satisfactory cognitive development are mobility skills, self-help skills, and the child's perception of his body parts, as well as the growth of a good self-concept. The child must have an identity separate from other people and objects in his environment (Bell, 1975). If a child with a visual impairment, strabismus, for example, is untreated, he may become blind (Lipton, 1970).

Frequent hospitalizations of visually impaired children are often necessary for medical and surgical attention to the visual problem. Nurses need to be able to adequately assess the level of cognitive and physical development of these children to be able to adopt a nursing-care plan to meet the particular needs of the child. The nurse can then establish goals for the child and the child's family.

Nursing can help meet the needs of parents with visually impaired children in several ways. The sustenal imperatives of nurturance, protection, and stimulation proposed by the Johnson model are basic for the support needed by the parents of these children. It is possible to look at all eight subsystems that this model embraces and relate them to the visually impaired child and his family. Johnson delineates these behavioral subsystems or parts of the human system as the core of the model.

The birth of a visually impaired infant can be emotionally disturbing to parents and other family members. The nurse must be supportive and assist in dispelling fears and erroneous attitudes concerning the infant. Eye contact, so important in maternal infant bonding (Rubin, 1961), may be missing, but the nurse can encourage the mother to substitute extra touching and more vocalization to secure this bonding.

The nurse is seen in the nurturing role when an infant is born with a visual anomaly. The nurse needs to provide support to the parents' dependency and restorative subsystems by the encouragement of effective and discouragement of ineffective behaviors. The nurse will assist the parents with the stress, guilt, and disbelief that accompany the birth of a less than normal child. A nurse with the knowledge of genetic counseling will sustain the parents' dependency subsystem if their child is born with an inherited blinding disease. In reviewing the literature, Butani (1974) recognized that the mother feels the birth of her defective infant to be personal failure. The goals the mother had set for her unborn child, fantasies regarding the child, and idealizations of this child are destroyed.

After helping the parents work through the grief process and reach a successful adaptation to the crisis, the nurse can further assist the parents and the child through anticipatory guidance. One area of guidance that is needed encompasses parental attitudes toward their visually impaired child. Attitudes of parents with blind children have been investigated and five categories have been identified. These feelings include acceptance, denial, overprotectiveness, disguised rejection, and overt rejection (Monbeck, 1974). The nurturing role of the nurse lends support to the parents' affiliative subsystem in order that the parent will be able to accept the child. The nurse can also stimulate the sexual subsystems of the parents and the child so that adequate bonding can take place. A healthy maternal (and paternal) infant attachment will assure the parents that they are capable of love, and the child that he is loved.

The parents need to know that visual impairment may affect the child's behavior. For example, the nurse can help the parents in regulating the home environment to minimize any behavioral deviations. This sustenance augments the parents' achievement subsystem. This gives necessary control to their own life. However, nursing interventions must include consideration of inherent cultural variations from family to familiy. Some behavior control for the visually impaired child can be established by an adequate stimulation program. The parents need to be encouraged to stimulate the child's residual (functional) vision. The emphasis needs to be placed on the vision the child does possess, not on the loss of vision (Barraga, 1976). Nurses can instruct mothers in the importance of the child's exploration of objects, toys, and the environment early in life. The visually impaired child demands stimulation through all the sensory modalities. This child needs visual stimulation to make optimum use of any vision he might possess. The child requires stimulation through extra touching by others and additional amounts of body contact. He needs to be introduced to all textures to be touched. Also necessary is increased auditory input (voices, music) and tastes and smells that are taken for granted by the normally sighted (Carolan, 1973).

The nurse should be cognizant of the community resources and agencies available to the visually impaired child for educational purposes. The community nurse can give psychologic and physical support to the parents' restoration subsystem through a continuing assessment of the family and the child. Nurses equipped with knowledge of visual impairment can be sources for early case finding and referral. By using serial and sequential observations of the visually impaired child, the nurse can detect possible developmental lags. Health teaching and health maintenance, in the form of primary preventive measures and anticipatory guidance, can be instituted and directed toward the enrichment of the visually impaired child's environment. The nurse is aware that each family has its own conceptualization of what its particular state of wellness should be. She uses this knowledge to provide protection for the parents' developmental subsystem.

Following a complete assessment, and continuing with the process, the nurse makes her diagnoses. Once a problem is identified, she will establish the methods of intervention (sustenal imperatives). Long- and short-term goals of intervention are predictive of expected outcomes. These goals are set in the form of behavioral objectives. One example of a short-term goal of a family and a visually impaired child would be to see evidence of an affiliative bond between the child and the mother. The mother is observed holding the infant close to her body while touching the infant's hands and speaking in a soft voice. The infant responds to her mother with smiling and cooing.

Another example would be indications that the father and other siblings are involved in the child's care. The infant's father is observed changing a soiled diaper with some obvious expertise. The father appears comfortable in this role. He calls to the four-year-old sibling to watch and to help him with this task. These examples represent a tie of the affiliative subsystem with the familial variable.

One possible outcome (observable patient responses) is the parents' and the child's adjustment to a particular situation (the visual impairment) (Grubbs, 1980). Both parents appear to the nurse to accept the child as he is. The child is encouraged in self-help skills however inept he might be with minimal parental interference. Although visually impaired, he is encouraged to feed himself when another's feeding him might facilitate mealtime im-measurably.

The other outcome is the parents' adaptation to the stress of the disability (behavior stability and effective coping mechanisms) (Grubbs, 1980). The parents are able to verbalize their feelings concerning the birth of their less than perfect infant. They express confidence in their ability to manage behavior problems associated with visual impairment. They have gone beyond the stages of guilt and denial. They are able to accept their child and the support and help offered by the nurse and others.

The nurse assessing the visually impaired child, diagnosing and identifying problems, planning intervention measures, and evaluating goals must consider the child's feelings, needs, and desires along with those of the family. The Johnson nursing model encompasses these parameters for nursing practice and is a practical tool for implementing all phases of the nursing process.

REFERENCES

Barraga N: Visual Handicaps and Learning: A Developmental Approach. Belmont, Ca., Wadsworth, 1976

Bell V H: An educator's approach to assessing preschool visually handicapped children. Educ Visually Handicapped 7:3:84, 1975

Butani P: Reactions of mothers to the birth of an anomalous infant: a review of the literature. Maternal-Child Nurs J 3: 1: 59, 1974

Carolan R: Sensory stimulation and blind infant. New Outlook for the Blind 67:3: 119, 1973

Grubbs J: The Johnson behavioral system model. In Riehl JP and Roy C (eds): Conceptual Models for Nursing Practice, 2d ed. New York, Appleton, 1980, pp 217–254

Holaday B: Implementing the Johnson model for nursing practice. In Riehl JP and Roy C (eds): Conceptual Models for Nursing Practice, 2d ed. New York, Appleton, 1980, pp 255—263

Lipton E: A study of psychological effects of strabismus. In Eissler RS (ed): The Psychoanalytical Study of the Child 25. New York, International University, 1970, pp 146–174

Marlow D: Textbook of Pediatric Nursing. Philadelphia, Saunders, 1977

Monbeck M: The Meaning of Blindness. Bloomington, Indiana University, 1974

Piaget J: The Child and Reality. New York, Penguin, 1973

Piaget J, Inhelder B: The Psychology of the Child. New York, Basic Books, 1969

Rubin R: Basic maternal behavior. Nurs Outlook 9:683, 1961

Siegel S: Non-parametric Statistics for the Behavioral Sciences. New York, McGraw-Hill, 1956

Stephens B: Cognitive processing in the visually impaired. Educ Visually Handicapped 4:106, 1972

Uzgiris I, Hunt H M: Assessment in Infancy: Ordinal Scales of Psychological Development. Chicago, University of Illinois, 1975

Karla Damus

An Application of the Johnson Behavioral System Model for Nursing Practice

Nursing's research task ... is to identify and explain the behavioral system disorders which arise in connection with illness, and to develop the rationale for and means of management. (Johnson 1968)

Any science, or art, for that matter (and I believe nursing should be an example of both) is ultimately founded on theories, the viability of which depend upon whether they are found to be true or not when applied in the laboratory of real life. Nursing's research task, as defined by Johnson, is simply and eloquently stated. But can it be a productive task? Is it in fact a theory upon which practicing nurses can build and thereby gain insight into their profession and themselves? These questions are of necessity abstract, but testing them requires the rigorous proof of concrete experience. As Lord Kelvin (1891) remarked:

> When you can measure what you are speaking about, and can express it in numbers, you know something about it; but when you cannot express it in numbers, your knowledge is of a meager and unsatisfactory kind; it may be the beginning of knowledge, but you have scarcely, in your thoughts, advanced to the state of science.

The following study was undertaken utilizing the Johnson behavioral model for nursing in order (1) to test the validity of the theory in nursing practice and (2) to gather information on the nursing aspects of patients diagnosed as having a specific disease. Post-transfusion hepatitis was selected as the specific disease for this study.

Initially I intended to conduct a descriptive survey applying the Johnson Behavioral System Model to a small sample of five patients all of whom had post-transfusion hepatitis. The plan was to accumulate enough data to demonstrate some correlation between a single pathologic variables and specific nursing diagnoses. After a few months of work it became apparent that there existed more than a general correlation. In fact, physiologic disequilibrium seemed to coincide with behavioral disequilibrium. The study was then expanded to include ten patients who were followed over an eleven-month period. The objectives of the study were similarly enlarged to include the delineation of a relationship between selected physiologic disequilibria and behavioral disequilibria as well as the correlation of particular nursing diagnoses with effective nursing interventions.

In this paper a concise explication of the study will be presented by (1) relating the reasons for selecting patients with post-transfusion hepatitis to the Johnson behavioral model and elaborating on relevant concepts of the disease, (2) describing the methodologic approach, and (3) discussing the limitations, results, and conclusions.

RATIONALE FOR SAMPLE SELECTION

The decision to use patients with post-transfusion hepatitis was predicated on a number of factors, primarily related to those characteristics of the disease that facilitated the application of the Johnson behavioral model to the patients' nursing care.

1. In general, hepatitis has a benign prognosis with complications seen in less than 10 percent of the patients, thereby precluding any behavioral instability based solely on anticipated prognosis.
2. The therapy for hepatitis is consistent: a diet, void of alcohol, which is high in proteins, carbohydrates, and vitamins; and increased rest, which is dictated by the patient's fatigue or enzyme elevations. Such a treatment regimen minimizes the possibility of observing prescribed drug-influenced behaviors.
3. Due to unpredictable changes in the disease, patients with hepatitis should be seen regularly on an outpatient basis. These regular visits provide many opportunities for serial application of the Johnson behavioral model with concomitant data collection.
4. The most reliable indicator of hepatitis is elevations of alanine aminotransferase (serum glutamic pyruvic transaminase, SGPT). The value of this pathologic variable is easily compared to the number of nursing diagnoses, thereby providing a convenient mode for relating physiologic disequilibrium (SGPT elevations) and behavioral disequilibrium (number of nursing diagnoses).

Contemporary Epidemiological Concepts of Post-transfusion Hepatitis

The character of post-transfusion hepatitis has been evolving since its identification in the early 1940s. The appearance of this disease was attributed to the extensive wartime use of plasma for the management of battle casualties, thereby proposing a correlation between the use of blood products and the incidence of hepatitis. Subsequent observations and studies validated this correlation. Then in the 1960s, Allen and Sayman (1962) published their comprehensive study in Chicago, which reported that the incidence of post-transfusion hepatitis was 30 to 40 percent following transfusion of blood or blood products. Through their accumulated morbidity and mortality statistics, they proclaimed this disease as a major clinical and public-health problem. Studies that substantiated their findings and conclusions flooded the medical literature so that it became evident and well-accepted that there was a definite risk of viral hepatitis transmission during the transfusion of blood and/or blood products. The risk is predicated on such factors as the source of the blood, the blood-processing technique, the susceptibility of the recipients, the titer of the viral agent in the donor, the carrier rate in donors, and especially the sensitivity of the assay employed to screen the blood for the viral agent.

It is generally agreed that the agent of transmission of post-transfusion hepatitis, or at least the indicator of such an agent, is the hepatitis B antigen (HBAg). Since its discovery by Blumberg in 1963, assays of varying sensitivity have been developed to screen blood for the presence of HBAg. As yet, however, there is no known assay that can detect all of the existing HBAg and therefore no way to assure the absence of the antigen in blood or blood products. It has been shown, however, that blood screened by the less sensitive technique of counterelectrophoresis (CEP) may appear negative for HBAg, but on rescreening with the more sensitive radioimmune assay (RIA) be found actually to be HBAg positive (Gitnick, 1973). This knowledge gave impetus to a number of post-transfusion hepatitis studies in which all transfused CEP negative blood was prospectively rescreened by RIA. The recipients of any blood units found to be positive on rescreening were then followed to determine the incidence of post-transfusion hepatitis. One of the largest studies of this kind was conducted at the UCLA Medical Center from which the sample of patients for my study was randomly selected.

The typical clinical course of post-transfusion hepatitis is characterized by an abnormal SGPT of at least five times the normal occurring within 25 to 210 days following the transfusion of blood or blood products. This insidious rise in enzymes can attain peaks from 5 to 200 times the normal and remain elevated from 2 to 30 weeks. In addition, there may be elevations of other chemical parameters such as the serum glutamic oxaloacetic transaminase

(SGOT), the alkaline phosphatase, and both direct and tital bilirubin. These abnormalities are sometimes accompanied by one or more of the following signs and symptoms: fatigue, anorexia, nausea, vomiting, mylagias, arthralgias, dark urine, light stools, and jaundice. It is of interest that icteric hepatitis accounts for less than 10 percent of all hepatitis in the population and only one of the ten study patients developed icteric sclera, while none developed frank jaundice. Of additional significance is the lack of correlation between SGPT elevations and the patient's signs and symptoms. High elevations may be associated with hungry energetic patients, whereas minimal elevations may be associated with vomiting, arthralgias, or any combination of the possible signs and symptoms. This is especially true in the situation of subclinical post-transfusion hepatitis where the hepatitis is silent and only the laboratory values indicate that the patient has the disease.

In summary, post-transfusion hepatitis is a disease of increasing frequency, which is seen following the transfusion of blood or blood products. The agent of transmission is believed to be the hepatitis B antigen (HBAg), and since there is no available assay which can detect 100 percent of the antigen, the risk of developing this disease is ever-present, creating a serious clinical and health problem. Studies to evaluate the sensitivity of various assays have reported that counterelectrophoresis (CEP) will miss a number of HBAg positive units, which can be detected by rescreening with radioimmune assay (RIA). Finally, there is no apparent correlation between the elevations of the SGPT and how the patient feels; often the SGPT will be elevated but the patient will experience no signs or symptoms, and other times the converse will hold.

METHODOLOGY

As mentioned, blood transfused at the UCLA Medical Center that was initially screened by CEP was prospectively rescreened by RIA. This rescreening occurred within two weeks after the transfusion. As expected, a number of CEP negative units were found to be RIA positive. By utilizing the blood bank records, the recipients of these HBAg positive units were identified, and their respective medical charts were examined. If the patient had normal liver functions on the day of transfusion and if the patient had received transfusions exclusively at the UCLA Medical Center, every effort was made to locate the patient and inform him of the probable risk of his developing post-transfusion hepatitis. Once contacted, it was recommended to him that he be followed either by the study nurse and physician at UCLA or by his private physician. The recipient was further advised that he should be followed at least six months because of the incubation period of the disease. If the patient chose to be followed by his private physician, no further contacts were made. If, however, he demonstrated an interest in the UCLA study, he was told that the follow-up was complementary and included:

1. having a 10 cc blood specimen drawn on a biweekly basis for seven months (for SGPT, SGOT, Bilirubin-total/direct, and HBAg-HBAb titers)
2. being seen by the study nurse on a biweekly basis
3. being treated by the study physician if necessary

Voluntary consent to this follow-up completed the criteria for entrance of patients into the UCLA Prospective-Post-transfusion Hepatitis Study. It was from this prospective study sample of 150 patients that ten patients were randomly selected for my study. These ten patients participated in the same follow-up as those patients in the prospective study, the only difference being that the theoretical framework of the Johnson behavioral model was applied to their nursing care and they were seen monthly instead of biweekly during the last three months of their follow-up. Table 1 summarizes some salient information about the ten patients in this study.

All ten patients were Caucasian; six were males and four were females. Their ages ranged from 26 to 85 years with a mean age of 50.5 years. The number of blood units transfused to each patient varied from 3 to 18 with a mean of 8.5 units per patient. The date on which the HBAg positive unit was transfused was also listed, and for these ten patients this occurred sometime between August 1, 1972, and March 5, 1973. These dates were extremely significant since each follow-up visit and all the time intervals of comparison for the ten patients were based on the number of days following the transfusion of the HBAg positive unit of blood.

There were ten follow-up visits for every study patient. The first visit

TABLE 1. Summary of Patients

Patient	Age	Sex	No. Units Transfused	Date HBAg Unit Transfused
DS	26	M	7	12/20/72
GB	27	F	13	10/17/72
LR	28	M	10	8/31/72
CR	37	M	10	3/5/73
EP	52	M	5	2/26/73
BU	53	M	18	1/8/73
MA	55	F	5	11/2/72
CO	69	M	3	8/1/72
ES	73	F	6	9/12/72
MT	85	F	8	1/6/73

always occurred within thirty days (± 3) following the HBAg positive blood, with the other nine succeeding at appropriate intervals. A fifteen-day interval was scheduled between each of the first seven visits, with a thirty-day interval between each of the remaining three. Therefore every patient was seen on the 30th, 45th, 60th, 75th, 90th, 105th, 120th, 150th, 180th, and 210th day following transfusion, affording ten different visits for data comparison.

Each visit took place in my office at the UCLA Medical Center, and lasted between 20 and 97 minutes, with a mean length of 43 minutes. For the majority of visits only the patient attended, but occasionally in order to facilitate the implementation of a nursing intervention, I requested that a family member or friend be present. To control as many environmental factors as possible the following sequence was employed at each visit:

1. A 10 cc clot tube of blood was drawn from either the right or left antecubital fossa using the syringe technique.
2. Blood test results from preceding visits were discussed in depth.
3. Questions from the patient regarding his physiologic status were entertained.
4. Data were collected for the ongoing assessment state by the use of an assessment tool developed within the framework of the Johnson behavioral system model.
5. Nursing diagnoses were formulated and validation for these and previous diagnoses was sought.
6. Appropriate interventions were initiated or supplemented.
7. Evaluation of the assessment, diagnoses, and interventions from present and previous visits continued with the institution of necessary changes.

Directly following each visit, this ongoing implementation of the nursing process within the framework of the Johnson model was accurately recorded. Specifically cited were the observed behaviors, the complete assessment, nursing diagnoses, the selected interventions, and any relevant evaluation. These were immediately compared to previous visits and particular attention was given to ineffective interventions and to repetitive diagnoses.

To facilitate the interpretation of these data, the classification of nursing diagnoses, and the categories of interventions derived from the Johnson behavioral model that are used in this study will be briefly discussed. A thorough and detailed exposition of the Johnson behavioral model and the nursing process has already been presented by Grubbs in a previous chapter of this text.

There are four diagnostic classifications of behavioral disequilibrium: discrepancy, insufficiency, dominance, and incompatibility. Discrepancy and insufficiency apply to disorders originating within the subsystems. They may be the consequence of either functional or structural problems. Dominance and incompatibility are manifested in disorders originating between subsystems, representing control and conflict, respectively.

There are also four categories of interventions, and their definitions suggest the modes of implementation. These categories are as follows:

Category	Mode
Restrict	impose limits or external controls on behavior; supplement immature or ineffective control and regulating mechanisms
Defend	prevent damage from exposure to unnecessary stressors; cope with threats on the patient's behalf
Inhibit	suppress ineffective responses
Facilitate	expedite incorporation of new demands; increase the opportunity to use a behavior

For purposes of clarity, only the aforementioned diagnostic classifications and interventions will be used in the presentation of study results. I have developed some diagnostic subclassifications and several subcategories of interventions, but their incorporation would only serve to cloud the discussion.

Limitations of the Study

There are several limitations of this study, which warrant a brief discussion. None of these limitations, however, interfered with the validity of the study results.

First, there was limited experience in the application of the assessment tool. This, plus the pragmatic necessities engendered by the application of theory to real life situations, led to several revisions of the assessment tool as the study progressed. Although none of these changes can be considered major, they may have altered the behavior elicited from the study patients to some extent. The consistency of the correlations observed over many hundreds of different observations, however, is a tribute to the resiliency of the Johnson model, despite minor alterations in its application to the nursing process.

A more concrete objection might be raised concerning the second limitation, that of observer bias. Early in the study a correlation between biochemical manifestations of the disease and behavioral disequilibrium became apparent. Because of the study methodology, my knowledge of the patient's SGPT values for each visit was unavoidable. It is therefore conceivable that the anticipation of behavioral disorders, in light of elevated SGPT values, may have precipitated their identification.

The difficulty encountered when applying the model's four categories of interventions represents a final limitation of the study. Partly due to the newness of these categories and to my limited experience in their use, I tended to decide on a specific intervention prior to selecting one of the model's four categories of interventions. In other words, I would intervene and then attempt to categorize my intervention. This probably represents the most serious limitation of the study.

Results

The results of this study are best summarized in the following tables and graphs. They are ordered so that the data correlating physiologic and behavioral disequilibrium are presented first, followed by the data emphasizing a relationship between the number and classification of nursing diagnoses with post-transfusion hepatitis, and finally by the data suggesting a relationship between specific nursing diagnostic classifications and particular interventions.

A tabulation of SGPT values for every patient on each of the ten visits is given in Table 2. All of the SGPT assays were performed at the same clinical laboratory using the manual method of Karmen.

Values less than or equal to 24 international units (IU) are considered normal, and by definition those values greater than or equal to five times the normal (120 IU) are consistent with post-transfusion hepatitis. All ten patients did develop post-transfusion hepatitis, but the date of onset varied (from 30 to 180 days after the HBAg positive transfusion) as did the duration of the illness (between 30 and 135 days). The mean SGPT values for the ten patients on each visit are also given in Table 2, representing overall physiologic disequilibrium at given days after transfusion of the HBAg positive unit of blood.

The number of nursing diagnoses for each patient visit is recorded in Table 3. There is a total of 474 nursing diagnoses, with a range of one to nine nursing diagnoses for each visit and a mean of 4.7.

It is apparent that some of the patients experienced much more behavioral disequilibrium over a longer period of time than others. Variables such as underlying disease other than post-transfusion hepatitis, age, socioeconomic status, cultural background, or cognitive state may have contributed markedly to these differences, but the fluctuations, as represented by changes in the number of nursing diagnoses, were correlated to the changes in SGPT values. This was demonstrated by comparing the mean SGPT values for each visit (listed in Table 2) with the mean nursing diagnoses for each visit (listed in Table 3). This comparison is clearly represented by Figure 1. A rise in the SGPT values is closely approximated by a rise in the number of nursing diagnoses. Similarly, a decline in the SGPT is associated with a decline in the number of nursing diagnoses. This clearly supports the contention that physiologic disequilibrium is reflected by behavioral disequilibrium.

One point on the graph that deserves particular attention is that which

TABLE 2. SGPT Values (IU)/Patient/Visit

Patient	Number of Days Since HBAg+ Unit Transfused									
	30	45	60	75	90	105	120	150	180	210
DS	32	40	48	78	96	100	121	168	100	79
GB	10	40	55	101	320	187	86	40	22	12
LR	32	30	149	620	490	700	233	74	644	218
CR	35	1670	522	710	670	840	1272	1362	276	35
EP	31	26	62	82	109	234	344	242	168	120
BU	71	96	350	520	1230	276	210	132	100	88
MA	120	840	460	940	1140	330	158	210	105	46
CO	48	41	130	480	920	1180	600	410	132	474
ES	23	14	19	16	16	25	48	80	140	166
MT	14	112	804	460	460	68	29	42	56	25
Mean SGPT/ Visit	41.6	290.9	259.9	395.7	545.1	394.0	310.1	376	174.3	126.3

TABLE 3. The Number of Nursing Diagnoses/Visit/Patient

Patient	Number of Days Since HBAg+ Unit Transfused										Total ND/Pt/ Ten Visits	Mean ND/Pt/ Visit
	30	45	60	75	90	105	120	150	180	210		
DS	4	2	2	3	3	4	5	4	2	3	32	3.2
GB	5	2	3	6	8	7	4	4	3	3	45	4.5
LR	6	5	8	9	9	9	8	3	7	3	67	6.7
CR	6	8	9	9	8	8	8	7	4	4	71	7.1
EP	4	2	2	2	4	5	6	6	4	4	39	3.9
BU	6	4	8	7	6	6	4	3	2	2	48	4.8
MA	6	8	8	9	7	8	5	4	4	4	63	6.3
CO	4	3	3	4	5	6	6	5	3	5	44	4.4
ES	4	3	2	2	1	2	2	3	4	5	28	2.8
MT	4	3	5	6	6	5	2	2	2	2	37	3.7
Total ND/ ten pts/visit	49	40	50	57	57	60	50	41	35	35	474	Total ND/ 10 pts/10 visits)
Mean ND/pt/ specific visit	4.9	4.0	5.0	5.7	5.7	6.0	5.0	4.1	3.5	3.5		3.5

ND = nursing diagnosis.

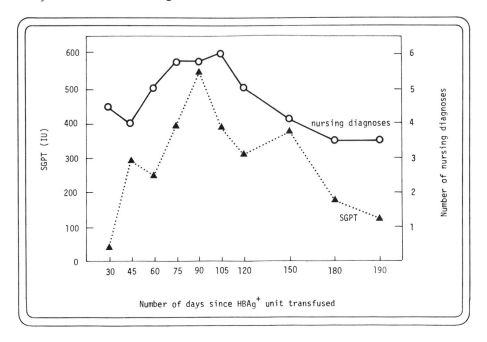

Figure 1 *A comparison of the mean SGPT and mean number of nursing diagnoses/visit for all ten patients.*

represents the number of nursing diagnoses on the 30th day following transfusion of the HBAg positive blood—the first follow-up visit. This point was consistently high on the individual graphs of all ten patients and is illustrated in Figure 2 of patient GB and Figure 3 of patient EP. Reasons for this elevation can only be postulated since the common nursing diagnosis on day 30 for all ten patients was dominance of the aggressive subsystem presumably due to anxiety. Hence, any one or a combination of the following factors may have precipitated this regularly identified behavioral disequilibrium on the first visit: the newness of the nurse-patient relationship, the method of contacting the patient, the venipuncture performed, the fear of developing post-transfusion hepatitis, the environment of the medical center, or the number of questions posed to the patient.

For further examination of the behavioral disequilibrium, all 474 nursing diagnoses were appropriately placed into the four classifications of insufficiency, discrepancy, incompatibility, and dominance.

Table 4 delineates the distribution of these classifications and indicates that almost 43 percent of all nursing diagnoses were labeled insufficiency, which reflects problems with the functional requirements (sustenal impera-

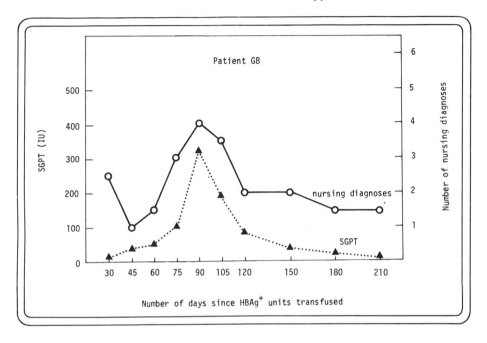

Figure 2 *Graph of the study patient GB demonstrating the increased number of nursing diagnoses on the first visit and the subsequent correlation of nursing diagnoses and SGPT values.*

tives) of the subsystems. Discrepancy due to structural problems represented 30 percent of the nursing diagnoses. Combining these two classifications, one finds that 345 or 72.8 percent of the 474 nursing diagnoses involve behavioral disequilibrium manifested within the subsystems, while only 129 or 27.2 percent represent behavioral disequilibrium between the subsystems.

TABLE 4. Distribution of Diagnostic Classifications for the 474 Nursing Diagnoses of the Study

Diagnostic Classification	No. of Nursing Diagnoses/ Classification	% of Total Nursing Diagnoses
Insufficiency	203	42.8
Discrepancy	142	30.0
Incompatibility	46	9.7
Dominance	83	17.5
Total	474	100%

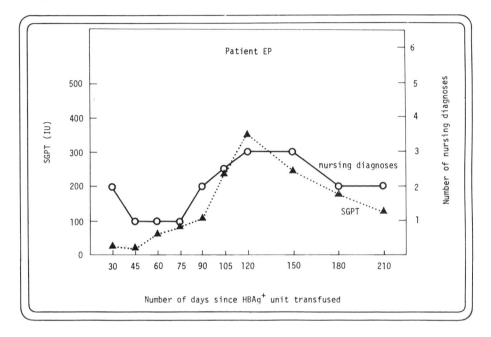

Figure 3 *Graph of study patient EP demonstrating the increased number of nursing diagnoses on the first visit and the subsequent correlation of nursing diagnoses and SGPT values.*

For further characterization of the source of behavioral disequilibrium, the classifications of the diagnoses were correlated with each of the eight subsystems. These results are given in Tables 5 and 6. They show that although each subsystem experienced instability, the achievement, sexual, and restorative subsystems were affected more often than the others. The least affected subsystem was the eliminative subsystem.

As expected, dominance of the aggressive and restorative subsystems represented about 60 percent of all diagnosed dominance. This can best be attributed to the observable anxiety, fear, and fatigue of many patients with hepatitis. The pathogenesis of hepatitis also helps to explain why there is so much incompatibility of the achievement/dependency subsystems and the ingestive/restorative subsystems, as does the knowledge that choices and actions of the achievement subsystem are narrowed, the sustenal requirements are dramatically increased, the drive strength for the goal of the ingestive subsystem is decreased, and the set of the restorative subsystem is altered. Thus although the recorded statistics for all 474 nursing diagnoses is a

TABLE 5.   The Number of Diagnostic
Classifications/Subsystem for Disorders
Within Each Subsystem/474 Nursing
Diagnoses

Subsystem	Insufficiency	Discrepancy
Achievement	36	26
Affiliative	18	19
Aggressive	37	17
Dependency	10	19
Eliminative	7	9
Ingestive	22	12
Restorative	41	14
Sexual	32	26
Total	203	142

convenient mode of summarizing copious amounts of data, the amount of energy and time that this study represents must be realized.

The remaining results are presented in Tables 7 and 8. They pertain to the nursing interventions implemented and were based on the nursing diagnoses. Each nursing diagnosis evoked a nursing intervention. Thus, the nurse had to select 474 interventions from the four categories: restrict, defend, inhibit, facilitate. Table 7 shows that 178 or 37.6 percent of all interventions were to facilitate, 131 or 27.6 percent to inhibit, 87 or 18.3 percent to defend, and 78 or 16.5 percent to restrict the patient's behavior.

Since the most common diagnosis was insufficiency, which defines a problem with the sustenal imperatives of nurturance, protection, or stimulation, it was predictable that the most common intervention would be to

TABLE 6.   The Number of Diagnostic Classifications/Subsystem for
Disorders *Between* Subsystems/474 Nursing Diagnoses

Subsystem	Dominance	Subsystem	Incompatibility
Achievement	2	Achievement/Dependency	13
Affiliative	4	Affiliative/Aggressive	7
Aggressive	29	Aggressive/Dependency	8
Dependency	17	Ingestive/Restorative	10
Eliminative	3	Restorative/Sexual	8
Ingestive	4		
Restorative	21	Total	46
Sexual	3		
Total	83		

TABLE 7. Distribution of Intervention Categories for the 474 Interventions of the Study

Intervention Category	No. of Interventions/ Category	% of Total Interventions
Restrict	78	16.5
Defend	87	18.3
Inhibit	131	27.6
Facilitate	178	37.6
Total	474	100%

facilitate, which includes supplying nurturance and stimulation. It also seemed reasonable to suspect other correlations between specific nursing diagnoses and particular nursing interventions. This led to the construction of Table 8 which relates the percentage of interventions in each category of intervention to the four diagnostic classifications. For example, if a diagnosis of insufficiency was made, 50.8 percent of the interventions were to facilitate, 23.6 percent to inhibit, 19.2 percent to defend, and only 6.4 percent to restrict. For a diagnosis of discrepancy, the most frequent intervention was to facilitate (35.9 percent) followed by 31.6 percent to inhibit and 23.3 percent to defend.

Diagnoses of behavioral disorders between subsystems usually resulted in the intervention to restrict as seen in 41.4 percent of all diagnoses of incompatibility and 39.8 percent of all diagnoses of dominance. In addition, when a diagnosis of incompatibility was made, 23.8 percent of the interventions were to defend, 19.6 percent to inhibit, and 15.2 percent to facilitate.

TABLE 8. Number (%) of Interventions/Category of Intervention/ Diagnostic Classification of 474 Nursing Diagnoses

Intervention Category	Insufficiency	Discrepancy	Incompatibility	Dominance	Intervention Totals
Restrict	13 (6.4%)	13 (9.2%)	19 (41.4%)	33 (39.8%)	78
Defend	39 (19.2%)	33 (23.3%)	11 (23.8%)	4 (4.8%)	87
Inhibit	48 (23.6%)	45 (31.6%)	9 (19.6%)	29 (35.0%)	131
Facilitate	103 (50.8%)	51 (35.9%)	7 (15.2%)	17 (20.4%)	178
Total	203	142	46	83	474

Dominance resulted in 35 percent of the interventions being to inhibit, 20.4 percent to facilitate, and only 4.8 percent to defend.

These results support the contention that not only is there a definitive correlation between behavioral and physiologic disequilibrium, but also a relation between specific nursing diagnoses and particular nursing interventions.

Conclusions

A number of definitive conclusions can be stated based on the specific study results. First, it is clear that the correlation between behavioral disequilibrium and physiologic disequilibrium is sound. Disorder in one will be reflected by disorder in the other. It is also apparent that there is a definite relationship between specific nursing diagnoses and particular nursing interventions. In fact, in patients with post-transfusion hepatitis, even the source of subsystem disorders can be identified and predicted. Finally, the data obtained unequivocally support the utility and practicality of applying the Johnson behavioral model in nursing practice. The success of its application is predicated on the nurse's comprehension of systems theory and the theoretical framework of the Johnson behavioral model as well as on her ability to integrate the model into every stage of the nursing process.

REFERENCES

Allen JG, Sayman WA: Serum hepatitis from transfusions of blood-epidemiologic study. JAMA 180:1079, 1962

Cossart YE: What determines the incidence of serum hepatitis after blood transfusion? Am J Dis Child 123:354, 1972

Gitnick GL: The clinical spectrum of hepatitis B antigen. Unpublished, UCLA, 1973

Johnson DE: One conceptual model of nursing. Paper presented April 25, 1968, at Vanderbilt Univ, Nashville, Tenn

Kelvin LWT: Popular Lectures and Addresses, 1891. In Bartlett J: Familiar Quotations, 14th ed. Boston, Little Brown & Co, 1968, p 723

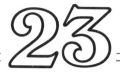

Claire G. Glennin

Formulation of Standards of Nursing Practice Using a Nursing Model

Formulation of standards for nursing practice is a necessary prerequisite to evaluation of the quality of care rendered by nurse practitioners. In the past, standards of performance of nursing practice were written from the perspective of the skill level of personnel performing nursing activities. The frame of reference for the standards presented in this paper is the nursing process via the Johnson Behavioral System Model. With each step in the nursing process used as a guide, standards were developed from various segments of the model. Before the undertaking of that task, it was necessary to consider some prerequisites. These will be presented prior to the discussion of standards.

PREREQUISITES TO DEVELOPMENT OF STANDARDS

Before standards can be developed, the type of nursing care to be evaluated must be specified. This is necessary because standards for judging quality of care should reflect specific variables embodied in the nursing-care situation. General categories of these variables include type of agency and scope of concern, units of care, aspects of care, and evaluation approaches (Donabedian, 1968). Several examples of specific variables related to each category are discussed below. In addition, those variables related to the type of nursing situation that might be evaluated by the standards formulated for this paper are identified in subsequent paragraphs.

The first category of variable, type of agency, refers to whether or not a health agency is a hospital, a public-health agency, a physician's office, or another form of health-care setting. Second, scope of concern pertains to the magnitude of health-service provision. For example, is the health-care situation concerned with patients on a one-to-one basis, small groups of patients, large groups of patients, or a whole patient community? Also, will standards focus on care provided by one professional group, a number of professional groups working together in one agency, or all the health disciplines that might be involved in provision of comprehensive community health care? In this paper, standards will focus on care provided for individual patients by professional registered nurses in a hospital setting.

Third, units of care encompass either episodic care or long-term care. Aspects of care may be preventive, acute, or restorative; and they may include such factors as social, psychologic, or physiologic management of health and illness. Standards in this paper were developed for patients receiving acute nursing care, with an emphasis on psychosocial management rather than on physiologic management.

Finally, a variety of evaluation approaches exist. Donabedian (1969) proposes that there are three such approaches: evaluation of process, of structure, and of outcome. Examiners using the process approach focus on the clinical decisions and actions of health practitioners. By comparison, evaluators using the structure approach are concerned with the properties of health-care facilities, equipment, manpower, and financing. Finally, assessment of outcomes consists of the appraisal of the end results of health care, specified in terms of patient health, welfare, and satisfaction. Patients' opinions, reactions, and behavior should be included within this third evaluation approach. Elements of the process and of the outcome approach are those used as bases for development of standards in this paper.

STANDARDS FOR NURSING PRACTICE

Standards for nursing practice are criteria against which the quality of practitioner performance may be judged. Quality of nursing care may be judged "good," "bad," or assigned some other rating according to the degree of conformity found between present standards, such as those presented in the following sections of this paper, and attributes of actual clinical nursing situations. Standards may consist of any of the elements of a health-care situation mentioned so far in relation to evaluation approaches. In reference to nursing care, they may include such factors as nursing-care facilities or equipment, nurse manpower, the sequences of actions taken by nurses in the care of patients, or patient outcomes. Standards formulated for this paper are based upon the nursing process approach, which is comprised of clinical nursing actions and patient outcomes. Phaneuf's (1972) definition of the nursing process was adopted for this paper.

> The nursing process encompasses all major steps taken in the care of the patient, with attention to their nature, purpose and rationale; their sequence;

and the degree to which they assist the patient to reach specific and attainable therapeutic and health goals.

The major steps in the nursing process identified for this paper were data gathering, assessment, diagnosis, prescription, implementation, and evaluation. Steps in the nursing process rather than nursing tasks were selected as the elements to be evaluated because well-thought-out steps in the nursing process are in line with nursing's emergence as an intellectual discipline that can define and manage health problems; the nursing process is under the direct control of nurses, whereas nursing tasks are often delegated by physicians; and the nursing process demonstrates a total picture of nursing care rather than the fragmented picture nursing tasks may depict (Phaneuf, 1972).

Data-Gathering Standards

The following approach was used for formulation of all standards. Each step in the nursing process was divided into several categories, all of which were related to the Johnson model in some way. In most cases, these categories were very similar to the categories of assumptions presented in the Johnson model. After the categories were identified, standards were formulated from various segments of the model.

Data gathering, the first step in the nursing process, entails gathering information that can be used to identify nursing problems. A nursing problem is defined as a patient situation that a nurse would attempt to change or maintain on the basis of whichever action she anticipated would attain her nursing goal.

The three categories of data gathering (Table 1) correspond to the model categories concerning man as a behavioral system. These are (1) structure and function of the behavioral system and subsystems and their interaction, (2) behavioral system balance, and (3) factors associated with change in the behavioral system and subsystems. Under the first data-gathering category, three standards were derived from the model in the following manner. The first standard states that it is necessary to obtain a complete history of behavioral subsystems and their interaction before the onset of illness. This was based upon the unit of patiency in the model, which implies that a change in patient behavior can be anticipated following illness. The second standard, which is based upon the same implication of the unit of patiency just discussed, states that one must make a complete current listing of behaviors indicative of the subsystems and their interactions, including a listing of physical, biologic, and social factors which might be significant in determining behavior. The standard contains this additional direction because a model assumption about man posits that behavior is influenced by the interactions of such factors. A nurse would need to identify these factors to assess possible

TABLE 1. Data-Gathering Standards for Nursing Practice

Categories	Standards
1. Structure and function of the behavioral system and subsystems and their interaction	a. Obtains a complete history of behavioral subsystems and their interactions before the onset of illness b. Makes a complete current listing of behaviors indicative of the subsystems and their interactions, including a listing of physical, biologic, and social factors which might be significant in determining behavior c. Gathers information about the patient's internalized values, beliefs, learning modes, and other control and regulatory mechanisms
2. Behavioral system balance	a. Observes and notes if the patient's behavior seems purposeful, orderly, and predictable b. Observes and notes approximate durations of periods of behavioral stability, when strong forces are required to disturb balance, and notes behavior related to adjustment and adaptation to changing conditions c. Collects data regarding the patient's personal preferences and requirements for nurturance, protection, and stimulation d. Observes and notes apparent level of energy expenditure, conformity of the patient's behavior with social demands, the quality of patient's interpersonal relations, and the patient's observable level of satisfaction with the hospital milieu e. Notes the patient's medical prognosis as an index of biologic survival
3. Factors associated with change in the behavioral system and subsystems	a. Gathers data concerning past and present factors related to inadequate drive satisfaction and lack of fulfillment of functional requirements of the subsystems b. Notes environmental conditions that might exceed the patient's capacity to adjust

causes of behavioral nursing problems. A third standard was formulated from the model assumption which states that regulatory and control mechanisms balance interaction within and between subsystems. Specific examples of control and regulatory mechanisms noted in model definitions of these mechanisms were incorporated into this standard, as explicit guides to nursing action.

Under the second category, standards were developed from each of the assumptions listed under the behavioral system balance category in the model. They were also derived from assumptions included under the model category dealing with functional consequences of efficient and effective behavioral system output, since these are related to behavioral system balance. The standards for the third category, factors associated with change, were similarly based upon assumptions included under the corresponding category in the model. The assumptions referred to here are explained in Grubb's paper on the Johnson model, which is included in this book.

Assessment Standards

Categories for assessment are exactly the same as data-gathering categories, and assessment standards were derived from many of the same model assumptions as those linked to data-gathering standards. However, the wording of assessment standards (Table 2) differs from that of data-gathering standards because requirements for the two steps in the nursing process differ.

TABLE 2.   Assessment Standards for Nursing Practice

Categories	Standards
1. Structure and function of the behavioral system and subsystems and their interaction	a. Notes current goal/drives, set, choice, and action and their interaction within the subsystems b. Compares current structure and function of the behavioral subsystems with past structure and function c. Assesses functional stress level by examining how adequately behavior within each subsystem achieves its professionally established goal d. Assesses structural stress level by examining discrepancies and insufficiencies within and between subsystems e. Analyzes efficiency and effectiveness of the operation of the regulatory and control mechanisms, including feedback mechanisms
2. Behavioral system balance	a. Assesses if imbalance exists in the behavioral system, based on findings related to purposefulness, orderliness, and predictability of behavior b. Assesses maximal durations of periods of behavioral stability, and examines the degree of adjustment and adaptation by means of nursing diagnostic exams constructed for this purpose c. Assesses requirements for nurturance, protection, and stimulation d. Assesses levels of energy expenditure, social adequacy, and patient satisfaction with hospitalization, based on evidence from appropriate laboratory examinations, observations of social behavior, and opinion questionnaires e. Assesses biologic survival outlook through findings of medical diagnostic examinations
3. Factors associated with change in the behavioral system and subsystems	a. Assesses specifics pertaining to inadequate drive satisfaction and inadequate fulfillment of functional requirements of the subsystems b. Identifies environmental conditions that exceed the patient's capacity to adjust

Collection of data requires only that complete inquiry be made and that information be recorded within certain areas prescribed by the model. On the other hand, assessment requires that all data be carefully examined, compared, and interpreted. For example, data gathering standard 1-b only requires that the nurse list all patient behavior that might be included within each subsystem, while the corresponding assessment standard 1-a requires that the nurse specify each structural element and its interaction within each subsystem. In addition, assessment may involve analysis of findings of diagnostic and psychologic tests and opinion questionnaires. Although it is not conventional for nurses to employ the use of diagnostic aids in formal nursing assessment procedures today, they may become commonplace in the future. Consequently, references to diagnostic aids are made in the assessment standards formulated from the Johnson model.

Diagnostic Standards

The nursing profession's task is the definition, explanation, and management of health problems that society accepts as appropriate (Johnson, 1972). Diagnosis encompasses the first two elements of the task: definition and explanation of nursing problems. According to the model, nursing problems involve behavioral system imbalance and instability, since these kinds of problems are at variance with the goal of action given by the model—behavioral system balance and stability.

The model implies three major categories of diagnostic standards: (1) classification and explanation of structural and functional problems within and between the behavioral subsystems, (2) classification and explanation of levels of behavioral system balance, and (3) definition of behavioral system objectives of nursing intervention (Table 3). The first two diagnostic categories correspond to the first two data gathering and assessment categories, since they were derived from similar model categories concerning man as a behavioral system. The third diagnostic category, dealing with objectives of intervention, involves an expansion of the model's goal of action to include several subgoals or objectives of nursing action.

Diagnostic standards were formulated from various sources associated with the model. Diagnostic standards in category 1 were developed from assumptions concerning man as a behavioral system and from one of the major units of the model. For example, diagnostic standard 1-a, denoting functional and dysfunctional behavior, is suggested by behavioral system assumptions that imply that behavior becomes functional or dysfunctional on the basis of goal-directedness. Diagnostic standard 1-b, denoting degrees and causes of structural and functional stress, was derived from the major unit of the model classified as the source of difficulty, which identifies structural and functional stress as causes of nursing problems. Diagnostic standards in category 2, which deal with behavioral system balance, were derived for the most

TABLE 3. **Diagnostic Standards for Nursing Practice**

Categories	Standards
1. Classification and explanation of structural and functional problems within and between the behavioral subsystems	a. Denotes functional and dysfunctional behavior b. Denotes degrees and causes of structural and functional stress c. Denotes defective system control and regulatory mechanisms d. Classifies all structural and functional problems within and between subsystems: dominance, incompatibility, discrepancy, and insufficiency e. Explains how problems in any subsystem affect functioning in other subsystems f. Explains how deficiency in one or more subsystems is compensated for in another or other subsystems
2. Classification and explanation of levels of behavioral system balance	a. Defines the "normal" state of behavioral system balance for the patient before illness b. Defines the level of behavioral system balance during illness as possible, desirable, or optimal
3. Definition of behavioral system objectives of nursing intervention	a. Defines objectives for the specific alterations in behavior that are appropriate for the patient within the limits of his social milieu and biologic and psychologic capacities b. Defines goals related to behavioral system stability and balance, integrity, adjustment, and adaptation c. Defines the level of behavioral system balance to be achieved through nursing intervention in a joint effort with the patient

part from the major unit of patiency as given in the model. According to the model, patiency is a situation in which the patient's usual patterns of behavior are threatened by loss of order because of illness. Therefore, a disturbed state of behavioral system balance during illness is expected. Consequently, diagnostic standards 2-a and 2-b are concerned with levels of behavioral system balance before and during illness. Diagnostic standards in category 3 were developed from major units and value assumptions of the model in a fashion similar to that used for derivation of standards associated with two other diagnostic categories.

Prescription Standards
Nursing prescription recommends nursing action designed to restore the client to health. The view of health dictated by the Johnson model as being appropriate for nurses and useful to society is behavioral system balance and stability. The first two prescription categories were formulated from the two intervention modes mentioned in the model (Table 4). These are (1) temporary imposition of external controls, and (2) fulfillment of subsystem functional requirements. Prescription standards concerned with the imposition of exter-

nal control and regulatory mechanisms were developed from examples of interventions given by Grubbs (1972) in reference to the Johnson model. Standards involving supplying conditions and resources for fulfilling subsystem functional requirements were based upon Johnson's (1972) suggestion that such requirements encompass nurturance, stimulation, and protection; and they reflect current methods used in nursing practice for supplying these requirements.

The third category for prescription was formulated directly from the diagnostic classifications of nursing problems recommended by Johnson (1972):

TABLE 4. Prescription Standards for Nursing Practice

Categories	Standards
1. Temporary imposition of external control and regulatory mechanisms	a. Provides protection by reducing or completely blocking external environmental stressors b. Provides functional outlets for emotions c. Reinforces functional behavior and extinguishes dysfunctional behavior to achieve overall behavioral system balance d. Controls the amount, kind, and frequency of succorance e. Sets outer limits for acceptable behavior f. Problem-solves with the patient
2. Supplying conditions and resources for fulfilling subsystem requirements	a. Provides nurturance by nourishing, cherishing, teaching, explaining, promoting the patient's development, supporting internal control and regulatory mechanisms, and by maintaining the patient in the best possible physical and mental condition b. Provides stimulation by providing opportunities for the patient's engaging in physical, mental, and social activities and by increasing the patient's general activity level
3. Diagnostic classifications Insufficiency problems Discrepancy problems Dominance problems Incompatibility problems	a. Provides the functional requirements of the subsystems b. Alters the goal, set, choice, and/or action within the subsystems until all elements work together in harmony c. Weakens the dominant subsystems by withholding their functional requirements, and strengthens the weaker subsystems through liberal provision of their functional requirements d. Shapes behavioral balance between the subsystems by modifying the conflicting behaviors until they are harmonious
4. Nursing-care plan for intervention	a. Writes a comprehensive nursing-care plan, listing all diagnoses, objectives of intervention, and intervention measures with their associated rationales b. Updates the nursing-care plan by means of continual assessment, diagnosis, and prescription

insufficiency, discrepancy, dominance, and incompatibility. It is not appropriate to state specific interventions to be included under these categories at the present time. There has not been enough study of the effects of specific nursing interventions used in the treatment of these problems to ascertain what kinds of ourcomes they lead to or what problems occur that are related to their implementation. Theory of this nature will evolve from the model as effects of interventions suggested by the model are analyzed in nursing practice. However, the general nature of the prescription for each problem is suggested by the classification of the problem itself. Associated categories and standards are (1) for insufficiency problems—provides the functional requirements of the subsystems; (2) for discrepancy problems—alters the goal, set, choice and/or the action within each subsystem until all elements work together in harmony; (3) for dominance problems—weakens the dominant subsystems by withholding their functional requirements, and strengthens the weaker subsystems through liberal provision of their functional requirements, and strengthens the weaker subsystems through liberal provision of their functional requirements; (4) for incompatibility problems—shapes behavioral balance between the subsystems by modifying the conflicting behaviors until they are harmonious.

The final category for prescription entails the writing of a nursing care plan for intervention. This category involves a summarization of all prescription measures and their rationale. Prescription standards included under this category are concerned with initial formulation of the nursing-care plan and the updating of the plan. This last category and its associated standards were not derived directly from the model. However, reason dictates that a complete listing and updating of all suggested interventions and their rationales must be available to practitioners in some form if prescription is to be implemented in a comprehensive manner.

Implementation Standards

The implementation step in the nursing process deals with how, when, and under what circumstances prescription measures are to be carried out. Implementation categories in this paper were formulated from value assumptions in the model and from criteria for social acceptance associated with the model (Johnson, 1972). The first implementation category directs the nurse to implement prescription in a manner congruent with the optimal level of behavioral functioning possible for and desired by the patient (Table 5). This category was developed from parts of the three following value assumptions in the model: (1) Nurses seek the achievement of the highest possible level of behavioral functioning by all individuals, (2) the level of behavioral balance achieved is judged always in the light of the individual's specific social milieu and biologic and psychologic capacities, and (3) the final judgment of a desired level is the right of the individual. The second implementation category directs the nurse to implement prescription in a manner that is useful and

TABLE 5. Implementation Standards for Nursing Practice

Categories	Standards
1. Manner of implementation congruent with the optimal level of behavorial functioning possible for and desired by the patient	a. Acts as an external regulatory and control force to try to balance the behavioral system and subsystems b. Validates diagnoses with the patient, checks with the patient to ascertain if the prescribed interventions meet with his approval, and modifies nursing action accordingly c. Meets the patient's requirements and personal preferences for nursing care when the patient needs intervention and, whenever possible, when the patient is receptive to intervention d. Continues to carry out only those prescriptions that assist the patient to achieve behavioral system balance and stability e. Does not carry out prescriptions that threaten biologic or social survival or that the patient refuses, unless, in the latter case, the behavior exceeds society's limits for tolerated behavior
2. Manner of implementation which is useful and congruent with social expectations and values	a. Avoids undue cost of treatment b. Carries out prescription in a professional manner acceptable to society c. Does not support behavior that exceeds society's limits for tolerated behavior d. Keeps complete and accurate nursing records

congruent with societal expectations and values. This category was derived from such criteria for social acceptance of the model as social congruence, significance, and utility.

Implementation standards included in category 1 were formulated from the major unit of the actor's role in the model and from model value assumptions. To illustrate, the major unit concerned with the actor's role states that the nurse should act as a regulatory and control force. Therefore, standard 1-a directs the nurse to consult with the patient about his nursing diagnoses and prescribed nursing care, is based upon the model value assumption that the final judgment regarding a desired level of behavioral system balance is the right of the patient. Standards associated with implementation category 2, which deals with social usefulness, values, and expectations, include current social values thought to be important by this author, since the model does not specify what these values are.

Evaluation Standards

Patient outcomes related to nursing action serve as the bases for formulation of evaluation categories and standards (Table 6). Desirable outcomes are those that reflect desired levels of patient health, welfare, and satisfaction.

The first two evaluation categories were derived from the two model

TABLE 6. **Evaluation Standards for Nursing Practice**

Categories	Standards
1. Level of behavioral system balance and stability achieved through nursing intervention	a. Observes if the behavior of the patient is purposeful, orderly, and predictable b. Observes the number and strengths of the stressful stimuli it takes to disturb behavioral system balance c. Observes how well the patient adjusts to changing conditions by evaluating how fast behavioral balance is restored d. Observes the patient's state of adaptedness by evaluating how much energy the patient can focus on situations other than on his own problems
2. Efficiency and effectiveness of behavioral output in achieving the goals of the system and subsystems, which are related to functional consequences of output	a. Observes the amount of energy the patient expends b. Examines the patient's record for notations regarding his medical prognosis, relative to assessing his outlook for biologic survival c. Examines the patient's record for accounts of the number of visitors and statements about the patient's interpersonal relations to evaluate his social adequacy d. Asks the patient to rate his satisfaction with nursing care
3. Correlation between the actual outcomes of care and the intended and unintended consequences of nursing care	a. Examines the patient's record to appraise the degree of correlation between preset objectives for alterations in behavior and actual behavioral changes b. Examines the patient's record to see if intended consequences of intervention have been realized—behavioral integrity, adjustment, and adaptation c. Examines the patient's record for specific positive and negative effects of unintended consequences of nursing care
4. Behavioral outcomes of nursing care matched against the value system of the model	a. Examines the patient's record to evaluate if behavior is within the social limits tolerated by society b. Observes if the optimal level of behavioral system balance has been reached c. Verifies with the patient that he desires the level of behavioral functioning that he is being helped to achieve

categories that are concerned with behavioral system balance and with functional consequences of effective and efficient behavioral system output. Evaluation category 3 was based upon the major units of the model concerned with intended and unintended consequences. Category 4 is linked to the value system category presented in the model.

Evaluation standards were formulated from major units, definitions, and various assumptions included in the model, many of which have been discussed previously. One additional point, pertaining to evaluation standards, should be mentioned. There are several sources of information the nurse could use to identify patient outcomes. These include direct observation, patients' records, and subjective evidence from patients. An appropriate source to use, relevant to the particular standard formulated, is indicated within the word structure of each evaluation standard.

SUMMARY

An attempt has been made to derive categories and standards of nursing practice from the concepts of the Johnson Behavioral System Model. Findings of this paper indicate that the model serves as a systematic guide for formulation of nursing practice standards. In addition, the model provides a basis for a comprehensive listing of many of the standards that would be needed to carry out each step in the nursing process.

A criticism of this presentation may be that in some instances several criteria have been grouped together in a single standard. For example, in data-gathering standard 2-d there are three separate criteria that would have to be measured: level of energy expenditure, social behavior, and patient satisfaction. For purposes of a nursing audit, specific standards would have to be divided into their separate components, or a system of quantification would have to be used that would take each separate factor into account. A major value of this paper, besides provision of a comprehensive listing of standards for nursing practice, is the fact that the approach used in formulation of standards from the Johnson model could serve as a guide to derivation of standards for other nursing practice models.

REFERENCES

Donabedian A: Promoting quality through evaluating the process of patient care. Med Care 6:3:181, 1968

Donabedian A: Problems of measurement. Part 2 of Some issues in evaluating the quality of nursing care. Am J Public Health 59:10:1833, 1969

Grubbs J: Operationalization of the Johnson Behavioral System Model for nursing, UCLA, class lecture, 1972

Johnson D: Behavioral system model—nursing practice. UCLA, class handout, 1972

Johnson D: The Johnson Behavioral System Model for nursing, UCLA, class lecture, 1972

Phaneuf M: The Nursing Audit. New York, Appleton, 1972

Joan M. Caley, Marilyn Dirksen,
Maryln Engalla, and
Mary L. Hennrich

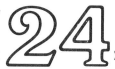

The Orem Self-Care
Nursing Model

This chapter presents first a theoretical discussion of the Orem self-care nursing model, then an example of the use of the model in practice. The theoretical discussion includes an historical perspective, definitions, and the elements of the model. The case study illustrates the use of the model with one psychiatric patient.

HISTORICAL PERSPECTIVE

Dorothea Orem's concept of nursing was first published in 1959. She describes nursing as "the giving of direct assistance to a person, as required, because of a person's specific inabilities in self-care, resulting from a situation of personal health" (Orem, 1959). She states that as persons are able to direct their own self-care, their requirements for nursing are modified and eventually eliminated. By self-care, Orem means the practice of activities that individuals personally initiate and perform on their own behalf in maintaining life, health, and well-being. Self-care is an adult's personal, continuous contribution to his own health and well-being. (Orem, 1971).

A more formalized development of the Orem model of nursing was initiated in April, 1965, by the Nursing-Model Committee of the School of Nursing Faculty of the Catholic University of America. Dorothea Orem was the leader of this group, whose task was to develop a model that would express the foundations for, and characteristics of, research in nursing. Members of this committee were concerned with the lack of specification of, and agreement about, the general elements of nursing that give direction to (1) the isolation of problems that are specifically nursing problems and (2) the organization of knowledge accruing from research in problem areas. (Nursing Development Conference Group, 1973). This committee developed, reviewed, and tested several tentative generalizations about nursing and submitted its final report to the School of Nursing in May, 1968.

Dorothea Orem published her second book, *Nursing: Concepts of Practice,* in 1971, after completing her work on the Nursing-Model Committee, while involved in the Nursing Development Conference Group. She provided a basic structural framework based on her concepts of nursing and self-care for the developing body of knowledge on the art and science of nursing. Orem states that "nursing has as its special concern man's need for self-care action and the provision and management of it on a continuous basis in order to sustain life and health, recover from disease or injury, and cope with their effects" (Orem, 1971). She related that self-care is a requirement of every person, and that nursing has its foundation in helping people meet this requirement.

The work begun by the Nursing-Model Committee was continued in 1968 by a group of eleven nurses of different backgrounds and areas of practice, who formed the Nursing Development Conference Group (NDCG). These nurses came together because of their dissatisfaction and the lack of an organizing framework for nursing knowledge. They believed that a concept of nursing would help to develop that framework. They held a series of meetings and cooperatively developed an approach to the structuring of nursing knowledge within a nursing framework (model). The concept of nursing as formalized by the NDCG was published in 1973 in *Concept Formalization: Process and Product.* This text clearly outlines the basic assumptions of the model concerning nursing and self-care.

DEFINITIONS RELATIVE TO THE OREM MODEL

In order to understand the elements of the Orem self-care model, the following definitions, drawn from the NDCG's work, are offered to the reader as a frame of reference.

Man is a psychophysiologic organism with rational powers. As a biologic organism, man exists, and responds both as organism and object, in an environment with physical and biologic components. As a rationally functioning being man formulates purposes about and acts upon self, others, and the environment.

Nursing is the giving of direct assistance to a person when he is unable to meet his own self-care needs. Requirements for nursing are modified and eventually eliminated when there is progressive favorable change in the state of health of the individual, or when he learns to be self-directing in daily self-care. The nurse (1) works directly with the needs of the patient, in close relation to his total living situation; (2) provides for direct need fulfillment—physiologic, interpersonal, and sociocultural—insofar as the patient, is incapable of self-care; and (3) functions on a basis of a holistic philosophy in assessing the areas of need, identifying, and utilizing resources for need fulfillment.

Action is behavior that is deliberate and intended to effect something to which it is directed, to alter its condition. It is particular to the person who endeavors to change or prevent change or preserve the state of something.

System is a set of objects, together with the relationships between the objects, and their attributes. The objects constituting the system behave together as a whole; changes in any part affect the whole.

Progress is a continuous and regular action taking place or carried on in a definite manner.

Patient is an individual who is in need of assistance in meeting his health-care demands because of lack of knowledge, skills, motivation, or orientation. The individual, with subsets of self-care agency and therapeutic self-care demand, requires nursing because of some health-related self-care deficits.

Self-Care Agency is the capacity of the person to engage in self-care. It is deliberate or voluntary behavior, and may involve habit. It is described in terms of abilities and limitations and refers to actions based on culturally or scientifically derived practices freely performed by individuals (or their agents). It is directed toward themselves or to conditions or objects in their environments in the interest of their own life, health, or well-being.

Therapeutic Self-care demand is a complex set of objectively established requirements for actions that assist a person with the maintenance of present states of health or well-being, or with movement toward estimated desirable states. Requirements can be of internal or external origin.

Orem (1971) further defines two types of therapeutic self-care demand: *Universal Self-care* is universally required by man and includes (1) adequate intake of air, water, food, (2) care related to excrements, (3) balance of activity and rest, (4) balance of solitude and social interaction, (5) prevention of hazards to life and well-being, and, (6) being normal.

Health-Deviation Self-care is required only in the event of illness, injury, or disease, including changes in (1) human structure (e.g., edematous extremities, tumors, amputation), (2) physical functioning (e.g., limited motion, colostomy), and (3) behavior and habits of daily living (e.g., loss of interest in life, sudden changes in mood).

Self-care Deficit is the qualitative or quantitative inadequacy of the self-care agency as related to therapeutic self-care demand. It exists when therapeutic self-care demand cannot be met entirely by the self-care agent (patient). The self-care deficit may be actual or potential (for example, in the case of a premature birth, the actual infant-care deficit may be the parents' lack of knowledge of how to provide physical care for the pre-term infant. A potential infant-care deficit could be the increased risk of parental engagement in infant abuse or neglect.). The self-care deficit or care deficit for another is the reason why nursing is needed; Nursing actions seek to overcome self-care deficits and to enhance and/or prevent loss of self-care capacities, and to enhance care capacities for significant and dependent others.

Nursing Agency is a complex set of qualities of a person acquired through specialized study and experiences in real-world nursing situations. NURSING SYSTEMS are the approaches nurses use to assist patients with deficits in self-care due to a condition of health. The nursing system for a particular patient in the Orem model may be wholly compensatory, partly compensatory, or educative-developmental.

Wholly compensatory system: The patient has no active role in the performance of his care. The nurse acts for and does for the patient (for example, patient is unconscious, or is totally incapacitated).

Partly Compensatory system: Both the nurse and the patient perform care measures requiring manipulative tasks or ambulation. Distribution of responsibility for performance of care varies with the patient's actual physical or medically prescribed limitations, scientific or technical knowledge required, and the patient's psychologic readiness to perform, or to learn to perform specific activities.

Educative-developmental system: The patient is able to perform, or can and should learn to perform, required measures of therapeutic self-care but cannot do so without assistance. The nurse's role in this system may be consultive only.

ELEMENTS OF THE MODEL

The Orem model focuses on nursing and self-care and employs an action system approach. This model can be analyzed using the elements of a nursing model as described by Johnson (1975). These elements include goal of action, patiency, actor's role, source of difficulty, intervention focus, or mode, and the intended and unintended consequences.

Goal of Action

The goals of action for the Orem model are as follows:

1. Accomplish the patient's self-care demand.
2. Move the patient toward responsible action in matters of self-care. The

patient either moves toward increased independence in self-care or adapts to interruptions in his capacities, or adapts to steadily declining capacities for self-care action.

3. Involve and transfer responsibility to members of the patient's family or significant others who attend the patient. As they become increasingly competent in making decisions about the continuing daily personalized care of the patient, or in providing and managing the patient's care, the amount of nursing supervision required may be decreased. Nursing consultation only may be required.

One or all the tools of nursing action may be appropriate in specific nursing situations. The outcomes of nursing are measurable in terms of the patient's or family's performance of self-care, according to established goals and/or standards. The goal of nursing is to keep the system in balance as the patient moves from health to illness or illness to health along the health-illness continuum.

Patiency

Nursing becomes involved when the therapeutic self-care demands exceed the assets of the self-care agency of an individual or group. To keep the system in balance, the patient requires the assistance of one or more nurses, who act wholly or partly, or educative-developmentally, on the self-care agency of the patient. According to Bachscheider (1974), "A deficit in the self-care agency establishes a need for the exercise of nursing agency."

The individual, with his own self-care agency and therapeutic self-care demand, requires nursing because of some health-related self-care deficit. This individual validly requires nursing assistance in specific aspects of his therapeutic self-care demand because his self-care agency in these aspects of care is limited in certain specific ways (therapeutic self-care demand→self-care agency→need for nursing system).

Actor's Role

The action, as previously defined, is undertaken by the nurse and/or the patient acting on the self-care deficit, or acting to meet the therapeutic self-care demand, which promotes balance in the system. The actual or potential difference between the self-care agency and the therapeutic self-care demand is the self-care deficit. According to Allison (1976), self-care deficit is the reason why nursing is needed, and nursing actions work to overcome self-care deficits and to enhance and/or prevent the loss of self-care capacities. The nurse also meets the therapeutic self-care demand. The actor in the Orem model is a combination of the patient and the nurse. There are in reality two actors in this model. The role of the patient as actor is to be responsible for his continuing self-care. The role of the nurse, according to NDCG (1973) is to help the patient

1. in the immediate exercise of self-care agency
2. in determining constituting parts of self-care demand and relations among the parts, and keeping therapeutic self-care demand adjusted to changes in the person or in the environment
3. in evaluating the characteristics of the individual's self-care system, with respect to adequacy, as related to an objectively established therapeutic self-care demand
4. in designing and assisting with institution and management of self-care systems that relate various abilities within the patient to self-care demand,
5. in designing and providing systems of assistance that substitute for the total or partial absence of self-care agency, and that compensate for specific inadequacies of self-care agency

Source of Difficulty

Quite simply, the source of difficulty in the Orem self-care model is a change in the health state, or some demand that self-care behaviors are not adequate to meet. In other words, the source of difficulty arises when the therapeutic self-care demand exceeds the self-care agency, resulting in a self-care deficit. For example, when a patient with a CVA is unable to keep his joints mobile, the nurse assesses the patient's self-care agency and determines that she must assist the patient in passive range of motion to prevent contractures. Another example of the source of difficulty is that of a newly diagnosed diabetic patient who is now unable to select his proper diet. The nurse assesses his self-care agency, determines he is lacking in knowledge related to his health deviation self-care, and selects his diet for him while she teaches him to do this for himself as soon as possible.

Intervention Focus/Mode

Briefly, the intervention focus deals with the self-care agency—the patient's knowledge, skills, and motivation. The intervention mode deals with the nursing agency—the partly compensatory, wholly compensatory, and educative-developmental systems that the nurse can use.

The intervention focus is on the "person as self-care agent". According to Orem (1971), unless the patient is able to face his own burden, and to struggle to live under it or improve his condition, he will not be effective in his role as patient.

The intervention mode utilizes the nursing process that Orem (1971) outlines as follows:

1. Determine why a person requires nursing.
   a. Determine the therapeutic self-care demand.
   b. Assess potential for self-care agency.
   c. Determine the self-care deficit in quality and quantity in relation to therapeutic-self care demand.
2. Design a system of assistance with therapeutic self-care and assisting components and plan for delivery of nursing according to the designed system. This nursing system is based on the patient's needs and capacities and designed in relation to the roles of patient and nurse as wholly compensatory, partly compensatory, or educative-developmental.
3. Initiate, conduct, and control assisting actions to achieve nursing results that are related to the identified therapeutic self-care requirements and to self-care limitations and abilities. Assistance can be provided by the nurse, family, friends, and/or community. Orem describes five general ways of assisting:
   a. Acting for
   b. Teaching
   c. Guiding
   d. Supporting
   e. Providing a developmental environment

Consequences: Intended/Unintended

The intended consequence of the Orem model is self-care, that the patient can realize self-management and provide continuing daily therapeutic self-care. Anger (1975) states in relation to a population of ambulatory adults, that "nursing's task is not to promote health, or to return an individual to a former and better state of health. Its task, instead, is to promote the individual's capabilities for rendering needed care to self in the service of his health state goals." Another intended consequence is that the Orem model helps establish boundaries of nursing practice.

Possible unintended consequences might be that when everyone is competent to manage their own care, there may be little or no further need for nursing. The patient may also choose not to engage in self-care.

THE OREM MODEL IN PRACTICE: A CASE STUDY

A twenty-three-year-old white female patient was admitted, somnolent but responsive, to an urban general hospital room after attempting suicide by ingesting an overdose of a tranquilizer and an unknown quantity of wine.

The emergency room admitting note stated that she was currently having serious marital problems, and that she stated that repeated attempts to seek help from friends that night were thwarted. She had made two previous unsuccessful suicide attempts. Mrs. B was found coincidently by her sister-in-law, who brought her to the hospital. A suicide note was found with the patient. Mrs. B told the admitting ER nurse that she would attempt to repeat the act.

Vomiting was induced and the patient was subsequently transferred to the hospital's inpatient psychiatric unit with an initial diagnosis of severe depression with serious suicide attempt.

In formulating the nursing-care plan according to Orem's model (1971), the admitting nurse on the psychiatric unit utilizes the steps of the nursing process as follows:

1. Determines why the patient needs nursing based on her therapeutic self-care demand, both universal and health deviation self-care status; her potential for self-care agency based on her knowledge, skills, motivation, and orientation; and the resultant self-care deficit, both quality and quantity.
2. Designs a system of assistance that is wholly compensatory, partly compensatory, or educative-developmental based on the patient's defined self-care deficit.
3. Initiates, conducts and controls assisting actions to achieve nursing results that are related to the identified therapeutic self-care demand and limitations of the patient's self-care agency.

Assessment of Therapeutic Self-Care Demand

The first task of the nurse is to gather information from which to determine the patient's need for nursing. Is the patient a legitimate patient?

To assess Mrs. B's universal self-care and health deviation self-care status the nurse elicited information from several sources: through patient interview and patient observation, from current and previous medical records, from other members of the health-care team, and from family members as appropriate. The universal self-care status specific to Mrs. B was assessed as follows:

1. Air, water, food: appears well nourished (5 feet 3 inches, 115 lbs); recognizes need for good nutrition, but often skips meals.
2. Excrements: eliminative functions essentially normal; past history of intermittent diarrhea and constipation; inactive hemorrhoid.
3. Activity and rest: expends extreme amount of energy ineffectually trying to cope with life stresses; difficulty sleeping when alone.
4. Hazards to life and well-being: enjoys alcohol and smoking cigarettes and using marijuana.

5. Being normal: neatly dressed, well-groomed according to accepted norms; utilizes preventive health practices, i.e., had physical exam two months ago; recognizes need for help and sought out marriage counseling; family role-models have exhibited deviant behaviors relating to use of violence and self-abuse, i.e., mother attempted suicide, father was alcoholic and physically abusive to wife and children; makes frequent self-deprecating comments; claims "embarrassment" as frequent emotion; feels at times that she deserved beating from husband and previous husband.

6. Solitude and social interaction: gainfully employed as dental assistant for past five weeks; enjoys job; does not like being alone; attempted to elicit help from friends before suicide attempt; does not want to terminate relationship with husband.

The health deviation self-care status specific to Mrs. B was assessed as follows:

1. Changes in human structure: none observed.
2. Changes in physical functioning: anorexia; weight loss in past two weeks; currently in menses, experiences pre-menstrual tension and heavy bleeding; currently taking antibiotic for treatment of diagnosed strep throat; diarrhea this a.m.
3. Changes in behavior and habits of daily living: loss of interest in life as evidenced by suicide note and drug overdose; insomnia; inconsistent food intake for past two weeks.

Assessment of Self-Care Agency

The nurse in determining the patient's self-care agency and his ability to maintain life, health, and well-being, assesses his repertoire of knowledge, skills, motivation, and orientation. The nurse then correlates these attributes with certain parameters that also affect his self-care agency. These include age, sex, health state, developmental state, and sociocultural factors.

Twenty-three-year-old Mrs. B appeared her stated age, and was physically mature without observable physiological defect or disease. She was employed, married with no children, having marital problems, the youngest of three sisters; she had friends. She was emotionally unstable. Her parental role models contributed to her poor self-image.

Assessment of Self-Care Deficit

The nurse determined that a self-care deficit existed because Mrs. B's therapeutic self-care demand exceeded the potential of her self-care agency to meet it.

I. Knowledge deficits
   A. Knowledge about physical and social environment
      1. Normal psychological responses to stress
      2. Coping mechanisms
      3. Conflict resolution without resorting to physical violence
   B. Knowledge about self-care goals and practices
      1. Motivational deficit rather than knowledge deficit
   C. Knowledge about scientifically derived health information
      1. Physiologic and psychologic effects of drug abuse
      2. Facts about cancer and hypertension relative to her personal risk status
II. Skills deficits
   A. Skills in utilizing available resources
      1. Skill in identifying and utilizing support sources available
      2. Skill in identifying personal cues alerting self to needs
   B. Skills in interaction with others
      1. Effective communication techniques
   C. Skills in activities of daily living
      1. Internal: control of behavior
         a) Specific techniques for coping with stress
         b) Diversional skills
      2. External: control of environment
         a) Independent living skills
III. Motivation deficits
   A. Psychologic maturity
      1. Maintenance of physiologic health despite emotional state
   B. Self-concept
      1. Formulation of personal goals
      2. Formulation of life goals
      3. Development of personal integrity
      4. Internalization of knowledge about self-care goals and practices
IV. Orientation deficits
   A. Culturally derived roles and practices
      1. Relationships with men
   B. Placement in family
      1. Youngest of three sisters (identifiable characteristic: no intervention possible)
   C. Membership in social groups
      (inadequate data available at initial assessment)
   D. Developmental maturity
      (no physical deviations noted; psychologic maturity deficits noted under motivational deficits)

Design of Nursing System

Once the nurse and Mrs. B identified the patient's self-care deficit, the nurse designed her interventions based on the specific knowledge, skills, motivation, and orientation deficits. Most of the interventions were related to the deficits in knowledge, skills, and motivation, as orientation deficits are more descriptive and oftentimes nursing and/or patient intervention cannot change these predetermined characteristics.

At this state of the nursing process, the nurse recognized Mrs. B's inability completely to meet her therapeutic self-care demand through her own self-care agency. The nurse recognized that Mrs. B did have some strengths in her self-care agency, but the health deviation self-care demands resulting from her psychiatric illness exceeded her self-care agency resources. The nurse therefore designed a partly compensatory nursing system to supplement Mrs. B's self-care agency and to overcome the identified self-care deficit.

Implementing the Nursing System

The interventions in the partly compensatory model are based on the identified deficits. Orem identifies the following categories of possible nursing actions: (1) acting for, (2) teaching, (3) guiding, (4) supporting, and (5) providing developmental environment. In implementing the nursing system, the nurse may use one or a combination of these actions (Orem, 1971). For purposes of this case study, the nurse prioritized the identified deficits and planned nursing action for the admission phase of Mrs. B's hospitalization.

Intervention Focus	Intervention Mode

1. Maintain physiologic health despite emotional state (Motivation deficit)	1. Guide and provide a developmental environment
	  a. Orient to unit
	  b. Daily suicide prevention contract
	  c. Diet as tolerated with snacks
	  d. Comfort measures for rest
	  e. Recreational and occupational therapy
	  f. Continued antibiotic therapy

2. Identify personal needs and support sources available (Skills deficit)	2. Teach, support and provide a developmental environment
	  a. One-to-one counseling p.r.n. to learn to identify and utilize support sources
	  b. Group therapy to learn to identify and utilize support sources
	  c. Develop list of strengths and weaknesses

3. Formulate personal goals (short-term) (Motivation deficit)	3. Act for and guide
	  a. Provide for regular meals with choices within structured times
	  b. Provide for socialization at appointed time with some choice involved
	  c. Provide for balance of rest and activity
	  d. Provide for choice situations/verbal contracts

Intervention Focus	Intervention Mode
4. Appropriate action based on identified needs (Skills deficit)	4. Teach, support, and provide developmental situation a. Teach patient to identify feelings b. Encourage patient to ventilate feelings c. Teach and permit patient to externalize anger d. Teach patient to effectively communicate feelings
5. Relationships with men (Orientation deficit)	5. Guide, provide developmental environment a. Provide male role models on unit, e.g., nurse, therapist b. Encourage interaction with males on unit, e.g., therapist, patients.

The nurse utilized knowledge, skills, and motivation in her nursing agency as she performed the above nursing actions. Although she acted for the patient in some situations, it was apparent that she chose a way of assisting the patient in learning new ways of meeting her therapeutic self-care demands whenever possible. In this way she increased Mrs. B's self-care agency and decreased the amount of time and quantity of nursing intervention Mrs. B would require in the future. She helped Mrs. B decrease her self-care deficit.

As Mrs. B's self-care deficit continued to decrease throughout the admission, treatment, and discharge phases of her hospitalization, and with her return to the community, her self-care agency increased and the need for nursing moved from a partly compensatory to an educative-developmental mode. She moved from a health deviation self-care state to a universal self-care state. The identified deficits in the self-care agency were acted upon as the patient progressed from illness to health. Additional characteristics of the self-care agency and therapeutic self-care demand could be identified at any time as the patient moved along the health-illness continuum.

REFERENCES

Allison SE: A framework for nursing action in a nurse-conducted diabetic management clinic. J Nurs Admin 3:53, 1973

Allison SE: Inpatient nursing: what is and what ought to be. The Alumni Magazine of the Johns Hopkins School of Nursing, Vol 75:1: 15–18, 1976

Anger MR, Komorski C: Components of a nursing program for patients in chronic pain. The Alumni Magazine of the Johns Hopkins Hospital School of Nursing

Backscheider JE: Self-care requirements, self-care capabilities, and nursing systems in the diabetic management clinic. Am J Public Health 64:12: 1138–1146, 1974

Backscheider JE: The Use of self as the essence of clinical supervision in ambulatory patient care. Nurs Clin North Am 6:4: 785–794, 1971

Crews J: Nurse-managed cardiac clinics. Cardiovasc Nurs 8:4: 15–18, 1972

Kinlein ML: Independent Nursing Practice with Clients. Philadelphia, Lippincott, 1977

Kinlein ML: The self-care concept. Am J Nurs 77:4: 598–601, 1977

Nursing Development Conference Group. Concept Formalization in Nursing: Process and Product. Boston, Little, Brown, 1973

Orem DE: Guides for Developing Curricula for the Education of Practical Nurses. Washington, D.C. US Dept of Health, Education and Welfare, Office of Education, US Govt, Printing Office, 1959

Orem DE: "Levels of Nursing Education and Practice," Alumni Magazine of the Johns Hopkins Hospital School of Nursing, 68:1: 2–6, 1969

Orem DE: Nursing: Concepts of Practice. New York, McGraw-Hill, 1971

Pridham KF: Instruction of a school-age child with chronic illness for increased responsibility in self-care, using diabetes mellitus as an example. Int J Nurs Stud 8: 237–246, 1971

Riehl JP, Roy C: Conceptual Models for Nursing Practice. New York, Appleton, 1974

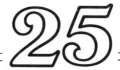

Leatrice J. Coleman

Orem's Self-Care Concept of Nursing

This chapter is presented in two parts. In the first section Orem's self-care concept of nursing is summarized in terms of the theoretical concepts that might be most useful within the nursing service department of a hospital. This summary includes the general concept of nursing and its elements, the classification systems for patients, the techniques essential for nursing practice, and the development and utilization of nursing personnel. In the second part of this paper, an application of Orem's concept of nursing is presented.

GENERAL CONCEPT OF NURSING

Nursing, according to Orem, is a specific type of health-care service based on the values of self-help and help to others. The goal of the health-care services is the health and well-being of individuals, families, and communities. Each health-care service has a particular role and a special focus for the activities it contributes to the achievement of this goal. The focus of nursing is to help the individual achieve health results through therapeutic self-care. Nursing practice is based upon the concept of self-care activities.

Orem defines self-care as the practice of activities that individuals personally initiate and perform on their own behalf in maintaining life, health, and well-being. Self-care action is the practical response of an individual to an experienced demand to attend to himself. The ability to perform self-care action reflects the individual's power of agency. To engage in self-care activities, the individual must have the ability and skills to initiate and sustain self-care efforts as well as the knowledge and understanding of self-care practices and their relationship to health and disease. The successful performance of self-care depends upon "the individual's level of maturity, depth of knowledge, life experiences, habits of thought and bodily, as well as mental health, state" (Orem, 1971). For self-care to be therapeutic, it must help to sustain life processes, promote normal growth and development, and prevent or control disease and disability and their effects.

CATEGORIES OF SELF-CARE

Orem identifies two categories of self-care demands and responses: universal self-care and health deviation self-care. Universal self-care is focused on integrated human functioning and human development. This category, often referred to as "meeting basic human needs," includes all those universally experienced demands that cause people to initiate actions. The universal self-care category consists of six subcategories:

1. Air, water, food—resources vital to the continuation of life, to growth and development, repair of body tissue, and to normal integrated human functioning.
2. Excrements—materials processed or produced by the body that are eliminated for physiologic purposes.
3. Activity and rest—patterns of energy expenditure and reserve required for optimal human functioning.
4. Solitude and social interaction—conditions of being alone or being with people, which are required for normal human development.
5. Hazards to life and well-being—conditions or situations that threaten or endanger the life and well-being of individuals or groups.
6. Being normal—efforts of the individual to conform to the norm of what is considered human relevant to current fashions, current scientific theories and facts, and cultural beliefs and practices.

Health-deviation self-care is focused on those demands and actions that the individual makes and requires only when there is obvious change in human structure, change in physical functioning, or change in behavior and habits of daily living. This category consists of the following two subcategories: (1) disease derived—changes due to disease, injury, disfigurement, and disability—and (2) medically derived—change due to the measures used in the medical diagnosis and treatment.

NEEDS FOR ASSISTANCE

Any interference with the individual's ability to perform adequately self-care activities decreases his power of agency and gives rise to a demand for assistance. When the reasons for such deficits are related to the individual's health state, this indicates that the person needs nursing. This need for compensatory action or action to help in the development of self-care activities is the basis for a nursing relationship. From the patient's perspective, nursing is assistance from a qualified person; from the nurse's perspective, nursing care involves "caring for, assisting with, or doing something for the patient to achieve the health results sought for him" (Orem, 1971). Ideally, the nurse works with the patient and his significant others to establish the nursing goals within the health care situation. These nursing goals direct nursing action and provide the basis for measuring nursing effectiveness.

NURSING PROCESS

For Orem, nursing practice involves a process of actions related to the nursing goals. This series of actions, referred to as the nursing process, includes determining why a person needs nursing; designing an appropriate system of nursing assistance based upon this determination; and planning, providing and controlling the delivery of the specified nursing assistance. The three steps of the nursing process are summarized below.

Obtaining the Nursing Focus: Assessment and Diagnosis

The first step of the nursing process involves assessing the patient's health situation, gaining a nursing perspective, and making a nursing diagnosis. Information is obtained about six factors: (1) the patient's health state, (2) the physician's perspective of the patient's health situation, (3) the patient's perspective of his health situation, (4) the health results sought for the patient and their relationship to the patient's life, health, and effective living, (5) the patient's requirements for therapeutic self-care, and (6) the patient's abilities and inabilities to perform therapeutic self-care.

This segment of the nursing process provides an accurate description of why a patient needs nursing care and determines the kind of nursing required. It entails "four phases: (1) communication and observation, including eliciting of information from the patient, his physician, and his family, which results in (2) a flow of information for (3) evaluation, analysis, and interpretation in light of the nurses' general fund of nursing knowledge, and (4) organization into relevant categories of information" (Orem, 1971). It may take hours or even days for the nursing personnel to obtain the information needed to provide the basis for understanding why a patient requires nursing care and to determine the most appropriate care for him.

Designing and Planning a System
of Nursing Assistance

The second step of the nursing process involves the designing and planning of a system of nursing assistance. Designing a nursing system is essentially a process of selecting valid ways of providing nursing assistance for a patient once his self-care requirements and limitations are identified and described. Orem suggests three basic designs of nursing assistance from which the nurse can select that system or that combination of systems that will most effectively aid in achieving the desired results for the patient. These three basic systems are described as follows:

1. Wholly compensatory system: The patient has no active role in the performance of self-care. The nurse assists by acting for and doing for the patient.
2. Supportive-educative (developmental) systems: The patient is unable to perform or can and should learn required measures of therapeutic self-care but cannot do so without assistance. The nurse assists the patient by supporting, guiding, teaching, or providing the developmental environment needed by the patient.
3. Partly-compensatory systems: The patient and the nurse both perform therapeutic self-care measures. The distribution of responsibilities for performance of care measures to patient or nurse varies with the situation. The nurse assists the patient by acting for and doing for the patient, supporting, guiding, teaching, or providing the developmental environment required by the patient. This particular system may take many forms.

The basic design of each nursing system indicates the kinds of techniques that nurses need to use in providing assistance. Although some techniques are useful in all systems, other techniques are specific to a given system.

Planning for the delivery of nursing according to the designed nursing system is the second part of step 2 of the nursing process. The nursing plan includes specifications for care measures, resources and coordinating activities, as well as the schedule of activities to be performed by the nurse, the patient, or others. Essentially the nursing plan is the starting point for the primarily practical phase of the nursing process, in which the methods selected for reaching the nursing goals are described in details of who, what, when, and where. The designed system of nursing assistance and the details of the nursing-care plan serve as guides for the nursing personnel during Step 3 of the nursing process.

Providing and Controlling the Delivery of Nursing Assistance

Step 3 of the nursing process involves the initiation, delivery, and control of nursing care according to the designed system of nursing assistance and the details of the nursing-care plan. This step is a cycle of assisting, checking, adjusting, and evaluating activities. Step 3 is the practical phase of the nursing process, which includes checking whether or not nursing actions have been performed, determining the results of nursing action, and gathering data essential for redesigning or readjusting the system of nursing assistance or the plan for delivery of nursing for the patient on an ongoing basis.

Each of these steps in the nursing process has many parts. Many actions are required to complete each step and provide sequential continuity between them. Although step 1 should be in process prior to or concurrent with steps 2 and 3, the use of these steps depends upon the nursing situation. In emergency or acute situations, the steps can enable the nurse to make rapid observations, judgments and decisions and to take immediate nursing action. However, in order to meet the nursing needs of a patient over time, each of the steps of the nursing process must be systematically performed relative to the immediate and the future nursing requirements of the patient.

CLASSIFICATION OF PATIENTS

Orem suggests two ways of organizing patients from a nursing point of view. One approach involves classifying persons from a health perspective as related to nursing care. The other approach entails grouping patients according to the three systems of nursing assistance.

Classification of Persons in Need of Nursing Care

According to Orem, a patient classification system organized and named according to nursing situations would be more useful to nurses than the present classification systems, which are organized and named according to medical concepts, such as specific medical fields or disease entities. In Orem's classification system nursing situations are divided into six groupings according to the orientation of the health focus for the patient. These groupings are summarized below.

Group 1—Life cycle. The health focus is oriented to the life cycle, and care is planned for the promotion of health and for protection against specific diseases and injuries. The life cycle focus is inherent in the health focus of the other groups.

Group 2—Recovery stage. The focus of health care is oriented . . . recovery from disease, injury, or a functional disorder.

Group 3—Illness of undetermined origin. The health focus is oriented to illness or disorder of undetermined origin. Health care is concerned with the degree of illness, specific effects of the disorder, and effects of specific diagnostic or therapeutic measures used.

Group 4—Genetic and developmental defects and biologic immunity. The health focus is oriented to the care and treatment of patients with structural and functional defects or a state of immaturity present at birth.

Group 5—Cure or control. The health focus is oriented to the active treatment of a disease, disorder, or injury of undetermined origin with concern for the degree of illness, the specific effects of the condition, and the specific effects of the therapeutic measures used.

Group 6—Stabilization of integrated functioning. The health focus is oriented to the resoration, stabilization, or control of integrated functioning. Health care is concerned with stabilizing and controlling the vital processes disrupted by the disease processes or by injury.

Classification of Patients According to Nursing Systems

Orem's three nursing systems provide a structure for organizing patients according to their nursing situation. Any given patient population can be grouped in terms of (1) the compensatory, (2) the partly compensatory, and (3) the supportive-educative nursing systems once its individual nursing requirements have been defined. This classification of patients is useful in planning for the number and kinds of nursing personnel needed to provide adequate nursing service for a given patient population.

TECHNIQUES ESSENTIAL FOR NURSING PRACTICE

Orem defines techniques as formalized methods for the performance of specific actions to achieve some particular result. Nursing utilizes a number of assisting techniques to achieve nursing results. The kinds of techniques needed are indicated by the basic designs of the nursing systems. Although those techniques related to universal and health-deviation self-care measures are basic to all nursing systems, each system requires specific and sometimes different kinds of assisting techniques. For instance, the assisting techniques required for compensatory systems differ from those required for supportive-developmental systems, but techniques from both these systems may be used in the partly compensatory systems.

Nurses should be proficient in the basic assisting skills essential for nursing practice. To function effectively within all systems, the nurse must understand and be able to utilize universal and health-deviation self-care measures. When compensatory systems are used, the nurse is the provider of care, but in supportive and developmental situations the nurse and the patient share in the provision of care. Therefore, assisting techniques must be developed that can be used by either the nurse or the patient in the performance of care.

Orem suggests that four types of assisting techniques be developed for the partly compensatory and supportive-developmental systems. These include helping the patient (1) perform care measures, (2) identify requirements for assistance, (3) obtain resources, and (4) integrate the required self-care measures within the system of daily living. Other assisting techniques include those used in (1) initiating, maintaining and terminating the nurse-patient relationship, (2) defining the role of the patient and the role of the nurse in the nursing situation, and (3) adjusting and adapting both nurse and patient to role changes as they occur within the situation.

UTILIZATION OF NURSING PERSONNEL

According to Orem, the steps of the nursing process are pertinent to both the delivery of nursing care to patients and the utilization and direction of nursing staff. Within the hospital setting, nursing service is usually provided by a nursing team comprised of a number of different types of nursing personnel, who are prepared to function at different levels. These types include the professional, technical, and vocational nurses, as well as aides, orderlies, and attendants. The complexity of the nursing situation determines which nurses are needed to meet the patients' requirements for nursing care. Some nurses are qualified to design, establish, and maintain valid systems of nursing for patients and to supervise members of the nursing team in their delivery of this care. Other nurses are qualified to function as team members who care for patients in accordance with established nursing systems. The qualifications for practice at these various levels are determined by the nurses' educational backgrounds and experience. With this many types of nursing personnel involved, it is essential that the hospital define and standardize the nursing functions and responsibilities for each level as they relate to the steps of the nursing process. These activities and responsibilities should be clearly specified in written position descriptions.

Orem emphasizes the need for planning and coordination of the activities of the nursing team. When nursing activities for the same patient or groups of patients are distributed to a number of nurses and non-nurses, communication and organization among these individuals is essential. Both the design for the nursing system and the communication activities of the team members can facilitate team effort. The patient-care plans provide guidelines for the assignation of nursing activity among team members. The requirements for nursing detailed in this plan determine which nurses are qualified to assist the patient and how the nursing assistance is to be distributed. For instance, the registered professional nurse may be responsible for assessing the patients' requirements for nursing assistance and for evaluating the results of the nursing care. The licensed practical nurse may be delegated the responsibility for providing the required assistance and for reporting to the registered nurse any observations pertinent to these care requirements. Each member of the nursing team must have specific information in order to provide the nursing assistance required by the patient. This information should include the patient's (1) nursing diagnosis, (2) designed system of nursing assistance, and (3) nursing-care plan detailed according to the designed system. Team efforts of the different tours of duty must be coordinated in order to insure the provision of continuous nursing care for patients. The activities necessary for the provision of such care must be specified for the nurses on the different tours of duty and an effective system of communication must be established among them.

Adequate staff development programs must be offered to prepare nurses who can perform the various steps of the nursing process, especially steps 1 and 2. Such programs should focus on the systematic use of the nursing process in the nurse's assistance of individual patients, as well as on enabling nurses to introduce adequate agency systems for the design and delivery of personalized nursing to groups of patients within a health-care institution.

APPLICATION OF OREM'S CONCEPT OF NURSING

This part of the paper addresses the application of Orem's self-care nursing concept as a guide for the nursing activities within a hospital nursing service. It describes the plans, the processes and some of the problems dealt with in an extant situation in which the director of nursing was converting a "theoryless" nursing practice to a self-care theory-based practice. The setting was a large major metropolitan hospital.

Once Orem's model was selected, the director of nursing and her staff formulated a two-fold administrative and educational plan for implementing the theoretical concepts throughout the nursing organization. The administrative plan entailed analysis and revision of the operational documents of the nursing service according to the elements of Orem's concept. The educational plan involved preparation of the nursing staff to understand and to use Orem's concepts for nursing practice.

Revision of Operational Documents

The primary function of the operational documents of the nursing service department is to direct activity within that department. The philosophy, purpose, and objectives of the department provide the framework for all further plans and activities. The philosophy of nursing expresses those values and beliefs that influence the practice of nursing in this particular setting. The purpose, which states the reason for the existence of the department, is elaborated into a number of permanent objectives, which are distributed downward through the entire organization and translated into objectives at the unit level. To effectively implement Orem's model, it was essential that the model's concepts be reflected in the department's operational documents and subsequently dispensed throughout the nursing service.

Department Philosophy and Goals

The director of nursing appointed an ad hoc committee representative of all nursing service personnel to analyze and to revise the departmental operational documents as related to Orem's concepts. Logically, these revisions began with the department philosophy. Since the current statement of the department's philosophy was compatible with Orem's concept, that statement was retained. The following statements were added to the philosophy to indicate commitment to Orem's nursing concept:

> Nursing is a specific type of human service based upon the values of self-care and care to others. Nursing services and activities are guided by Orem's self-care nursing concept.

After the committee had revised the statement of nursing philosophy, they began to rework the goals for the department in terms of Orem's model. Major changes among the goals involved incorporating Orem's concepts such as patient agency, nurse agency, nursing assistance, and the nursing process. The following examples illustrate some of these changes.

Example A

Original goal: The patients' physical, emotional and social needs are met by the highest possible level of professional nurse competence and understanding.

Analysis: This statement is incompatible with Orem's concept of nursing assistance. The phrase "patient's physical, emotional, and social needs are met" implies that the patient is being manipulated by the nursing staff rather than participating in the decisions and activities related to his requirements for nursing assistance. Rather than "patient's needs," Orem discusses the patient's requirements for therapeutic self-care as they relate to patient agency and nurse agency. Decisions regarding the nursing assistance required by the patient involve mutual contributions from the patient and the nurse wherever possible.

Revised goal: The patients' systems of nursing assistance are designed, planned for, and delivered with a high level of professional competence by appropriately prepared nursing personnel.

Example B

Original goal: To develop comprehensive techniques for obtaining complete history and information about the patient, together with individualized nursing-care plans, in order to determine and assess patient's total needs.

Analysis: This statement also focuses on "patient's needs" rather than on the concepts of therapeutic self-care, patient agency, and nurse agency. Instead of "comprehensive techniques . . . to determine and assess patient's total needs," the statement should indicate the use of Orem's nursing process as a guide for the provision of nursing assistance.

Revised Goal: Orem's nursing process is systematically utilized by the professional nurse for obtaining the nursing perspective and making the nursing diagnosis, for designing and planning the system of nursing assistance, and for providing and controlling the delivery of the nursing assistance required by patients.

Example C

Additional Goal: Orem's self-care nursing concept is to be implemented and employed as a guide for nursing practice within the nursing service department.

Analysis: This statement represents an additional goal rather than a revision of another goal. It was included in the departmental goals to ensure the utilization of Orem's nursing concept as the basis for nursing practice throughout the department.

Departmental Policies

Policies of the nursing service department function as broad general guides to organizational behavior. Clearly stated policies reflect the basic departmental philosophy, facilitate the achievement of departmental objectives, and provide the basic means for coordinating and integrating organizational processes. Therefore, it was necessary for the committee to review and revise these policies according to Orem's nursing model. For instance, the following statement was added to the orientation policy in the *Procedure Manual* for the nursing department: "Each new employee is oriented to Orem's nursing concept as a guide for nursing activities."

Divisional Philosophy and Objectives

Various committees were also formed at the divisional and unit levels for the purpose of revising their philosophy and objectives in terms of Orem's model. The following excerpts from the revised documents of the surgical division reflect the incorporation of Orem's concepts. The first deals with the division's philosophy, the second with its goals.

> Nursing is a specific type of human service which focuses on helping the individual achieve health results through therapeutic self-care. The concept of self-care activities is the focus of nursing practice. Underlying this concept is a basic commitment to caring for and about one's fellow man.

> To analyze and revise all divisional documents relative to Orem's self-care nursing concept.
>
> To provide the educational programs required for the nursing personnel to understand and to effectively use Orem's concepts of nursing as a guide for nursing activities.
>
> To establish standards of nursing practice relative to the surgical patient that reflect Orem's nursing concepts.

Position Descriptions

The divisional and unit committees were also responsible for carrying out the objective of analyzing and revising all nursing service documents and tools according to Orem's nursing model. For example, position descriptions for the nursing personnel required revision in terms of Orem's concepts. According to Orem these position descriptions should be developed in relation to the steps of the nursing process and the demands of various types of health-care situations. The following excerpts from the revised position description for Clinical Nurse II illustrates the changes that were made in order that it conform to Orem's concepts.

> Duties of the position:
> Utilizes the steps of the nursing process in the provision of nursing care for patients on admission and throughout their hospital stay.
> A. Gathers information to gain a nursing perspective and to make a nursing diagnosis; designs and plans appropriate systems of nursing assistance; provides and controls the delivery of the nursing assistance system by checking, adjusting, and evaluating nursing activities.
> B. Maintains preestablished nursing systems of assistance for assigned patients.
> C. Elicits full participation and contribution of members of nursing team.

Nursing Tools

The nursing admission and assessment sheet and the nursing-care plan were among the nursing tools revised by the committees. Both of these tools were crucial to the utilization of Orem's nursing process as a guide for the nursing practice throughout the organization. The nursing admission and assessment sheet functions as an aide to the nurse in gathering pertinent information about the patient that provides the framework for designing the required system of nursing assistance and for formulating the nursing-care plan. The revised tool facilitates this information-gathering process. For example, the format of the nursing admission and assessment sheet was redesigned to include space for the obtaining of data in the following categories:

1. Patient's perspectives of his health situation
2. Patient's state of health
3. Health results sought for patient
   a. Life
   b. Normal or near normal functioning
   c. Effective living despite disability
4. Patient's capacity as an agent of his self-care
   a. Present abilities to engage in self-care
   b. Health-related disabilities in giving self-care
5. Patient's requirements for therapeutic self-care
   a. Universal self-care
   b. Health deviation self-care

Guidelines constructed by the committee to accompany this particular tool contain questions the nurse might ask the patient in relation to each of these categories.

Revisions of the nursing-care plan included an enlarging of the form to provide space for the following elements of Orem's concept: (1) nursing goals, (2) requirements for self-care in terms of patient agency and nurse agency, (3) specification of the techniques, resources, and nursing activities necessary for the accomplishment of self-care measures. In fact, the nursing-care plan form is under ongoing scrutiny in order that a more effective, efficient tool might be developed.

Nursing-Care Evaluation Instruments

Instruments used for the evaluation of nursing care were examined and revised in light of Orem's concepts. The kind of change that was indicated can best be illustrated by an examination of the major objective of the *Standards of Nursing For The Pre-Operative Patient*. This objective was originally stated as follows:

> The major objective of pre-operative care is to attain the best possible condition of the patient for surgery. The means of achieving this goal are determined by the needs of the individual patient.

This statement is inconsistent with Orem's approach. The revised objective incorporates Orem's concepts such as patient agency, nurse agency, therapeutic self-care, and the nursing process.

> The major goal of pre-operative nursing care is to assist the patient in achieving the best possible condition of health for surgery. This goal is achieved by designing, planning for, and delivering the nursing assistance required by the individual patient.

Preparation of the Nursing Personnel

The nursing staff was prepared to understand and to use Orem's concepts through formal classes and structured clinical experience. Since the concept of self-care activities as the focus of nursing practice is the core of Orem's model, this concept was used as the base for the educational activities of nursing staff at all levels. Nursing personnel were expected to become conversant with Orem's terminology and to develop competency in utilizing the basic concepts, such as universal self-care, health deviation self-care, therapeutic self-care, nursing assistance and assisting techniques, as well as the nursing process. Professional nurses were prepared to perform the various steps of the nursing process by special staff development programs. These nurses were expected to make nursing assessments and nursing diagnoses; to design and plan systems of nursing assistance; and to initiate, deliver and control nursing care relative to the designed system and the nursing-care plan for each patient within a given patient population.

Change Process

The implementation of Orem's self-care nursing concept within the nursing service involved change. Therefore, it was essential that the nurse administrator consider the important factors of the change process, such as the time needed to effect the change, the resistance to the change, and the resources for implementing the change. Both the informational and the emotional aspects of change were addressed. For example, a system of communication was established to ensure that everyone was informed about the change process. Plans for following up the implementation process focused on maintaining changes and on evaluating the change project.

Currently, implementation of Orem's model is underway on several units within the medical and surgical divisions of the nursing department. Plans for expanding the use of the model will be activated once the model has been established in these areas.

SUMMARY

This chapter has demonstrated the usefulness of Orem's self-care concept of nursing in a hospital nursing service department. It has illustrated how the model is implemented through the nursing process, and how it is employed in classifying patients and in utilizing nursing personnel. In addition, the chapter has presented a specific instance of the implementation of Orem's concept in a large metropolitan hospital.

REFERENCES

Davis K: Human Behavior at Work—Human Relations and Organizational Behavior. New York, McGraw-Hill, 1972

Donnelly PR: Guide for Developing A Hospital Administrative Policy Manual. St Louis, The Catholic Hospital Association, 1973

Glaser BD, Straus AL: The Discovery of Grounded Theory—Strategies for Qualitative Research. Chicago, Aldine, 1967

Nursing Development Conference Group: Concept Formalization in Nursing— Process and Product. Boston, Little, Brown, 1973

Orem DE: Nursing—Concepts of Practice. New York, McGraw-Hill, 1971

Pigors P, Myers CA: Personnel Administration—A Point of View and A Method. New York, McGraw-Hill, 1973

Stevens BS: The Nurse As Executive. Wakefield, Massachusetts, Contemporary Publishing, 1975

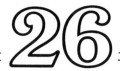

Martha E. Rogers

Nursing: A Science of Unitary Man

The explication of an organized body of abstract knowledge specific to nursing is indispensable to nursing's transition from pre-science to science. The need for such a body of knowledge can be identified in an escalation of science and technology coordinate with public demands for health services of a nature and in an amount scarcely envisioned by either the askers or the providers.

Traditionally nursing's goals have encompassed both the sick and the well, and the consideration of environmental factors has also been integral to nursing's efforts. Education and practice in nursing have been, without interruption, directed toward maintenance and promotion of health, prevention of illness, and care and rehabilitation of the sick and disabled. Recognition that people are more than and different from their parts has characterized nursing from the time of Florence Nightingale to the present.

Nursing as a learned profession is both a science and an art. A science may be defined as an organized body of abstract knowledge arrived at by scientific research and logical analysis. The art of nursing is the utilization of the science of nursing for human betterment, and its fulfillment is a lifetime endeavor. Historically the term *nursing* has been used as a verb signifying "to do." Perceived as a science the term *nursing* becomes a noun signifying "to know." The education of nurses requires the transmission of nursing's body of theoretical knowledge. The practice of nursing is the use of this body of knowledge in service to people. Research in nursing is the study of the phenomenon central to nursing's concern.

The uniqueness of nursing, like that of other sciences, lies in the phenomenon by which nursing's focus is identified. The focus of the science of nursing, unitary man, is a logical outgrowth of nurses' long established pre-scientific interest in people. Moreover in a universe of open systems (to be discussed later in this chapter) consideration of the environment must be deemed integral with the study of unitary man. Specifically then, the science of nursing seeks to study the nature and direction of unitary human development integral with the environment and to evolve the descriptive, explanatory, and predictive principles basic to knowledgable practice in nursing. No other science or learned professional field deals with unitary man as a synergistic phenomenon whose behaviors cannot be predicted by knowledge of the parts.

A conceptual system constitutes tbe substantive base of a science of nursing. Such a system is arrived at by the creative synthesis of facts and ideas and is an emergent—a new product. Theories derive from the conceptual system and are tested in the real world. The findings of research are fed back into the system, and the system undergoes continuous alteration, revision, and change commensurate with the new knowledge. A science is open-ended. The elaboration of a science emerges out of scholarly research.

DEVELOPING A CONCEPTUAL SYSTEM FOR UNITARY MAN AND ENVIRONMENT

Four building blocks are essential in the development of the conceptual system presented in this paper, (1) energy fields, (2) universe of open systems, (3) pattern and organization, and (4) four dimensionality. A brief discussion of each of these areas follows.

Energy Fields

Energy fields have been noted in the literature for several decades as constituting the fundamental unit of both the living and the non-living. *Field* is a unifying concept. Energy signifies the dynamic nature of the field. Energy fields extend to infinity. They have no real boundaries. However for purposes of study of a given phenomenon one may specify imaginary boundaries according to arbitrary criteria. This conceptual system is concerned with two energy fields: (1) the human field and (2) the environmental field. More specifically, man and environment *are* energy fields. They *do not have* energy fields. A field has meaning only in its entirety. It is indivisible. The unitary human field is not a biologic field or a physical field or a social field or a psychologic field, each of which deal with only a part of unitary man. The human field is more than and different from the sum of its parts. Unitary man cannot be understood by knowledge of his parts anymore than ordinary table salt can be predicted by a knowledge of sodium and chlorine. Unitary man has his own integrity. One cannot generalize from parts to a whole. The characteristics and behaviors of unitary man are specific to unitary man. The science of unitary man is a new product. Moreover the phrase *matter and energy* is redundant. Matter is energy manifesting itself in dynamic wave patterns. An energy field is the fundamental unit of unitary man and of environment.

Openness

Energy fields extend to infinity. Consequently they are open—not a little bit open, not sometimes open, but continuously open. The long-established view of the universe as an entropic, closed system is rapidly losing ground. Proposals that living systems were open systems led Von Bertalanffy to postulate that living systems manifested negative entropy. Evidence has continued to accumulate in support of a universe of open systems. The closed-system model of the universe is contradicted and obsolescence of such concepts as steady-state, adaptation, equilibrium and the like is made explicit.

Pattern and Organization

Pattern and organization identify an energy field. These are continuously changing. Moreover in a universe of open systems change is always creative and innovative. Human and environmental fields are continuously characterized by wave pattern and organization but the nature of the pattern and organization is always novel, always emerging, always more diverse.

Four-Dimensionality

The human and environmental fields are postulated to be four-dimensional. When Einstein proposed that the three coordinates of space and the coordinate of time be synthesized to arrive at a new dimension—the fourth—and postulated the theory of relativity, the universe took on an entirely new look, Newtonian absolutism was contradicted. The concept of four-dimensionality postulated a world of neither space nor time. Unfortunately words are as yet inadequate to communicate the scope and depth of this concept. A useful analogy of this difficulty can be found in Edwin A. Abbott's book titled *Flatland* (1952). This four-dimensionality is not a spatial dimension nor is it to be confused with fourth dimensions being proposed by other disciplines such as mathematics and psychology. A four-dimensional world is clearly different from a three-dimensional world. Efforts to schematize four-dimensionality require substantial abstract thinking. In spite of the risk of oversimplification and potential error the following sketch (Figure 1) may be useful. Imagine unitary man as a four-dimensional energy field embedded in a four-dimensional environmental field.

The four-dimensional human field is characterized by continuously fluc-

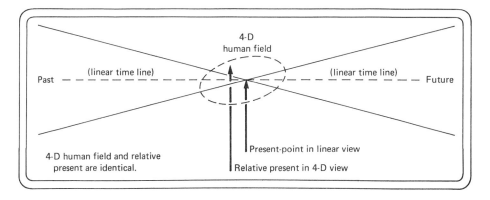

Figure 1 *4-D Environmental Field*

tuating imaginary boundaries. The present as a point in time is not relevant to a 4-D model. Rather the four-dimensional human field is the 'relative present' for any individual. Some implications for the explanation of paranormal events come into view. Four-dimensional reality is perceived as a synthesis of nonlinear coordinates from which innovative change continuously and evolutionally emerges.

The building blocks presented above are integral to the imaginative synthesis out of which a conceptual system emerges. Definitions of unitary man and environment give specificity to the conceptual system and are stated as follows:

Unitary Man: a four-dimensional, negentropic energy field identified by pattern and organization and manifesting characteristics and behaviors that are different from those of the parts and which cannot be predicted from knowledge of the parts.

Environment: a four-dimensional, negentropic energy field identified by pattern and organization and encompassing all that outside any given human field.

Each human field is unique, and so too is each person's environmental field. The human field and its environment field are coextensive with the universe. Unitary man and environment are integral with one another. Further, this system is postulated to be a humanistic model and not a mechanistic one. Human behavior manifests reason and feelings. Further it is postulated that man has the capacity to participate knowingly and probabilistically in the process of change.

Principles of Homeodynamics

Principles and theories derive from the organized conceptual system. First to be discussed are the principles of homeodynamics. These are broad generalizations that postulate the nature and direction of unitary human development. They are stated as follows:

Principle of helicy: The nature and direction of human and environmental change is continuously innovative, probabilistic, and characterized by increasing diversity of human field and environmental field pattern and organization emerging out of the continuous, mutual, simultaneous interaction between the human and environmental fields and manifesting nonrepeating rhythmicities.

Principle of resonancy: The human field and the environmental field are identified by wave pattern and organization manifesting continuous change from lower-frequency, longer wave patterns to higher-frequency, shorter wave patterns.

Principle of complementarity: The interaction between human and environmental fields is continuous, mutual, simultaneous.

These principles have validity only within the context of this conceptual system of unitary man. Their meaning has specificity within their definitions and provides for unambiguous communication. The principle of complementarity is in actuality subsumed within the principle of helicy. However for purposes of clarity as well as to emphasize the significance of mutual simultaneity and its contradiction of highly cherished "causality," it seems important to identify it specifically.

Reality "is" according to one's perception of it. How one perceives it depends on the conceptual model one holds of the world. What we see, how they see it, and the questions they ask differ according to their conceptual models. Within the context of this conceptual system, then, unitary man and his environment are in continuous, mutual, simultaneous interaction, evolving toward increased differentiation and diversity of field pattern and organization. Change is always innovative. There is no going back, no repetition. Causality is contradicted. Living and Dying are developmental processes. This is an optimistic science but not a utopian one.

The illusion of causality is one that many persons, including scientists, have great difficulty relinquishing. J. T. Fraser (1975) notes that "since Aristotle, Western thought has held causality and its corollary, lawfullness, almost sacrosanct." Heisenberg's principle of uncertainty, Plancks' quantum theory, and Einstein's relativity, introduced early in this century shook the physical world. Later Bertrand Russell (1953) pointed out, "The reason physics has ceased to look for causes is that, in fact, there are no such things. The law of causality is a relic of a bygone age, surviving, like the monarchy, only because it is erroneously supposed to do no harm." The appearance of causality is an illusion, a mirage. History tells us of persons burned at the stake for declaring the earth revolved around the sun. Michael Polanyi's (1958) comment that "almost every major systematic error which has deluded men for thousands of years relied on practical experience" is worthy of note. The appearance of causality does not make it so. In a universe of open systems mutual simultaneity is explicit.

Theories deriving from the conceptual system provide a means of describing, explaining, and predicting . . . unitary man. Only a few such theories will be presented in this paper. Their implications for better understanding unitary man and for determining the nature and direction of nursing intervention will be discussed briefly.

Theory of Accelerating Evolution

Change is postulated to proceed in the direction of higher wave frequency field pattern and of organization characterized by growing diversity. Higher frequencies portend acceleration. Multiple references of the past decade or so, including the best seller *Future Shock* by Alvin Toffler, testify to a speeding up of change. Simple forms change more rapidly than complex ones. Developmental norms of 30 to 40 years are no longer valid. People are sleeping less and living longer. The nature of motion common in today's world changes and its speed increases by leaps and bounds. SSTs and rockets to the moon are only a beginning. The Rand Corporation is currently developing a very high speed transit "tubecraft" that will whisk people across the country by electromagnetic waves at approximately 14,000 miles per hour. Travel time from New York City to Los Angeles is expected to be 21 minutes. Homes are filled with electrical equipment. Increasingly higher frequency waves are identified in atmospheric changes and radiation increments as well as in the practicalities of ultraviolet rays and ultrasonics. Man and environment evolve and change together. The doom sayers who propose that man is destroying himself are in quicksand. On the contrary there is a population explosion, increased longevity, escalating levels of science and technology and multiple other evidences of man's developmental potentials in the process of actualization.

One would anticipate that new norms might very probably include higher blood pressure readings and increasingly active children. *Normal* means average and average means a majority of the population. What is "normal" for one person need not be "normal" for another. What was normal 40 years ago would not be normal today. Large numbers of the public at *every* age are, today, reported to manifest blood pressure readings higher than the norms established some years back. Blood pressure is itself a rhythmical phenomenon. Accelerating change characterized by higher wave frequency field pattern and organization might be expected to manifest itself in new norms for blood pressure readings plus a wider range of distribution of differences among individuals. Similarly one might anticipate a speeding up of evolutionary development currently noted in the large number of children who are being labeled hyperactive.

Explaining Paranormal Events

Consider the point made earlier that "human field" and "relative present" are identical. Moreover what is a relative present for one person is different from that for someone else. Examine the implications for explaining precognition, deja vu, clairvoyance and the like. Clairvoyance, for example, is rational in a four-dimentional human field in continuous mutual, simultaneous interaction with a four-dimensional environmental field. So too are such events as psychometry, therapeutic touch, telepathy, and a wide range of other phenomena. Within this conceptual system such behaviors become "normal" rather than "paranormal."

Rhythmical Correlates of Change

Human field rhythms are not to be confused with biologic rhythms or psychologic rhythms or similar particulate phenomena. Human field rhythms are manifestations of the whole. Sleep/wake patterns when perceived as field behaviors point up both developmental emergence from sleeping to waking and signify evolutionary potentials of "beyond waking." Not only is there substantial evidence that man is sleeping less today (at all age levels) but that the sleep/wake pattern has changed.

In many studies in a range of disciplines increased physical motion has been noted to be associated with biologic, physical, and psychosocial development. But what about human field motion? Are the pragmatics of "taking a slow boat to China" or of comments such as "my motor is running too fast" (or too slow) or "stop the world I want to get off" suggestive of changing patterns of human field motion? What about the "multi-stimuli" classrooms in which many children seem to prosper? Validation of postulated indices of human field motion and developmental evolution is being sought in investigations currently in progress in the Division of Nursing at New York University.

When perceived as rhythmical developmental processes, living and dying take on different meanings. Perception of time's passing is clearly different from time estimation. Evolution from the pragmatic to the visionary bespeaks the fulfillment of new potentials and growing diversity.

IMPLICATIONS FOR PRACTICE

The implications of such theories for human service must be examined if the goals of a learned profession are to be met. There is nothing in this conceptual model that predicts man will be freed from all "disease" and live happily every after. So-called disease and pathology are value terms applied when the human field manifests behaviors that may be deemed undesirable. Values are continuously changing. Errors are often introduced. New knowledge revises old views. A few examples of changes in nursing practice based on the science of unitary man are presented below.

The Aging Process

Aging is a process that is continuous from conception thru dying. *Aged* is a term used to identify persons generally according to some established arbitrary chronologic decision. In this conceptual system aging is a developmental process. Moreover aging is a continuously creative process directed toward growing diversity of field pattern and organization. It is *not* a running down. The aged need less sleep and the patterned frequencies of sleep/wake are more diverse. A liking for sharp tastes among the aged bespeaks rather than deteriorating taste buds more likely an appreciation of the complexities of a range of taste phenomena. Cognitive skills are reported to increase with aging. Color preferences change in the direction of higher wave frequencies. Aging is not a disease. New life-styles are being promulgated by the aged themselves. Nursing's role in maintaining and promoting the health of the aged requires major changes in attitudes and nursing practice.

Hypertension and Hyperactivity

These behaviors are properly viewed as manifestations of evolutionary emergence. The mass marketing of iatrogenesis needs to cease. Why are third-graders being taught to use sphygmomanometers? What is the significance of mushrooming numbers of sphygmomanometers in multiple shopping centers? What is the meaning of a society of drug takers (and I am not referring to illegal use of hard drugs)? What is the relationship between labels and hypochondriasis and other forms of behavior? Change is developmental. Diversity is to be valued. True, parents whose indoctrination and wave patterns proclaim they need 8 hours of sleep in every 24 hours may have difficulty with their healthy three-year-old who refuses to sleep more than 4 hours in each 24-hour period. A nurse must demonstrate imagination and ingenuity in helping such parents to accept the "normality" of their child and to design ways of enabling both parents and child to fulfill their different rhythmic patterns without either's being condemned. New relative norms with marked flexibility and open-endedness must be initiated. A positive attitude toward changing diversity is imperative.

The use of this conceptual system as a basis for description, explanation, and prediction is far-reaching. Broad principles to guide practice must replace rule-of-thumb. The unitary human being is different from the sum of his parts. Principles drawn from the biologic, physical, and psychosocial sciences, no matter how excellent they may be in their own respective fields, cannot be used to describe, explain, or predict about unitary man. Calling nursing science a science of unitary man signifies nursing's potential for fulfillment of its social responsibility in human service.

REFERENCES

Abbott EA: Flatland. New York, Dover, 1952

Fraser JT: Of Time, Passion, and Knowledge. New York, Braziller, 1975, p 40

Polanyi M: Personal Knowledge. Chicago, The University of Chicago Press, 1958, p 183

Russell B: On the notion of cause, with applications to the free-will problem. In Feigl H, Brodbeck M (eds): Readings in the Philosophy of Science. New York, Appleton, 1953, p 387; cited in Kerlinger, Fred, *Foundations of Behavioral Research.* New York: Holt, Rinehart, and Winston, Inc. 1964

Toffler A: Future Shock. New York, Random House, 1970

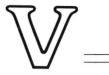

Interaction Models
for Nursing Practice

The topics of the four chapters in this section display considerable variety. In the first chapter Brink presents a systematic analysis of health-care delivery from the perspective of a natural triad. She offers a resume of Freilich's model in kinship systems and in acute-care settings, shows that the model is based upon normative role-performance, and discusses the inadequacies of the model in the areas of role enactment, prediction of triad development in new groups, and cross-cultural applicability.

The chapters by Riehl and Wood are presented as a pair. In Chapter 27, Riehl bases a model on symbolic interactionism, some of the theory of which is included in the paper by Rose in Part II of this text. Riehl discusses the assumptions, definitions, and concepts of the theory that are employed in the model and illustrates its implementation by examples throughout the paper and by a brief discussion of its applicability to the nursing process. In the second of these two articles, Wood reviews how the Riehl model can be implemented in nursing administration.

Chapter 29 by Preisner, is the last in this series. Although she uses a systems concept as a theoretical base, it is subsumed under an interaction model. This becomes evident in the focus of the model, which utilizes an eclectic approach to what transpires between the nurse therapist and her client, and, to some extent, in Preisner's unit of analysis for collected data, which is based upon her client's interpersonal life-style. In this chapter, she also relates her framework to the nursing process in order to illustrate how the two are integrated.

Pamela J. Brink

27

Systems Analysis of Health-Care Delivery: The Case of the Natural Triad

Models, such as the natural triad, are not particularly new to anthropology. In fact, prior to the impact of cybernetics and its application to social sciences (Bertalanffy, 1968), anthropology was using systems analysis as an approach to the study of culture groups. Since anthropologists were interested in whole cultures, usually island groups or isolated populations, they were forced into seeing how the various parts of the culture interacted to form the whole. The structural-functional approaches used basic systems analysis—a conceptualization of a whole with parts in interaction. Although systems analysis and model building were not unknown, cybernetics provided the specifications, or formula, by which a model could be built and its relation to social systems analysed.

The purpose of this paper is to discuss the natural triad (Freilich, 1964) as a model per se, as well as its application in kinship systems and in the health-care delivery system of the United States. The model appears to be based upon either expected or normative role-performance in traditional or authoritarian settings.

THE NATURAL TRIAD

Freilich designed the natural triad to explain the mother's brother's role. In certain patrilinear societies the mother's brother was a kindly uncle who had a warm, affectionate relationship with his nephew. The role of the mother's brother was just the opposite in matrilinear societies. Here the maternal uncle was a powerful figure who had full control over his sister's son. It was the mother's brother who was the decision maker, who gave or withdrew permission for certain activities, who was essentially the authority in the family. These seemingly opposing roles intrigued Freilich enough to examine them for any consistency.

What Freilich found was that there was a pattern of interaction that was repetitive in all these systems. In every society he examined, he found three roles represented: (1) a high-status authority figure (HSA), (2) a high-status friend figure (HSF), and (3) a low-status subordinate (LSS). The HSA was the individual who had the position of control or decision making. He was the authority in the relationship. Either the father ot the mother's brother could fill this role. The HSF was the warm, loving individual, close to the nephew or son. The LSS was always the individual in a subordinate position to the authority figure—either the son or sister's son. The basic structure of the triad involved one person of a low status and two persons of a higher status, an authority/subordinate relationship, and a friend or protector relationship.

On further examination of the sample, Freilich found an unanticipated relationship between the HSA and the HSF. The behavior required in the kinship system between the father and the mother's brother, regardless of which person filled the HSA or HSF role, was that of formality or avoidance. This would imply, or suggest, friction between the parties involved. The relationship was standardized in all situations.

Freilich diagramed the model (Figure 1) to denote the positions and relationships of the Natural Triad. The HSA and HSF were located in a position above the LSS in a status heirarchy. The authority interaction between HSA and LSS was designated by a minus ($-$) sign, signifying a basically negative type of relationship. The interaction between the HSF and LSS was designated by a plus ($+$) sign, signifying a basically positive type of relationship. The relationship between the HSA and the HSF was designated by a zero over a minus sign ($\underline{0}$) to signify negative or formal interaction or a total absence of contact through avoidance. The triad, therefore, was composed of one positive and two negative relationships.

The primary relationship within the triad was between the HSA and the LSS. Freilich, therefore, determined that there were "role protectors" to maintain the HSA in his position relative to the LSS. These were stated as follows: formal terms of address or reference; a limited rate of interaction; and a form of interaction designed to raise, maintain, or produce tension between the two parties. The relationship between the HSF and the LSS was secondary to that of the HSA/LSS. In the HSF/LSS relationship the interaction pattern involved informal terms of reference or address, a high rate of interaction and behaviors (on the part of the HSF) designed to reduce tension for the LSS. The tertiary relationship within the triad was between the HSA/HSF. Here the interaction pattern included formal terms of address and reference or avoidance of address, a minimal rate of interaction or total avoidance, and tension.

This was the basic structure and pattern of interaction of the natural triad designed to clarify the role of the mother's brother. The model was based upon an analysis of unilinear kinship systems in which the mother's brother was mentioned.

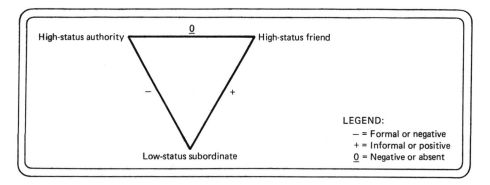

Figure 1 *The natural triad.*

THE NATURAL TRIAD IN ACUTE HEALTH CARE

The natural triad, as designed and tested by Freilich for the mother's brother, was tested in the acute-care setting of the American hospital system (Brink, 1972). The triad, as described by Freilich, was found to exist.

Within the American hospital system, the natural triad was formed by the physician as the HSA, the patient as the LSS, and the nurse as the HSF. The primary relationship of HSA to LSS existed, as described, between the physician and the patient with similar "role protectors." The patient addressed the physician by the title of "doctor" and often referred to the physician as "my doctor." The rate of interaction between physician and patient was limited. The physician visited the patient at least once daily either to chat, change dressings, or discuss treatment plans. Tension production occurred through the withholding of information such as diagnosis, prognosis or treatment plans, through lack of information on the above, or through the physician's being unavailable when the patient wanted to see him. Since the physician had full authority over the patient's hospital stay and made decisions for the patient in relation to his health and freedom of movement, he was the high-status authority for the patient. By virtue of the bureaucratic structure of the hospital, the patient was of low status and subordinate to the physician. The relationship could be described as formal, distancing and, therefore, negative.

The secondary relationship of high-status friend to low-status subordinate was fulfilled by the nurse/patient relationship. Terms of address or reference of patient to nurse were either the less formal title of *Miss* or *Mrs.* or the first name. The rate of interaction between nurse and patient was greater than that between physician and patient, and the role of the nurse was often that of a "buffer" between patient and physician. Frequently the patient asked the nurse to explain what the physician had said or done or to intervene between the patient and physician. In this sense, the nurse functioned to reduce tension for the patient.

The tertiary relationship between physician, as HSA, and nurse, as HSF, was also found to exist with the predicted qualities. By virtue of their separate relationships with the patient, the nurse and the physician often held conflicting opinions on issues of the patient's care such as information giving, frequency of medications, adequacy of orders for the patient's comfort and so on. Interaction was often formal as seen in the terms of address or reference, limited to exchanges over orders on the chart, or totally absent except for telephone conversations.

The setting in which the natural triad existed in its pure form was that of the lineal, status hierarchy of a bureaucratic hospital system. The major departure from the triad model described by Freilich for the mother's brother was that of a bisexual role relationship. In the American health-care system, although the physician can be of either sex, physicians are usually male. Nurses, on the other hand, are usually female. Only the patient as LSS can be of either sex with no change in status within the hierarchy.

The natural triad was also found to exist within the nursing hierarchy, with the head nurse functioning as the HSA and the staff nurse, licensed vocational nurse or nurse's aide functioning as the HSF to the patient, who clearly remained in the LSS position. In this case, role protectors remained much the same, and the role relationships between members of the triad were in the predicted directions.

The natural triad was found to exist in a bisexual form within a lineal system of authority. In addition, there were a variety of triads within the hospital system itself, apart from the primary triad of nurse/patient/physician. Each health discipline within the hospital could form triadic relationships with the patient as LSS or could form cross-discipline triadic relationships such as that between physicians and nurses. The decision as to which discipline or individual fulfilled which position in the triad could be determined by an examination of the role protectors used and by whom.

CRITIQUE OF THE MODEL

In Freilich's original article on the natural triad, he tried to extend the model to the American nuclear family. The attempt to transpose a model based on a unilinear kinship system and a unisexual construct met with little success in a bilateral, bisexual system of relationships. The natural triad of the mother's brother was based upon the following:

1. The mother's brother triad was found in traditional unilinear kinship groups. Freilich did not analyze the mother's brother in bilateral kinship systems.

2. The mother's brother triad was based on a unisexual construct. Freilich did not extend or examine the relationships between mother's brother, mother, and daughter/son.
3. The status hierarchy of the original triad was based on generation. Freilich did not describe factors other than generation.
4. The model was developed from ethnographic accounts of the normative or expected role-performance of the members of the triad. Freilich had no way of knowing whether or not these accounts actually represented a mean distribution of actual role performances or what, if any, deviant behaviors occurred. No description was given of conflicts that arose as a result of nonconformity with the role prescriptions.

For a model of human behavior to be successfully applied to areas other than that for which it was designed, the rules by which the model was developed must be clearly specified. In addition, since a model is simply a diagrammatic schema representing the system under analysis, the rules for systems analysis should be adhered to. Let us examine the model of the natural triad from the systems analysis approach.

A system is simply a conceptualization of a whole, composed of parts in interaction. Once a particular system has been isolated for study, the boundaries of the system should be identified to distinguish that system from other systems and from the environment from which it has been isolated. We can accept, on principle, that the natural triad is indeed a system with parts in interaction. The three parts to the system (HSA, HSF, and LSS) form an isolable group within a kinship system. As described, however, the natural triad exists in either matrilineal or patrilineal kinship systems only. If the natural triad is to be examined within the kinship system, as the macrosystem or the environment, then all forms of descent groups must be incorporated into the analysis.

The second rule of systems analysis is that all systems interact with their environment in the form of input, transformation, and feedback. The relationship between the system under analysis and its environment should, therefore, be clearly specified. We cannot find the environment within which the natural triad subsists and to which it is in closest juxtaposition. From where does the mother's brother relationship receive its input, from the family, the household, the lineage system, the value system, the economic system or the political system? If we can speculate that the interaction within the triad fits the criteria for the process of transformation, we are still left with the question of feedback. To what environment does the triad feed back, to a system other than the one from which it received input, the same system, or to the environment as a whole?

Systems are usually designated as *open* or *closed*. The definition of open or closed that I prefer places the system on a continuum. The more closed a system, the less interaction occurs between the system and its environment and the more predictable the feedback. Conversely, the more open the system, the more interaction occurs between the system and its environment, the more variables must be accounted for, and the less predictable is the feedback as a result of the variation of possible equations in the transformation process. The natural triad, as originally conceived, appears to be a relatively closed system. There seems to be either minimal or no interaction with the environment and, consequently, highly predictable feedback. Although the rules for human behavior may be quite clearly specified for a particular social system and its subsystems, individual humans may or may not behave according to the rules. Therefore analysis of the behavioral system should delineate whether it is dealing with the closed system of the rules for behavior or the infinitely more open system of how the individual actually behaves. The mother's brother triad seems to be based upon the *rules* of interaction between the members of the lineage, rather than how the individual behaved in every instance of interaction within the triadic situation.

The analysis of a system should include the concepts of *entropy* and *equilibrium*. The concept of a system involves energy. A system receives energy from the environment, transforms that energy into a usable form, and then discharges unused energy as well as transformed energy back into the environment. As the system moves through these processes, it uses up its available supply of energy, so is in a state of flux, disorganization, energy loss or entropy. In order to survive (i.e., remain intact) systems tend toward homeostasis. In other words, to counteract the effects of entropy, systems constantly attempt to equilibrate themselves through a balancing of energy resources. For example, if a system is receiving low energy input, the rate of transformation and energy use must also slow down. The output of energy from the system is therefore reduced. In the event that a system receives too much energy at any given time, the system must transform the energy at a higher rate, convert some of the energy for storage purposes, and/or eliminate at a higher rate transformed or unused energy in order to maintain its own functioning. In his original article Freilich (1964) stated that the system "tended toward" equilibrium through the balancing of the negative and positive aspects of the interaction forms, but he did not deal with the concept of entropy.

Since all parts of a system interact with one another, a change in one part will affect all other parts of the system. Parts of a system are always in process, adjusting to the changes that are taking place. The more open the system (the more variables that must be incorporated into the system), the more change is taking place and the greater the rate of adjustment. Freilich does not deal with this. Yet any model of human behavior should incorporate this principle in order to allow for change. Freilich's discussion of the American nuclear family would have been enhanced had he incorporated this concept in his paper. In the bilateral American kinship system, the explicitly stated rule of behavior (or value system, if you will) is that the father is the head of the family. The "rule," therefore, for behavior within the father/mother/child triad is that the father is the HSA, the mother is the HSF, and the child is the LSS. How does the triad adjust if the mother takes on the HSA role in some situations and the father remains HSA in others? How does the triad adjust to the situation in which the parents confer the HSA position on the child? Freilich's hesitancy in discussing this area arose from his initial designation of the natural triad as a closed system based upon the normative rules of behavior. Since his experience with American nuclear families did not always fit the rules, he was restricted by his own model. Without the incorporation of this one basic principle, Freilich's model remains an analysis of a closed system of behavioral rules rather than a model for predicting human behavior within a situational context.

When I attempted to extend the natural triad into the American health-care delivery system, I ran into the same difficulties as did Freilich in the nuclear family situation. The model simply does not fit open systems of behavior in which individuals have a choice of interaction patterns. In the acute-care setting of the hospital situation, the patient is expected to behave as an LSS. What happens when the patient refuses to behave according to the rules? Many patients today are questioning their physicians about their diagnoses, treatment, medications, and even the lengths of their hospital stays. Some patients are demanding a higher rate of interaction with their physicians, are using informal terms of address and reference, and are very well read on their own diagnosis. In essence, the patient is refusing to acknowledge the authority of the physician and is reducing his status. Many patients are refusing to turn to the nurses as the buffering agent between themselves and the physician and are going to the physician directly. These nonadherence behaviors to the traditional rules for patient behavior are more clearly represented by the path consistency construct (Sweetser, 1967). Sweetser challenged Freilich's natural triad model from that point of view in her paper.

When hospital situations outside of the United States were examined for the natural triad, there were problems in those settings as well. Prior to the 1960s, in many Central American countries, the nurse was the LSS. Nurses were of the same status as housekeepers or the cooks. In fact, when a young woman with no experience applied for a position in a hospital, She was offered one of these three jobs. The education of nurses has changed since that time so that the possibility of the existence of the natural triad is greater today than it was then.

In the British system, the ward matron is the high-status authority on her ward, and all persons (including the physician) are expected to defer to her decisions on ward matters. In other situations, the physician is the HSA.

These examples present problems for analysis closely akin to the dilemma in which Freilich found himself when he was analysing the American nuclear family.

The last area in which I found myself experiencing difficulties with the model was that of prediction. In a newly forming group, how does the theorist predict the development of the triad? If we take the situation of the community mental health centers that are proliferating in the United States, the problem is apparent. These centers employ therapists from a variety of disciplines—medicine, psychology, nursing, and social work. The client (as the patient is termed) walks into the center and is assigned a therapist. The therapist is obviously the high-status authority and the client is again the low-status subordinate. Who then fills the position of the high-status friend? Even if the therapist requests consultation with a colleague or is under supervision for his case load, the client never meets these other professionals. Since the formal organization of these mental health centers is not lineal in nature but rather collateral, the possibility exists that the natural triad as a model is restricted to lineal hierarchical organizations. In addition, the model is best applied in traditional settings in which behavioral rules have been set, rather than in developing organizations.

A final point needs to be made about the model. Freilich used small, isolated or well-defined social systems for the development of the triad. In these societies, all members of the group understood the rules of behavior for given situations and for given status positions. In essence, the smallness of the societies enhanced the ability of the members to share similar or identical cognitive maps of their social system. This is not true of exceedingly large, complex systems such as the United States. Therefore the expectation that each member of a natural triad in the health-care system sees his role relationships in opposition to each other in the same way is pure fantasy. Members of the same health discipline do not interpret their roles identically in relation either to their peers or to allied fields. Therefore, an analysis of the natural triad would have to be based on normative, repetitive behaviors within situated activity systems (Goffman, 1961) rather than on a shared system of rules of behavior.

CONCLUSIONS

This paper has attempted to apply Freilich's model of the natural triad to the American health-care delivery system. The model was found to be useful when applied to traditional role sets that had been in existence over time. The model was also useful in predicting role strain or conflict between persons who fill the positions of HSA and HSF. This delineation of role strain or role conflict between the HSA and the HSF is a significant contribution to role theory. The model was found to be more of a closed system than an open system with the boundary-maintaining mechanisms operating rigidly and inflexibly toward environmental interaction. The model was also found to be limited to normative situations and was not readily applicable to situated activity systems or to actual role performances. In addition, as a predictor of future triad development, the model falls short. Testing of the model in the field would probably provide guidelines for the incorporation of these limitations and should be expedited.

A model is a mechanical schema based upon past interactions. The larger and more open the system to the environment, the more variables are present, and therefore the more change is likely to take place. A model is expected to simplify and present in a diagrammatic way the basic nature of the parts in interaction. Therefore a model of human behavior must be derived from the arithmetic mean of repetitive social interactions or the normative rules of behavior. To open a model to deviants at either end of the normal curve threatens the simplicity of the construct.

As a model, the natural triad exemplifies the limitations of most models of human behavior. A behavioral model is a post hoc description of behavioral rules or at best normative or expected behavioral patterns. The model allows for the existence of one role set at a time, in which one individual fills only one position at a time. The person occupying the position cannot be described in relation to his attitude or sentiment toward his position. Finally, models are limited in their predictive value. Since a model is set, it can only predict future behaviors based upon past behaviors that occurred within the specified formula. Models are unable to predict change within the system if one part fails to function or changes its function. The strength of models lies in their ability to organize and simplify descriptive data.

ACKNOWLEDGMENT

I wish to acknowledge Morris Freilich for providing me with the idea for the original application of his model to the health-care delivery system.

REFERENCES

Bertalanffy L: General systems theory. A critical review. In Buckley W (ed): Modern Systems Research for the Behavioral Scientist. Chicago, Aldine, 1968

Brink PJ: Natural triad in health care. Am J Nurs 72:897−899, 1972

Freilich M: The natural triad in kinship and complex systems. Am Sociol Rev 29:529−540, 1964

Goffman E: Encounters. Indianapolis, Bobbs-Merrill, 1961

Sweetser DA: Path consistency in directed graphs and social structure. Am J Sociol 73:287−293, 1967

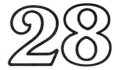

Joan P. Riehl

The Riehl Interaction Model

A review of nursing models indicates any given framework is based upon a theory and includes the basic assumptions, definitions, and concepts of the theory relevant to the model. These key factors will therefore be presented as the basic structure of the approach discussed in this chapter.

The underlying perspective for this model is symbolic interactionism (SI) which is based upon one approach to self-concept theory (Wells & Marwell, 1976). A basic premise is that the self-concept is the key element between behavior and the social organization to which the individual belongs. The self-concept (responding to oneself as an object) is essential for us to behave as human (i.e. to have minded behavior). One of several dichotomous issues in the SI approach to self theory is the concept of the self as a conscious versus an unconscious dimension. Symbolic interactionists, e.g., Mead and Blumer, define the self in terms of observable behavior and believe the self is only operative in self-conscious behavior. They view self behavior as thinking behavior. It is not an habitual process, nor does it include levels of consciousness as in the psychoanalytic model as advocated by Freud and his followers.

Although many have contributed to this theory, George Mead (1934) was an early writer to whom much of its content can be attributed. Herbert Blumer (1969) is a leading exponent of this theory today and defines SI as the interaction that occurs between human beings who interpret or define each other's actions instead of just reacting to them. Their responses are based on the meanings they attach to such actions. In SI, social action is lodged in the acting individuals, who fit their lines of action to one another through a process of interpretation. Group action is the collaborative action of these individuals. Arnold Rose (1962), whose article in this text is entitled "A Systematic Summary of Symbolic Interaction Theory," discusses the assumptions of this theory in analytical and generic terms. The generic focus is on the youngster and especially on the socialization of the child, while the analytical focus includes all other ages. These assumptions complement other theories well, such as Erikson's (1963) eight ages of man.

ANALYTIC ASSUMPTIONS

Since these assumptions are discussed in detail in the article by Rose, they will only be briefly reviewed here. The analytic assumptions with pertinent comments are as follows.

Assumption 1. *Man lives in a symbolic as well as in a physical environment and can be stimulated to act by symbols as well as by physical stimuli.*

Assumption 2. *Through symbols, man has the capacity to stimulate others in ways other than those in which he himself is stimulated.*
This important assumption includes a discussion on role taking, which is pertinent to nursing, and differentiates between significant symbols, which require interpretation, and natural signs, which are instinctive responses.

Assumption 3. *Through communication of symbols, man can learn huge numbers of meanings and values—and hence ways of acting—from other men.*
From this it is assumed that man's behavior is learned throughout his life. It is specifically learned through symbolic communication rather than through trial and error or conditioning, for example. As a result, man has a culture, which guides his behavior.

The general proposition, or deduction, that emerges from this assumption is that through the learning of a culture, or subculture, men are able to predict each other's behavior and gauge their own behavior accordingly.

Assumption 4. *The symbols—and the meanings and values to which they refer—do not occur in isolated bits, but in large and complex clusters.*
The latter refers to the term *role,* that which guides an individual's behavior, such as the nurse's role or the patient's role. A general proposition of this assumption is that the individual defines himself as well as other objects, actions, and characteristics. As defined by Mead, the self, whose structure is binary, consists of a role taker called a "me," and the perception of the person as a whole, which is called the "I," or self-concept. Since the "me" is made up of the attitudes of others, these others can take this role and predict an individual's behavior in a given capacity. Thus, in nursing, we have job

descriptions of positions that numerous persons can fill. However, since it takes a series of "me's" to make up an "I," each person in a given position behaves differently, with some more successful than others in a particular role.

There are two concepts using the term role that are often confused in the literature (Lindesmith and Strauss, 1949; Newcomb, 1950; Sergent, 1950). These concepts, *role-taking* and *role-playing,* have been clarified by Contu (1951). He points out that playing at a role represents role-taking on an elementary level and pretending to play a well-known role. Role-taking is a psychological concept instituted by George Mead which is a mental or cognitive activity (not overt behavior), and means the taking into oneself of another person's attitude, point of view, or perceptual field. Mead's usage of the term referred to the symbolic process in which a person puts himself in the other's place to gain insight, to anticipate another's behavior, and to act accordingly. Role-playing is a sociological concept that refers to behavior, performance, conduct, overt activity, or a socially prescribed way of behaving in particular situations. A man's occupying the position or status of parent, for example, is expected to play the role of father—which involves a series of role behaviors in regard to his child.

Assumption 5 *Thinking is the process by which possible symbolic solutions and other future courses of action are examined, assessed for their relative advantages and disadvantages in terms of the values of the individual, and chosen for action or rejected.*

This assumption covers the nursing process as it is often defined, i.e., the inclusive steps of nursing assessment, diagnosis, planned intervention, and evaluation of action. Closely related to this assumption are three premises identified by Blumer (1969): (1) Humans act toward things on the basis of the meaning things have for them; (2) the meaning of things arises from the social interaction one has with one's fellows; and (3) meanings are handled through an interpretive process by the person's dealing with the things he encounters. Since meaning arises in the process of interaction between two persons, and individuals differ, even the most carefully thought out plan may go awry. For example, Faris (1964) identifies four varieties of action: (1) immediate, which is infrahuman; (2) delayed, which is mediated by thought and conversation by humans; (3) frustrated, which too often happens; and (4) retrospective (hindsight), as meaning arises (insight, or the "aha" phenomenon) and self-appraisal occurs.

In SI much emphasis is placed on action. In fact, a cardinal principle is that any empirically oriented scheme of human society must respect the fact that human societies consist of people engaging in action. In addition to action, SI is grounded on a number of other basic ideas. They depict the nature of human groups or societies, social interaction, objects, human beings as actors, and the interconnection of the lines of action. In discussing actors, Blumer (1969) explores role taking. He points out that a human being can be an object of his own action, e.g., when he places himself in the position of others to obtain their viewpoint. And in regard to action, a key factor of SI is that one has to get inside of the defining process of the actor in order to understand his action. This is no small task but is essential to effect a behavioral change.

Blumer describes four central concepts of SI. (1) People, individually and collectively, are prepared to act on the basis of the meanings of objects that comprise their world. (2) The association of people is necessary as a process in which they make indications to one another and interpret each other's indications. (3) Social acts, whether individual or collective, are constructed through a process in which the actors note, interpret, and assess the situation confronting them. (4) The complex interlinkages of acts that comprise organizations, institutions, division of labor, and networks of interdependency are moving and not static affairs.

GENERIC ASSUMPTIONS

Rose identifies and discusses four generic assumptions.

Assumption 1. *Society—a network of interacting individuals—with its culture—the related meanings and values by means of which individuals interact—precedes any existing individual.*

Assumption 2. *The process by which socialization takes place can be thought of as occurring in three stages.*
(1) The infant is habituated to a certain sequence of behaviors and events through a psychogenic process, such as trial and error. (2) When the habit is blocked, the image of the incomplete act arises in the infant's mind and he thus learns to differentiate the object (e.g., *mother*) in that act by a symbol (the word *mother*). In time, the social behavior of the individual and his personality develop from his ongoing social acts. And, according to Mead, the individual's ability to use language is the nexus between the social process and his emergent personality. (3) As the infant acquires a number of meanings he uses them to designate to others, and to himself, what he is thinking.

Assumption 3. *The individual is socialized into the general culture and also into various subcultures.*

Assumption 4. *While some groups and personal meanings and values may be dropped or become lower on the reference-relationship scale, they are not lost or forgotten.*

METHOD

Social scientists and psychologists focus on the formation of social action as the product or the antecedent factors to explain the causes of behavior. The SI approach is different from these. Its methodological position is that social action must be studied in terms of how it is formed. The premise that social action is built up by the acting unit through the process of noting, interpreting, etc., implies how social action should be studied. According to Blumer (1969), in order to treat and analyze social action, one must observe the process by which it is constructed. To do this, it is necessary to trace the way the action is actually formed. This means that one must see the situation as it is seen by the actor.

THE ELEMENTS OF THE MODEL

The elements of the model are naturally derived from the assumptions. These consist of the goal and the method. The goal of action is based upon a key factor of SI, which is taking the role of the other. To accomplish this, three methods are employed, which are governed by the patiency or target of action (the role assumed by the patient), and by the actor's (nurse's) role with the patiency. One methodological approach is for the nurse to utilize role taking in order to see the situation as it is viewed by the patient. Since the role taker is equivalent to the "me" in any given role arrangement, role taking enables the nurse and others to study and understand the cause of the patient's behavior in segments, which makes the difficulty surmountable. Ultimately, the total person, the "I," or self-concept, may be analyzed. This may be necessary only in long-term care, while analysis of the "me's" may often be sufficient for short-term care. A second basic method employs the human factor of interpretation of actions. In this regard, three of the varieties described by Faris (1964) are utilized: delayed action by the nurse, which permits mediation of thought; reduction of frustration; and promotion of foresight and insight rather than of restrospective learning, which often occurs too late. The third and final method requires process recordings, at least initially, until the nurse is sufficiently adept to respond insightfully to the patient's behavior on the spot and when the cause of the patient's behavior is difficult to identify. Not only does the nurse role-take but she encourages patients and relatives to do so in order that each may understand the position of the other. These methods are not new, but they are effective and lend themselves well to the theoretical framework of symbolic interactionism.

Three additional elements must be included to meet the requirements of an effective conceptual model for nursing, namely, the source of difficulty, the intervention, and the consequences. The problem, or source of difficulty, refers to any deviation from the norm or desired condition. In an interaction model involving a patient and a nurse one very difficult problem that might occur is role reversal. In such a situation, the patient assumes the therapeutic role while the nurse becomes the recipient of care. When role reversal occurs it is unintended rather than planned. A third party would probably have to intervene to correct the situation. An example of another problem that would be less difficult to solve is evident when a patient is reluctant to part with the sick role. Intervention would require enlisting the aid of the family, friends, and community resources to assist the patient through rehabilitation and back to a normal life.

THE NURSING PROCESS

Utilizing the thinking process, the nurse examines and assesses the patient in each situation. As discussed in the article by Abbey, the nurse considers the central, proximal, and distal parameters as well as the six factors of FANCAP. If a patient has been admitted to an acute-care hospital, the nurse includes a review of all his medical data and utilizes this in the plan of care. For example, if the role the patient assumes is due, in part, to a nutritional problem (e.g., obesity), and he views himself as helpless, the nurse employs this knowledge in working with the patient, the dietitian, and the patient's family and other health personnel to resolve the problem. In addition to his medical status, the nurse determines what, if any, psychosocial (including economic) problems he has. In the assessment, the nurse ascertains the roles the patient has assumed in the past and those he currently holds, the patient's problem-solving ability, his adaptability, how he has resolved similar problems in the past, how he copes with his general environment and with crises, stress, etc. Most importantly, the nurse observes him and the role he takes in varied situations, such as with his doctor, his family, and with the nursing staff, to learn as much as possible about the defining process of this actor—the patient—which is essential to understanding him. The nurse utilizes this information in planning the intervention and in evaluating it. In general, it is easier for the patient to assume roles he has previously played in order to solve current problems, but it is sometimes necessary for a person to learn or accept a new role in order to survive.

Once the assessment process begins, some short-term nursing diagnoses may emerge and the problems are quickly resolved. But like symbolic interactionism, assessment is a dynamic process that is influenced by day-to-day input, and although the hospital nurse may identify some long-term problems, she may be able to do very little about them herself. Referral to rehabilitation facilities, public health, and other community agencies then becomes imperative.

In order to formulate a plan of care, execute an intervention, and evaluate its result, nurses create plateaus of assessment. Once initiated, the nursing process is circular, for as new information is evaluated it is also assessed, on an hourly, daily, weekly, or monthly basis.

CONCLUSION

If a diagram aids visualization of this model, the reader is referred to Figure 1—a schematic representation of the model—in the article by Josephine Preisner. As the input and feedback increase between the nurse and the patient, the two circles move closer together and begin to overlap. In addition, as the nurse has a wealth of developing knowledge, so has the patient. Thus, a similar schematic configuration has the patient at its center and is superimposed on this drawing. Prior to the first meeting of the patient and the nurse, the patient configuration and nurse configuration may be vastly different or highly similar, depending on their backgrounds. The more complementary (in the intended direction) the two roles are, the more successful the nurse-patient relationship will be. As these persons become more knowledgeable about each other, the two configurations begin to overlap and move toward an ecliptic formation. The eclipse should never be complete, however, because maintaining a certain distance is essential for the preservation of the individualality of each person. For the nurse this distance is crucial for her objectivity, which is required if she is to continue to assist the patient. For the patient, the distance is essential if he is to function independently on the road to recovery.

REFERENCES

Blumer H: Symbolic Interactionism: Perspective and Method. Englewood Cliffs, NJ, Prentice-Hall, 1969

Coutu W: "Role-Playing Vs. Role-Taking: An Appeal for Clarification." Amer Sociol Rev 16:180–187, 1951

Erikson EH: Childhood and Society. New York, Norton, 1963

Faris REL: Handbook of Modern Sociology. Chicago, Rand McNally, 1964

Lindesmith AR and Strauss AL: Social Psychology, Dryden Press, 1949

Mead GH: Mind, Self and Society. Chicago, University of Chicago, 1934

Newcomb TM: Social Psychology. Dryden Press, 1950

Rose AM: Human Behavior and Social Processes. Boston, Houghton Mifflin, 1962

Sergent SS: Social Psychology. New York, Ronald Press, 1950

Wells LE and Marwell J: Self Esteem. Its Conceptualization and Measurement. Beverly Hills, Sage Publications, 1976

Marilynn J. Wood

29

Implementing the Riehl Interaction Model in Nursing Administration

The practice of nursing in hospital settings has long been fraught with problems, some of which are related to the management of nursing service within the hospital. Hospitals themselves have been burdened with antiquated bureaucratic structures, which are seen by professionals as creating insurmountable obstacles and labyrinths of red tape, thus interfering with or even preventing professional practice. These problems are most acute for nursing.

One might ask, "Why nursing rather than any other professional group in the hospital?"

During this century hospital nursing has moved out of the realm of independent practice, in which services are contracted and paid for by patients, and has become a service provided to patients by the hospital. Thus nurses and nursing services are an integral part of the hospital organization. Physicians, on the other hand, generally have maintained independent practice as the basic organization for medicine, and thus in most cases medical practice is still contracted and paid for by patients.

Within the hospital, nursing administration has had a difficult time maintaining goals congruent with professional nursing practice. The patient is not always the focus of nursing practice in hospitals. Instead the focus has become that of maintenance of the system by nurses. This focus on the system, rather than on the patient, has been fostered by the hospital organization itself, as nurses have been relied upon by others to "fill in" any and all gaps in the system's 24-hour-a-day operation. Nurses provide not only service "after hours" and on weekends in many areas other than nursing (pharmacy, clinical lab, X-ray, etc.) but also a basic network of support to the hospital system. Thus nurses are often responsible for transporting patients and equipment among hospital departments, keeping the patient units stocked with supplies, providing most of the record keeping upon which the system depends, as well as giving handmaiden service to the physician. Is it any wonder that nursing is unable to focus its goals on meeting the patients' needs?

By focusing on meeting the needs of the system instead of the patient, nursing has abandoned the patient advocate role that should be central to nursing practice. Thus head nurses are often interested primarily in keeping physicians happy; critical care nurses are often more interested in monitoring complex equipment than in the patient attached to the equipment; and staff nurses resent being asked to give direct patient care, which they consider "aides' work." All of these demonstrate the result of years of focus on the system rather than on the patient.

At a time when the medical model of independent practice is subject to serious public disillusionment, it does not seem appropriate for nursing to attempt to solve its problems by converting to independent practice. However, if nursing is to survive as a profession within inpatient settings, nurses must assume the patient advocate role, making the patient the central focus for nursing care, as would be the case in independent practice. A new approach is needed, and it is suggested here that this new approach be based on a conceptual model that provides a framework for both the practice of nursing and the delivery of nursing services.

Although there are many conceptual models used by nurses to facilitate the nursing process, the Riehl Interaction Model seems most appropriate for nursing administration since it focuses on roles. Based on symbolic interaction theory, the model focuses on the response of people to the meanings they attach to the actions of others. Much emphasis is placed on *action,* and the key factor in symbolic interactionism is that a person has to "get inside" the defining process of another in order to understand the action of that other person. This is also the key to good management.

Riehl has explained how the interaction model can be used as a basis for the nursing process. This paper will examine its use in the organization and delivery of nursing services by focusing on the roles of patients and nurses. The discussion is centered around the four assumptions of symbolic interactionism presented by Riehl in Chapter 26.

Assumption 1 *Man lives in a symbolic as well as physical environment and can be stimulated to act by symbols as well as by physical stimuli.*
Within the health-care professions there are many shared meanings and values by which individuals and groups are stimulated to act. These "norms" are not, however, shared with the patient. Since patients are not part of the health-care delivery system, the responsibility for teaching the patient how to behave in a world of unfamiliar symbols lies with the nurse. The patient cannot teach the nurse to behave according to his or her norms, but the nurse can be brought to understand what the patient's norms are, and thus ease the patient's transition into the health-care system. This concept is central to the

patient advocate role of the nurse. Since it is vital to begin this process with patients as soon as they enter the hospital system, this function must be a high priority for nurses upon a patient's admission to the hospital. Thus the person making the initial assessment of the patient must be a nurse capable of performing this function. The concept of primary nursing is useful to the patient advocate role because of its emphasis on professional nurse's assumption of full responsibility for individual patients during an entire hospital stay. This method of organizing the delivery of nursing care would facilitate implementation of the Riehl model in nursing services.

Assumption 2 *Through symbols man has the capacity to stimulate others in ways other than those in which he himself is stimulated.*
Recognizing that patients initially do not respond to the norms of the health-care system, nurses are uniquely able, because of their close proximity to patients, to discover the stimuli to which individual patients respond. These stimuli might originate in a patient's cultural background where beliefs about health and illness tend to be learned. If a patient believes that his illness stems from a curse placed upon him by his mother-in-law, his response to a cardiac rehabilitation program might seem bizarre to the professional staff. The primary nurse is in a unique position to assess culturally based beliefs of the patient that might impede response to treatment, and interpret these to other members of the health team, thus enabling the use of appropriate stimuli for the patient. As part of patient assessment, nurses must identify cultural, social, and psychologic variables pertinent to the patient's responses and then through the process of role taking predict the patient's responses to the health-care system and interpret these responses for other members of the health-care team. This advocate function is particularly important during the initial period of a patient's adjustment to the hospital.

Assumption 3 *Through communication of symbols, man can learn huge numbers of meanings and values—and hence ways of acting—from other men.*
Eventually patients learn by trial and error what the expected patient role is in the health care system. Normally people learn new roles rapidly through symbolic communication, as they see which of their behaviors evoke positive responses from others. However, when people are ill, their ability to learn new roles may be seriously hampered, since their attention must necessarily focus on personal changes related to the illness. Thus a patient's ability to assimilate cues through symbolic communication will be affected to varying degrees depending on the illness. Nurses can assist patients in interpreting cues from the environment and also can act as their advocates, when necessary, to prevent their bombardment with negative feedback when they fail to respond according to the norms governing expected patient behavior.

If an individual is a patient long enough, that person will become part of the culture of the health-care system. This process has been well documented through observation in long-term care facilities (Brink and Saunders; Goffman). However, in most acute-care facilities, patients do not become part of the system, but rather remain on the fringes—necessary for the system's survival, but not actively involved in it. Thus it is easy to see how the attention of the members of the system can become focused on their own roles in the system rather than on the patient, who is transitory. To change this critical situation, complete refocusing of the nurse's role is essential.

Assumption 4 *The symbols—and the meanings and values to which they refer—do not occur only in isolated bits, but often in clusters, sometimes large and complex.*

The term *role* as used throughout this paper, refers to a cluster of norms and values that guide and direct an individual's behavior in a given social setting. Patient role and nurse role are the two such clusters, seen as reciprocal and complementary. The major structural difference between them lies in the fact that the patient role is usually temporary, whereas the nurse role is a permanent part of that individual's life.

Within a culture or system, one of its most important facets will be the value placed on each role by others in the system. Typically roles develop into a hierarchy with those possessing the most positive value at the top. In the health-care system the patient role has a negative value, but because patients are not really part of the system, this role is usually not considered in the hierarchy at all. Nurses, on the other hand, are considered an integral part of the system, but since they are performing functions subservient to most others in the system, their role is not considered of high value by themselves or others.

There are instances in which nurses do occupy high-status roles (for example, critical-care nurses), and when they do, these roles are always relatively free of functions that are subservient to most others in the system. Thus the critical-care nurse is considered accountable only to the physician and performs many independent functions, whereas the general staff nurse is seen to be in a distant relationship to the physician and to perform many functions unrelated to those of medicine and often falling within the realm of such low-status roles as messengers and clerks.

By focusing on the patient advocate role, nurses would be relieved of many subservient functions, and their value in the system would immediately go up as they divorced themselves from low-status connections. Since increased status implies a more positive attitude toward the nurse role by others in the system, this would seem a necessary first step toward any change in the patient's status in the hospital.

This proposed change in the role of the nurse would undoubtably create many problems for current hospital organizations; however, none of these appear insurmountable. It has the decided advantage of according precisely with the stated purpose of every hospital, which is to meet the patient's health-care needs, and it seems an apt solution to many of the problems besetting both patients and nurses. The patient advocate role for nurses would effectively focus hospital nursing practice on the patient instead of on the system, while elevating the status of nursing by increasing its independence and decreasing its subservience. The patient, on the other hand, although still a stranger to the hospital culture, now would be represented by a member of the system who would know the norms and values and be able to communicate with and for the patient.

Organizational changes would include reassignment of non-nursing functions to others in the organization and redefinition of the professional nursing role to accord advocacy functions the highest priority. This latter would, of course, necessitate removing many supervisory functions from the professional nurse and might require a reduction in the numbers of non-professional nursing personnel utilized by the hospital. An organizational change to primary nursing might prove the most effective way of implementing the patient advocate role for nurses.

None of the ideas presented here is new and unique; all of the solutions have been offered before in other contexts. What is new and unique is the idea of looking at them in the interaction framework, which because of its emphasis on roles and relationships, is extremely workable as a model for nursing service.

Josephine M. Preisner

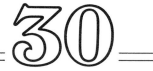

A Proposed Model for the Nurse Therapist

It is the purpose of this presentation to describe the model which guides my practice. The theoretical framework was developed during a supervised clinical experience at an outpatient psychiatric clinic. I was, at that time, a graduate student in community mental health nursing. The utility of the model in practice is illustrated here by a brief review of the care of one patient.

STRUCTURE AND ELEMENTS OF THE MODEL

Systems theory has been utilized as a theoretical base for the model. According to Parsons (1968) this theory embodies

> . . . the concept that refers both to a complex of interdependencies between parts, components, and processes that involve discernible regularities of relationship, and to a similar type of interdependency between such a complex and its surrounding environment.

My rationale for utilizing this theory is that I could benefit from increased understanding of relationships as a result of consideration of their multiple interdependencies. In addition, it is possible to view the interaction of this system with others, e.g., the medical model.

The schematic configuration of the model may be seen in Figure 1. The focus of action is directed toward the patient by the nurse therapist. Feedback from the patient sets into action the regulatory and control mechanisms of the system. This feedback, in the form of behavior, is the basis for the nurse to select or reject various approaches to therapy. As the patient's behavior changes, the nurse, in her regulatory role, reevaluates his state of equilibrium

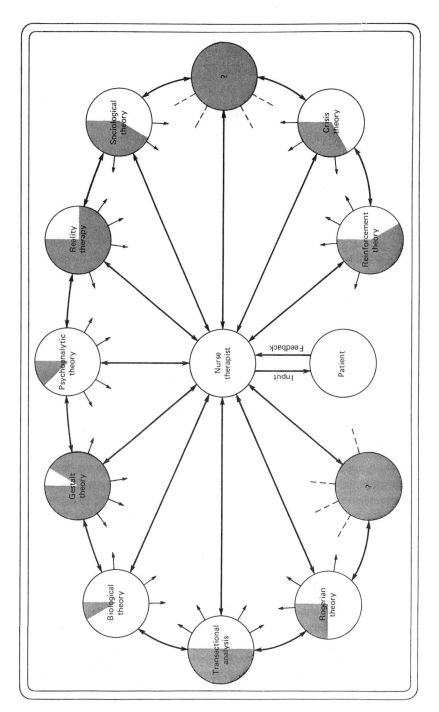

Figure 1 Schematic representation of model.

and again reviews her repertoire of interventions, rejecting those no longer useful and instituting those that seem to be appropriate. The system itself is dynamic, living, and open. New theories, techniques, and therapies can be brought into the system as they are developed or as the nurse therapist becomes aware of their existence. Thus, the major elements of the model are

1. The patient: an individual viewed as a bio-psycho-social being whose behavior system is threatened or actually out of balance due to excessive external forces or stress, lowered resistance, and/or failure to adjust to moderate forces (Johnson, 1968).
2. The nurse therapist: the practitioner who regulates and controls input and feedback mechanisms according to the patient's state of equilibrium. Practitioners may vary greatly in their level of expertise and their choice of techniques. A broad knowledge base provides for eclecticism in practice.
3. Goal: behavior that is functional for the patient and concurs with cultural norms and should result in a state of dynamic equilibrium.
4. Intervention: application of a broad range of therapeutic approaches to promote the goal.

In order to understand better the dynamic interaction of the elements of the model, we must look at Figure 1. The outer circles symbolize some of the better known approaches to therapy. First, the nurse therapist receives feedback from the patient. Next she reviews the approaches open to her. The broken lines in the figure lead to all of those approaches with which the nurse is not conversant; solid lines lead to approaches with which she has some acquaintance; shaded areas indicate parts of the underlying theory that she does not yet know or understand; the unshaded segments represent familiarity and understanding of underlying theory. The nurse therapist indicated in Figure 1 may therefore be seen to have a great deal of familiarity with psychoanalytic theory and a minimum of understanding of Gestalt theory. The therapist assesses the feedback that she has received from the patient, reviews the various approaches available, assesses their utility in the given situation, selects appropriate interventions, and applies them through the input channel to the patient.

One can readily see that a nurse therapist with a broad knowledge base will have a greater selection of interventions. This does not, however, eliminate the neophyte from practice. As her knowledge of the various theoretical approaches increases, the range of possible interventions that she may choose increases proportionately.

A look at the various approaches, shown in the schematic representation as a ring of circles, indicates some of the areas of knowledge from which the nurse therapist may draw interventions. Heavily shaded areas in all approaches except psychoanalytic theory indicate a practitioner who almost exclusively utilizes a psychoanalytic approach to therapy. Circles with question marks (there may be many more than shown here) indicate theoretical approaches not yet developed, not yet available to the nurse therapist's field of experience, or not available due to the restrictions imposed by the nurse's condition of licensure, e.g., prescribing medication.

THEORIES AND THERAPIES

The eclectic nature of this model reveals explicitly that the nurse therapist may select her therapeutic interventions from several sources. She will not be an advocate of any one approach, but will, based on her assessment of the patient or group, select that approach she considers to be most appropriate at that given point. She is free to add, combine, or reject approaches depending on her assessment of the patient's system and its state of equilibrium.

Although I do not purport to have knowledge of all of the known approaches to psychotherapy, I will briefly discuss here some of the theories and therapies that might well be selected by the nurse therapist utilizing an eclectic model for practice. A review of current psychotherapeutic literature, as well as the sources referred to in this section, is recommended to those readers interested in adding to their knowledge of these approaches.

Reality Therapy

This approach is based on the concept that patients commonly deny the reality of the world around them. Therapy is directed toward assisting the patient to recognize and accept reality so that he may work toward meeting his needs within its framework. Glaser (1965) calls this Reality Therapy. The two bassic needs that patients are assisted to fulfill are "the need to love and be loved and the need to feel that we are worthwhile to ourselves and to others."

Therapy does not probe events that have taken place in the past. The therapist becomes emotionally involved with the patient and helps him to perceive accurately the real world to the extent that he is able to fulfill his needs. In essence, the patient is assisted in moving from irresponsible to responsible behavior.

Psychoanalytic Therapy

The originator of the psychoanalytic approach to therapy was Sigmund Freud. His conceptualization of the organization and dynamics of personality forms the knowledge base upon which many modern analysts establish their practice. Theorists such as Alfred Adler and Harry Stack Sullivan have contributed much to supplement this knowledge.

The therapist utilizing the psychoanalytic approach will place emphasis on the "conscious control of behavior, without self-disapproval, to achieve satisfying consequences from the environment—to 'strengthen the ego'" (Ford and Urban, 1963). During the course of therapy, the patient's unconscious is probed and change is seen to take place through the development of insight. This insight is facilitated by the interpretation rather than the evaluation of behavior.

Crisis Theory

The individual who finds himself in a state of disequilibrium due to the application and failure of his usual problem-solving mechanisms when faced with a hazardous event may be considered to be in a state of crisis. Crisis theory, formulated by Gerald Caplan, provides a framework for assessment and intervention.

The form of therapy based on this theory is brief, usually lasting no longer than six weeks. The focus is on identifying the hazardous event and assisting the individual to solve problems so that equilibrium can be achieved. During therapy new coping mechanisms are developed that will help him to avoid disequilibrium in future hazardous situations (Caplan, 1964).

Gestalt Therapy

Frederick Perls is usually credited for the development of Gestalt therapy. The scientific body of knowledge upon which it is based includes Gestalt psychology, existential philosophy, and Freudian theory. Although an oversimplification, one might say that the goal of Gestalt therapy is to assist the individual to integrate and develop awareness of his feelings and emotions (Fagan and Shepherd, 1970).

As the patient's blocked awareness results in perceptual distortion of himself and his environment, responsible behavior is facilitated when these barriers are removed. The patient must work to get in touch with his own feeling so that he can experience and live in the real world.

Transactional Analysis

The transactional approach to psychotherapy was developed by Eric Berne. This form of structural analysis assists the therapist to maintain control over the situation and to achieve more rapid results than the conventional psychotherapies (Berne, 1961). An understanding of the theoretical base for this approach requires consideration of the structure of personality. This structure consists of three types of ego states, which Berne called Parent, Adult, and Child.

The first step in the approach is the analysis of the patient's personality structure. The therapist then assesses and makes diagnoses based on the ego state from which each symptom arises. With this knowledge, he proceeds with therapy and analyzes the transactions in which the patient is involved (Berne, 1961).

This framework may be seen as a means whereby the communication process, both verbal and nonverbal, is studied. The patient is assisted to identify the dominance of his ego states in various transactions so that he can consciously alter them in order to accomplish what he wants. Anxiety is reduced when he learns that he can achieve his goals through behavior alteration.

Rogerian Theory

The theory of therapy and personality change developed by Carl Rogers is frequently oversimplified and discussed in terms of the techniques that he proposes. Criticism of his theory is directed at the suggestion that it is a theory at all. Proponents of the Rogerian approach to therapy follow the process that he constructed based on his theory of personality development.

The goal of Rogerian therapy is to achieve personality and behavioral change. Rogers outlines certain conditions that must be met in order for this therapeutic process to occur. Basically, fulfillment of these conditions leads to the development of a genuine relationship between the therapist and patient. The psychotherapeutic process works toward releasing an already existing capacity in a potentially competent individual. Goal achievement in therapy can be measured by the degree of congruence that the individual reaches, the extent to which he is open to his experience, and the reduction of his utilization of defensive maneuvers. Each step that is taken toward this goal results in a more fully functioning person (Rogers, 1961).

Reinforcement Theory

Reinforcement, or stimulus-response theorists have developed a cluster of theories that purport to explain the development of behavior. This behavioral school of psychology is deeply concerned with the learning process. Although these theories have many similarities, they each have unique qualities (Hall and Lindzey, 1970).

For our purposes I will briefly present some background on the theory of Albert Bandura and Richard Walters. The therapeutic process which they propose is known as behavior modification. This theory of personality takes into consideration the social context in which behavior is acquired and performed. Traditional learning theory has been expanded and modified by the development of principles of social learning. These principles are the basis for the development of techniques to modify behavior (Hall and Lindzey, 1970). Thus behavior is considered to be learned socially, and change, or modification of behavior, must take into consideration such concepts as imitation and identification, social reinforcement, and self-reinforcement (Hall and Lindzey, 1970). Although most reinforcement theorists propose the modification of behavior, they have met with difficulty when attempting to remove their study from the laboratory setting.

This approach to behavioral change is currently receiving much attention. Experimental studies with animals have presented these researchers with clear concepts that are being applied to human subjects. A primary criticism of the reinforcement approach has been its failure to take into consideration the cognitive functioning of the individual. Yet the schools of psychologic thought which do propose emphasis on cognitive functioning have been criticized also. In essence, reinforcement theorists question the value of an approach that does not take into consideration the stimulus for behavior (Hall and Lindzey, 1970).

Sociologic Theory

Social scientists have helped us to develop some understanding of life, human relationships, and responses that we may expect from our fellow man (Wilson, 1966). Sociologic theory gives us ways to look at our world, helping us to interpret the social phenomena that occur and affect us. Frequently used concepts are culture, role, status, class, stratification, bureaucracy, attitude, mobility, structure, and institution (Wilson, 1966). Familiarity with these concepts allows us to see ourselves and others with more clarity. We become aware of the multiplicity of roles imposed upon the individual depending upon his status in society. And we are concerned with the resources within his family, among his friends, and within his community. Moreover, social and cultural norms may be considered through this approach. In short, sociologic research findings help us to predict the effects on the individual of life in the social world.

Biologic Theory

The biologic approach is natural and appropriate for consideration by the nurse. Her basic preparation is heavily weighted in this area. As she views her patient, she is concerned with his physical status, medications that he may be taking, and somatic symptoms that he experiences. Manifestations of organic disease are often seen in the patient with a metabolic disturbance, the alcoholic, the elderly, or the brain-damaged. Acute or chronic psychotic reactions may be seen based on organic disease of the brain (Hofling, et al., 1967).

An understanding of characteristic physiologic responses to stress is valuable in making an assessment and choosing effective interventions for patients, regardless of the setting or category of illness (Brunner, 1970). Knowledge of the development and functioning of body systems in health and illness is of particular value to the nurse therapist. In the event that she is able to see a correlation between her patient's physiologic and psychologic state of health, she is in a unique position to assist him, within his capacity, to achieve the highest possible level of wellness.

Advantages of the Model

A review of the model reveals some explicit as well as implicit advantages. Admittedly, my limited experience as a nurse therapist can be expected to influence my perception of both the advantages and disadvantages associated with the use of the model. At this time, no consideration has been given to the utility of the model in research; however, we may identify some aspects of its practicality in nursing practice and education. The model's advantages are as follows:

1. Man may be viewed as a bio-psycho-social being. This view is consistent with the nurse's basic orientation to the art and science of nursing.
2. The nurse may begin to function as a therapist during the earliest phase of her placement in any clinical setting and at any point in time. Therapy takes place during and within any nurse-patient relationship. Extraordinary expertise is neither expected nor necessary.
3. Growth of the therapist is encouraged and has no limits. Acquisition of knowledge increases range of possible interventions. It is not anticipated nor is it remotely possible that any one nurse therapist could, or would, wish to master all of the theories upon which the approaches are based.
4. The therapist may accept or reject approaches at will. She uses the eclectic approach to therapy. She may use any one or any combination of approaches that she wishes. The feedback and input mechanisms provide for reassessment at any point, and approaches that are no longer effective may be replaced.
5. As the system is open and dynamic, there may be interaction with other disciplines with unique and special expertise. For example, the social worker shares some of the approaches utilized by the nurse therapist. Input from the social worker reaches the nurse therapist through their shared approaches. This dynamic interaction is mutual and allows each

discipline the opportunity to seek and share knowledge. It may be seen that this interaction benefits both disciplines but does not threaten the integrity of either.

6. Research studies undertaken by any discipline may produce findings that contribute to the scientific body of knowledge underlying one of the known approaches. In this same manner, research may also open the path for the development of a new approach. Shared knowledge between disciplines may then broaden the repetoire of theory and therapy available to all.

7. The patient need not conform to any one approach. If he is in treatment with a therapist who uses a reality therapy approach exclusively, or almost exclusively, circumstances dictate that he achieve what is possible for him within the confines of the reality therapy model. It is possible that he could achieve more if, for example, more attention was paid to his biologic functioning, and if some components of behavior modification were utilized in his therapy.

8. Nursing faculty need not present a single view of therapy. Faculty members with special expertise in different theories of therapy will contribute their knowledge and indicate where, within the framework of the model, this knowledge is situated, and how it may be utilized.

9. The nurse therapist may function in a variety of settings, e.g., day treatment center, inpatient psychiatric unit, outpatient mental health clinic, general hospital, office setting, public or community health agency, voluntary agency, and school.

10. It is possible for the nurse therapist to develop and maintain close professional ties with members of other disciplines. They are, in at least some respects, treading a common ground.

Disadvantages of the Model

The disadvantages associated with use of the model have not been fully determined. It is expected that as the model is used, certain basic limitations will be observed. The only disadvantage that would seem to be readily apparent is the utility of the model in the treatment of the autistic child. Although no one approach has yet been found to deal with this condition, work currently being done indicates that consistency of therapeutic approach is necessary. This would involve in-depth knowledge of the approach and would not permit contamination by other techniques and theories. There may also be some question of the utility of the model in the treatment of the chronic schizophrenic. Some evidence leads to a biologic basis for the development of this disease entity.

Implications for the Therapist

The nurse therapist who functions at her best in a highly structured situation may well feel uncomfortable operating within this model. Should she be employed in a crisis intervention center, the agency itself may dictate the acceptable theory or theories upon which therapy is to be based. In-depth knowledge of one approach may be expected by the agency, and the nurse therapist may be placed in a position where it is necessary for her to meet these expectations if she wishes to keep her job. Nevertheless, in many cases she does have the option of selecting the eclectic model for practice. Whether or not she chooses it depends, in large measure, upon her basic philosophy of nursing, her flexibility, and her assumptions about man and his internal struggle for survival within his environment.

The Model in Use

During the period of time that I saw patients at the psychiatric outpatient clinic, the model was used as a guideline for practice. During the latter part of this student experience it became apparent to me that theory was an important part of my practice. It was also apparent that many theories were used to develop interventions, and that knowledge of theory in one area might easily be more extensive than in another. Although not a clinical practitioner with great expertise, I found that I was somewhat successful in my rendering of patient care. Yet was it possible to really accomplish anything worthwhile without the extensive, in-depth knowledge that the theorists themselves and most of the practitioners in the clinic seemed to feel was necessary for work with patients having emotional disorders? It was with some feelings of self-doubt that I proceeded to work with my patients. However, these feelings were mixed with a desire to prove that a graduate education focused on psychiatric and community mental health nursing was an appropriate background for a nurse therapist.

Louise

The patient who is presented here is Louise. I worked with her for ten weeks, and in some ways feel that I know her better than some members of my own family. She was thirty-three years of age and married for the second time. There were two children living in the home, a ten-year-old son by her first husband and a five-year-old daughter by her present husband. She was hospitalized for one month shortly after she remarried and received ECT for a diagnosis of depression. She had been treated by several therapists including one psychiatrist. Her husband went with her for marriage counseling for several months after her discharge from the hospital.

Physically, Louise had been in good health except for a condition of hypoglycemia, which she controlled by diet. A chart-review conference at the clinic considered Louise and the problems that she presented in her intake interview. She was diagnosed as having an anxiety neurosis and was referred to an orientation group until an individual therapist could be found for her. After several weeks as a member of this group, she was referred to me for individual therapy.

Instead of a thorough discussion and description of my work with the patient, for purposes of this presentation I will briefly describe the utility of the model in assessing and selecting appropriate interventions to use with her.

1. I found the Rogerian theory to be a valuable approach to therapy with this patient. I attempted to fulfill the conditions that Rogers stated must be met if the therapeutic process is to occur. One specific condition, that of holding the patient in unconditional positive regard, was of particular value throughout our relationship. During the first few weeks Louise would test me with comments like "I'll bet you've never known anyone as bad as me," or "I'm always complaining, how can anyone stand to be around me?" At times like these I expressed unconditional acceptance and positive regard for her both verbally and nonverbally. This method of testing me was used throughout our ten weeks together but gradually decreased in frequency. Thus, I was able to assess her level of trust and the state of our relationship through the feedback that she gave me. My hope here was to build her self-esteem within our relationship so that she could carry positive feelings about herself into other relationships. Already I could see that she was using fewer defensive maneuvers and was more open to her experience. Louise's anxiety level was usually very high at the beginning of each session, and I found that I was able to help her to bring herself under control by using the Rogerian approach. Again, through the feedback mechanism, I was able to assess continually the effectiveness of the approach. Louise began to experience a greater degree of positive self-regard, and, as the weeks went by, our relationship was strengthened.

2. Reinforcement theory, specifically behavior modification, became a useful approach with Louise as our relationship took on greater meaning for her. Social reinforcers were used here. In one instance, I recall being frustrated with her for not expressing her

feelings. I told her that it would be helpful to me if she would use terms such as *angry, happy, sad,* etc., when I asked her how she felt. This was difficult for her at first; however, each time she expressed a feeling as I had requested, I gave positive reinforcement, e.g., "It really helps me to understand your feelings when you express yourself that way," or "I understand," and later on, merely smiling and nodding. I was able to assess the value of this type of intervention when she told me that she could hardly wait to get to our session to tell me how well she had managed to deal with a stressful situation at home. It was apparent that she wanted my approval and was willing to modify her behavior in order to get it. Gradually she discovered that she was able to cope more effectively with her problems with these new behaviors. Thus it was possible for her to reinforce herself when she experienced the positive effects of her new behaviors. On one occasion she announced, "I was really proud of myself for keeping my head."

3. The sociologic approach was particularly useful in viewing Louise's strengths. She saw herself as a spineless, weak, and worthless being, totally dependent on her husband. Focus on her social relationships revealed that it was Louise who made and maintained the friendships with others for the family. She was well-liked on her job, enjoyed parties, and would have liked to entertain in her home if the financial situation had been better. Use of this approach permitted me to fill in information about her relationships with others. In addition to the benefit to me, as therapist making an assessment, it was helpful to Louise to review these relationships and to help identify them as resources and strengths. In the past she had considered these friendships as examples of her extreme dependence on others. It seemed to surprise her when I said that people choose their friends and that it seemed apparent that her friends wanted to maintain their relationships with her. There was no reason for them to continue to see her if they were offended by her dependence on them. Reviewing this, we were able to see that, in some instances, she was seen as the 'strong' half of the relationship. During our last weeks together, Louise joined a Bible study group. This was something that she had long wished to do but had previously avoided because her husband had refused to go with her. Thus another strength was revealed and Louise achieved a higher level of independence.

4. Hypoglycemia was not a condition with which I had great familiarity. However, I pursued the biologic approach when I asked the

patient about treatment for this condition. I found that she was supposed to be on a high-protein diet but rarely kept to it. She felt that protein foods were too costly and could not be managed on her restricted budget. I failed to act in this area as I might have wished. All high-protein foods are not out of her price range, and I could have spent more time discussing this with her. The acute discomfort that she was experiencing with her family situation led me to set priorities, and disposition of the hypoglycemia was placed low on my list. This may not have been a wise decision, as it might well have been helpful, in terms of relieving her lethargy, if she were on the prescribed diet. Increased energy might well have helped her to deal with the stresses in her life. She referred to herself as 'weak,' and this view of herself might have contributed to her low self-esteem. She often wished that she was 'strong like other women.' This, of course, might have been a rationalization, and all of the strength of an Amazon could well have failed her if she continued to live in a chaotic and stressful environment.

5. My course work at the university involved readings and discussion of the crisis model during the time that I first met and began to work with Louise. I was anxious to have a 'crisis' patient and tried to fit her into the paradigm. This was a fruitless task. I was frustrated, as I wanted to be able to use this theory in my practice. It didn't seem fair that my interviews with Louise failed to elicit even a hint of the hazardous event. Several times I asked her what it was that brought her to the clinic on the first day. Try as I would, crisis theory did not seem to fit.

6. During the last few weeks of therapy, I became aware of the ways in which Louise attempted to communicate with others. She related situations to me that allowed me to make use of the transactional approach. The dominant ego state was quite obviously her "child" in most of her transactions with others. She was concerned and interested to discover that her "child" often evoked her husband's "parent." We were able to look at ways in which she could consciously alter the dominance of her own ego state. With this new position, the "adult" would not necessarily bring instant gratification, but Louise was able to try it on for size. She saw this as a way to change some of the responses that she evoked from others. She was, at first, impatient with her failure to obtain immediate results. This was overcome when we reviewed her expectations and examined the "adult" position. She began to develop greater patience. It became possible for her to identify the "child" responses in others without responding in kind.

Interaction of the Elements

Perhaps it is possible to view the dynamic interaction of the model elements more clearly now that we have reviewed some of the approaches used by this therapist. If we refer to the schematic representation of the model (Figure 1), it may be seen that there is no single dominant element.* Every theoretical approach holds a position within the system that is capable of interacting with the patient system through the nurse therapist.

Assessment

As the nurse therapist selects a therapeutic approach based on her assessment of the patient's state of equilibrium, we can see that her choice of approaches is limited only by her knowledge base and the feedback that she receives from the patient. Accurate interpretation of this feedback is vital if she is to select interventions that will promote a state of dynamic equilibrium for the patient. It is the feedback, in the form of behavior, that must be assessed. In the case study presented, we could see that Louise did not hold herself in high esteem. The therapist, having some knowledge of Rogerian theory, chose this approach with its specific techniques for increasing the patient's feelings of self-worth.

As the therapist became aware, again through the feedback mechanism, that Louise's communications with others did not bring her satisfaction, the various therapeutic approaches available were reviewed. Selection of the transactional approach was based on this particular therapist's knowledge base. Assessment of the effectiveness of this approach was possible because the therapist did have an understanding of the goals of therapy in the transactional paradigm.

It would seem appropriate at this point to present the reader with an assessment tool to facilitate diagnosis and intervention selection. Unfortunately, a tool such as this has not yet been developed. As this writer has only recently developed the conceptual framework, many more questions seem to arise than answers. What kinds of data are needed? From what sources should information be solicited? What questions could be considered salient? What should be done with the information once it is obtained? There are, in fact, endless questions that arise when considering the construction of such an instrument. Indeed, it might be valuable to consider and debate the true worth of an assessment tool in light of the early stage of development of the model itself.

---

*No attempt has been made here to depict visually the areas of developed and undeveloped knowledge of this therapist. The schematic representation (Fig. 1), with its shaded and unshaded areas, merely demonstrates knowledge that has been developed in a nonexistent, and therefore entirely fictional, nurse therapist.

Perhaps we might simply view the patient in terms of the gains and losses he experiences as a result of the behavior he uses. Assessment of the effectiveness of the applied interventions could also focus on these gains and losses. What is it that the patient has to gain by continuing to use behavior that fails to achieve his goal? For example, why did Louise repeatedly tell the therapist that she was weak? It is possible that she was merely stating in advance what she feared the therapist thought about her. In this way she might have hoped to manipulate the therapist into stating, "No, you're wrong. I don't see you as a weak person." The therapist would then avoid looking at Louise's feelings about herself. The gain here would be protection from having to look closely at herself. Further, the therapist would not really get close enough to discover what a "terrible" person Louise really was. Finally, the therapist would not reject her. The loss that Louise might have experienced was an opportunity to learn more about herself. Taking a risk by not hiding behind this defensive behavior may have been ego strengthening for her. Perhaps she felt that she did not deserve acceptance from others and that the most important loss was the opportunity to experience the absence of criteria dictating 'conditions' of worth.

So, for Louise, we could assess the gain as an opportunity to validate her own feelings of worthlessness and to avoid rejection. The loss would then be acceptance and an opportunity to see herself in a better light. Whether or not there would always be a parellel between gains and losses is questionable. Certainly it might be worthwhile to consider this aspect as efforts are made to further refine the model.

A View of the Components

Consideration of the examples presented indicates that there is dynamic interaction between each theoretical approach and the patient, by means of the nurse therapist. How then do the approaches themselves interact? In order to understand this we must consider their relationships with each other by viewing their multiple interdependencies.

Each therapeutic approach is made up of various components. Earlier in this paper, in the discussion of Gestalt therapy, it was stated that this approach is based on the scientific body of knowledge that includes Gestalt psychology, existential philosophy, and Freudian theory. And the contributors to the components of this body of knowledge are not restricted to the theorists who developed Gestalt therapy. For we know that Freudian theory is also utilized in the knowledge base of psychoanalytic therapists. And Gestalt psychology has contributed much to theories of learning, and many theorists make use of existential philosophy in formulating their own theories. It is, therefore, the interdependencies of the parts or components that must concern us. The logic upon which this concept is based has been clearly and simply stated by Pascal: "Just as the same thoughts differently arranged form a different discourse, so the same words differently arranged form different thoughts'' (Miller, 1950). Thus it can be seen that the components of the various theoretical approaches do have multiple interdependencies.

A Final Word

We can take nothing for granted. The above model needs to be subjected to critical scrutiny. Basic construction, roles, and relationships may require substantial refinement if the model is to be of value to the practitioner. Flaws not presently apparent to the writer may emerge as the model is scientifically investigated.

Nurses are not new to psychiatric settings. Patients with problems that disturb their emotional equilibrium are not strangers in the community. It seems that the question to answer is whether or not we see the nurse fulfilling the role of primary therapist. If, in fact, we do, then the proposed model may be of some assistance in helping her to organize her practice and to reduce any conflicts she may experience as she assumes her role. The degree to which these objectives are met, and the degree to which the goal of action is achieved, will determine the utility of this model for the nurse therapist.

REFERENCES

Berne E: Transactional Analysis in Psychotherapy. New York, Grove Press, 1961

Brunner LS, Emerson CP, Jr., Ferguson LK, Suddarth DS: Textbook of Medical-Surgical Nursing, 2nd ed. Philadelphia, Lippincott, 1970

Caplan G: Principles of Preventive Psychiatry. New York, Basic Books, 1964

Fagan J, Shepherd IL: Gestalt Therapy Now. Palo Alto, Science and Behavior Books, 1970

Ford DH, Urban HB: Systems of Psychotherapy. New York, Wiley, 1963

Glaser W: Reality Therapy. London, Harper, 1965

Hall CS, Lindzey G: Theories of Personality, 2nd ed. New York, Wiley, 1970

Hofling CK, Leininger MW, Bregg E: Basic Psychiatric Concepts in Nursing, 2nd ed. Philadelphia, Lippincott, 1967

Johnson DE: One conceptual model of nursing. Unpublished, April 28, 1968

Miller JG: In Gray W, Duhl FH, Risso ND (eds): General Systems Theory and Psychiatry. Boston, Little, 1969, Quoting Pascal's Pensees, original ed 1670. Translated by Stewart HF: New York, Pantheon, 1950

Parsons T: Systems analysis, social systems. International Encyclopedia of the Social Sciences, Macmillan, 1968

Rogers CR: Becoming a Person. Boston, Houghton, 1961

Wilson EK: Sociology: Rules, Roles, and Relationships. Homewood, Ill., The Dorsey Press, 1966

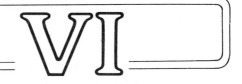

The Coalition of Nursing Models

This final section presents three papers with a similar theme: the coalition of nursing models. In the first of these, one case study is viewed from the perspective of several different models. In the second paper, the results of a survey of nursing models in current use are given. And finally, a unified model of nursing, which incorporates nursing knowledge now available, is reviewed.

Chapter 30 poses the following question: What is the relationship among the various nursing modes; ie., what are their similarities and differences? For an answer to this question, one case study is analyzed from the viewpoint of five models—one developmental, three systems, and one interaction. It was not possible to use all the models described in this text in this analysis. However, it was felt that the models used were representative. Chapter 30 thus views one patient situation from the perspective of the Peplau, Roy, Johnson, Orem, and Riehl models. Comments about the similarities and differences among the models are drawn from this analysis.

In Chapter 31, the results of a survey are presented. The need for this became evident during the planning of this edition. The first text included models known by the authors to be taught in schools of nursing. In the preparation of this book, an expanded input was desired and it was felt a survey would help accomplish this. The survey sought to ascertain which models were being taught in theory and which were implemented in clinical practice. The study indicates what conceptual frameworks are currently popular at what level of nursing education, as well as which ones will probably predominate in the near future.

In the first edition, it was suggested that nurses consider adopting a unified model. The last chapter of this text expands upon this idea. At this point there appears to be, in general, sufficient similarities in the several models' views of the recipient of nursing care and the goal of nursing care to warrant accepting these two as common basic structures. The two primary additional structures that complete a framework are the diagnostic and intervention modes. These two factors are influenced by nursing areas of specialization or orientation and, thus, are inherently more flexible and should remain so to allow for an expansion of the knowledge base. The accepted methodologic approach to nursing care is what is commonly called the nursing process. Both the structure and method of a unified model are explored and discussed in the final chapter.

A Case Study Viewed According to Different Models

Conceptual models affect the kind of practice in which a nurse will participate. In this text, the individual authors have explored the implications of their given models for each one's own practice. To further understand the implications of the basic kinds of models—systems, development, and interaction—the author felt it would be illustrative to analyze one patient situation from the viewpoint of representative nursing models.

A graduate student from the University of California at Los Angeles provided the case study. This patient example represents a commonly occurring situation in nursing practice. The case study was given to a group of graduate students at the University of Portland. Each group analyzed the case study according to their assigned model. This work was used as input in preparing an analysis of the data base, nursing diagnoses, goals, and interventions according to each model. The draft of the analysis of the patient situation, from the viewpoint of each model, was sent to the respective nurse theorists. Comments from the theorists were then incorporated into the revised analysis presented here.

A word should be said about two basic limitations of the procedure being used. Whenever a written case study provides the data for clinical judgments, the danger of incomplete data is present. Often in the real situation the first thing the nurse would do would be to elicit the additional data she needs to make her judgments regarding diagnoses, goals, and interventions. This limitation was apparent when the various models were used to describe the data base. Each model prescribes specific data to be collected. The case study gave only certain facts. Where it seemed appropriate some inferences were drawn from the data in the case study.

A second limitation of the process being used lies in the author's decision to use a single simplified format for the nursing-care plans based on the five nursing models. This decision was made to facilitate the comparison of models. However, it forces some of the models into a less appropriate or incomplete format. For example, a care plan for the interactionist model might be presented better with labels such as shared interpretation of need, intervention, validation of effectiveness.

Given these limitations, the following case study was analyzed as a starting point for comparing the implications of the basic kinds of nursing models for nursing practice. The analysis according to five nursing models is given below.

The Case of Dr. Ambrose

Dr. Horace Ambrose was admitted to the cardiac care unit five days ago, where the medical diagnosis of acute inferior myocardial infarction was established. Following an uncomplicated course with no chest pain past the initial episode, Dr. Ambrose was transferred on the sixth day to a private room on the medical unit.

Information from the chart and the nurse in the cardiac care unit revealed the following data. This was the first hospital admission for Dr. Ambrose, who presented himself at the hospital with the chief complaint of "crushing" severe substernal chest pain. Indeed, this forty-seven-year-old man stated he had "never experienced such pain." The patient had no prior history of illness that had required hospitalization. Dr. Ambrose expressed pride in his state of "excellent health" and gave an account of having regular check-ups, following a planned daily exercise schedule, participating in golf and tennis, watching his diet and weight, and abstaining from smoking. The nurse stated that on his last day in the unit he made comments during his bath such as, "I'm not feeling any pain, I can do that," and talked about being transferred from the unit as meaning he could soon resume his successful practice as a head and neck surgeon. The nurse also related that his wife Janice, age 42; daughter Julie, age 18; and son Paul, age 16, were frequent visitors and overtly expressed their concern about the patient. His mother Martha, age 70, who also lives in the household, was unable to come to the hospital due to her arthritis, but she called frequently about her son. The nurse revealed that the patient was an American Jew and that some of the concerns and behavior of the family may be related to this fact.

Today an aide reported that she had seen the patient go to the bathroom and she wondered if there had been a change in the orders. The team leader confirmed that he was still on commode privileges only. An L.V.N. entered his room and found him standing at the sink shaving. She said, "I told him to get back to bed. He replied that he felt well enough and that his activity could be extended safely. He certainly isn't asking for assistance like he should." The team leader noted that the patient's son had brought his father a chili cheeseburger (at Dr. Ambrose's request). Another aide reported that the patient asked to have a phone connected as soon as he was transferred to the medical unit. He immediately made a call to his office, stating he would be leaving the hospital in the near future and to start arranging surgery for one of his patients.

The nurse who gave Dr. Ambrose morning care charted that he was holding a newspaper and not using the bedside table as all myocardial infarction patients were instructed. She had found the patient very talkative and her interview had validated his interest in sports and his concern about returning to his practice. He mentioned that he had noticed some weakness in his extremities, which was new, but felt this might be due to his increased activity after five days of rest. During their conversation, Mrs. Ambrose entered the room. As the nurse was leaving she heard the patient ask his wife to keep him informed on all financial matters and decisions in the family, since he was feeling better now. Later, the wife told the nurse about her husband's interest in sports as a participant and expressed concern about how she was going to get him to slow down. "I keep telling him not to get out of bed and to take it easy. (pause) He just doesn't listen to me about such things."

THE ROY ADAPTATION MODEL—DATA BASE FOR CASE STUDY

In accordance with the Roy Adaptation Model of nursing, the nurse establishes a data base for her nursing diagnoses by observing patient behavior in each of the adaptive modes, and by describing the focal, contextual, and residual stimuli affecting these behaviors.

In the case of Dr. Ambrose, the only negative physiologic behavior is the weakness in extremities, which is secondary to his increased activity. The behavior of increased activity is discussed under another mode. Self-concept behaviors in regard to the physical self are all positive, that is, Dr. Ambrose takes pride in his excellent health and gives accounts of regular checkups, daily exercise, golf and tennis, watching diet and weight, and non-smoking.

The analysis of data in this case focuses on role-function and interdependence behaviors. Many of Dr. Ambrose's behaviors could be described as role behaviors. For example, in the secondary role of physician, he made a call to his office and stated he would be leaving the hospital soon and his staff should begin arranging his surgery schedule. In regard to his tertiary role of accepted illness, there are likewise a number of negative behaviors. For example, he stated that he felt well enough so that his activity could be extended, and he did such things as going to the bathroom to shave and holding a newspaper without the aid of a tray table. Yet these same behaviors could also be viewed as inappropriate independence behaviors.

Roy (1976) has described elsewhere that what often appears as a simple role problem turns out to be basically an underlying interdependence problem. The clue to this difficult differential diagnosis is the effect of the introduction of role cues and the requirements for adequate role performance. It is assumed that in this case Dr. Ambrose has already received the information he needs to perform the sick role adequately and that the requirements for success in that role are present, for example, willing care givers and others to care for his work and home roles. Thus, this case will be treated as an interdependence problem.

Dr. Ambrose's negative independent behaviors are identified as follows: going to the bathroom, shaving, failing to ask for assistance, having phone connected, holding newspaper, asking to be informed of financial and household matters, and not listening to his wife. The one dependent behavior he exhibits is asking his son to bring in food for him.

It is hypothesized that the focal stimulus immediately leading to this inappropriate independent behavior is the conflict between a high need for independence and the current demand for dependency during illness. The other factors that may be influencing the situation, that is, the contextual and residual stimuli, include the fact that he has basic knowledge of illness but does not see his activities as harmful, values own self-care, feels nurses are over-protective, avoids feelings about danger of illness, and focuses on activities of wellness.

The nursing diagnosis according to the Roy adaptation model is stated as the predominant behavior as influenced by the focal stimulus. The goal is a change in maladaptive behaviors or a reinforcement of adaptive behaviors. Nursing interventions are manipulation of the stimuli causing maladaptation. The plan for the nursing care for Dr. Ambrose, using the Roy Adaptation Model, can thus be summarized as follows:

Nursing Diagnosis	Goal	Intervention
Maladaptive independent behaviors related to conflict between a high need for independence and the	Patient will cognitively and affectively structure the situation to allow dependent behaviors such as	Assign clinical specialist to discuss behavioral conflict with patient and allow patient to control own con-

Nursing Diagnosis	Goal	Intervention
current demand for dependency due to sick role.	accepting help in self-care, allowing wife to accept family responsibilities, and postponing return to professional activities.	flict by (1) facilitating expression of feelings and perceptions involved in the conflict situation; (2) identifying and clarifying the perceived and actual conflict involved, (3) re-educating patient through teaching, translation, and interpretation of perceptual data, e.g., coming to new interpretation of meaning of being on medical unit—not just elimination of all restrictions, but need for self-restriction.

THE OREM SELF-CARE MODEL—DATA BASE FOR CASE STUDY

The data base for the nurse using the Orem self-care model involves an analysis of the therapeutic self-care demand and the self-care agency. Deficits are then identified in orientation, skills, knowledge, and motivation.

The therapeutic self-care demand can be described in terms of both universal and health-deviation self-care. Dr. Ambrose's universal self-care is generally positive. In the category "air, food, and water," it is noted that he is careful about diet and weight. There is no evidence of problems with excrement. Concerning activity and rest, he is an active participant in sports (golf, tennis) and exercises daily. His social interaction includes wife, mother, and two children living in the home, and he is the decision maker in the family. As to hazards to life and well-being, Dr. Ambrose is a nonsmoker and concerned about physical fitness, but may be unaware of stress points in his life. In regard to the last category, "being normal," he insists on keeping informed, is a successful surgeon, and has no prior history of illness.

The difficulty in Dr. Ambrose's case comes from his health- deviation self-care demands. His changes in human structure involve the physiologic changes related to acute myocardial infarction. Changes in physical functioning involve the medically imposed restrictions on activity. However, Dr. Ambrose is not abiding by these restrictions. Changes in behavior and habits of daily living are related to these changes in physical functioning. Dr. Ambrose's current physical condition requires extensive changes in his behavior and habits of daily living, yet he has not made these adjustments.

The self-care agency can be comprehended from the following description: a forty-seven-year-old male whose general health is excellent whose sociocultural factors include married, father, son, head of household, and American Jewish tradition.

Based on the limited case study data, it is assumed that there are no deficits in skills or orientation. However, Dr. Ambrose may have deficits in knowledge and motivation. These deficits are the nursing diagnoses. The goal is patient self-care. The nurse's role in the Orem model is to be compensatory, partly compensatory, or educative-developmental.

Using Orem's self-care model, the plan for nursing care then can be specified as follows:

Nursing Diagnosis	Goal: Self-Care by Patient	Interventions Mode: Partly Compensatory, Educative-Developmental
Knowledge Deficit —role of patient	Learn and accept role as patient.	Guide, teach, provide developmental environment review reason for patiency provide choice situations within restrictions; involve in own care teach, using role reversal situations consult with mother on useful techniques in modifying son's behavior.
—stress as a precipitating factor	Identify stress situations.	Guide, teach, provide developmental environment provide patient with pertinent literature relevant to deficit encourage verbalization on factors precipitating MI appraise health hazard (identify stress points) talk with family on identifying stress as precipitating factor in illness enlist wife and children's support in providing therapeutic environment.
Motivation Deficit —acceptance of limitations of illness	Incorporate limitations of illness into self-care agency.	Guide, support, provide developmental environment encourage verbalization about life goals, long- and short-term; sources of stress; identifying stress; sources of support; modifying life-style relative to illness approach nonjudgmentally.
—ability to relinquish control	Accept increase in therapeutic self-care demand.	Guide, support, provide developmental environment enlist respected colleague support and/or colleague with similar therapeutic self-care demand plan for joint counseling before discharge encourage psychiatric consultation p.r.n.

THE JOHNSON BEHAVIORAL SYSTEM MODEL—DATA BASE FOR CASE STUDY

In establishing a data base using the Johnson Behavioral System Model, the nurse examines the subsystem structural units of action, goal or drive, set, and choices, then looks at variables causing or influencing these units.

Basically it seems that in the case of Dr. Ambrose, the two subsystems involved are achievement and dependency. The actions, or observed behaviors, of the achievement subsystem are holding newspaper without using overbed table, standing at sink to shave, continuing business by telephone, and asking to be informed on family financial matters. The goal or drive of this behavior is a strong and significant need to achieve mastery and control. The set of this subsystem seems to be a fairly rigid determination to maintain his status of a self-sufficient and dominant individual. Dr. Ambrose's choices in the subsystem are limited. He can achieve only by performing his accustomed activities by himself regardless of the changed state of his health.

The dependency subsystem shows an absence of action or observed behaviors; that is, Dr. Ambrose is not asking for assistance when needed. It would seem that the goal or drive of this subsystem is very low in Dr. Ambrose. He does not aim to maintain environmental resources needed for obtaining help, assistance, attention, permission, reassurance, and security. His set is not in this direction and his range of choices does not include dependent behaviors.

The variables that may be influencing or causing the structural units of these two subsystems are as follows: developmental—forty-seven-years-old; cultural—American Jew; familial—wife, mother, son, and daughter in the home; sociologic—successful head and neck surgeon; pathologic—acute myocardial infarction; environmental—hospitalized for the first time.

Based on this data, the nurse can make a diagnosis. According to the Johnson model the major diagnostic classifications are insufficiency or discrepancy for disorders originating within one subsystem and incompatibility or dominance for disorders manifested within more than one subsystem. Goals will be stated in terms of behavioral system balance and dynamic stability. The general modes of intervention using the Johnson model are to stimulate and protect, to alter set or action, to add to choices, and to restrict, defend, inhibit, or facilitate.

Based on the Johnson model, we can thus outline the plan for the nursing care of Dr. Ambrose as follows:

Nursing Diagnosis	Goal	Intervention
Dominance of achievement subsystem due to rigid set and limited choice	Stabilize all subsystems by modifying their goal, set, or choices, with a resulting	Stimulate and protect dependent responses by being available to meet

Nursing Diagnosis	Goal	Intervention
Insufficiency of dependency subsystem due to lack of goal, set and choices	pattern of decreased activity level to that specified by the cardiologist and of verbalization of need for assistance in self-care and in family and work matters.	patient needs, rewarding initial dependent responses, and having patient express temporary need for these behaviors. Add choices of achievement behavior within restrictions, for example, ask advice on patient-care problem. Inhibit ineffective behaviors by relating their effect to evidence of cardiac status.

THE PEPLAU DEVELOPMENTAL MODEL—DATA BASE FOR CASE STUDY

The Peplau developmental model prescribes a data base for analysis of both the patient and nurse behavior in each of the phases of their relationship—orientation, identification, exploitation, and resolution. Needs or threats are identified along with the resulting tension and levels of satisfaction or security.

The nurse-patient relationship described in the Dr. Ambrose case is in the early stages of orientation and identification. The patient's behavior is largely independent, for example, his going to the bathroom and shaving at the sink. The vocational nurse assumes an authoritative role and tells the patient to go back to bed. Dr. Ambrose's independence is threatened by his illness, leading to the tension of anxiety. The nurse has similar anxiety due to her unmet need to be obeyed. Dr. Ambrose does not identify with the nursing staff, but maintains his identification with his roles of doctor and family man, for example, in having a phone connected, arranging surgery, asking wife to keep him informed of financial matters and family decisions. These role identifications are also threatened by the illness, thus leading to anxiety and his efforts to maintain what is threatened. The vocational nurse is further frustrated and remains anxious. There is little satisfaction or security for either patient or nurse.

The nursing diagnoses of the Peplau model are developmental problems based on physiologic demands or interpersonal conditions. Goals involve forward movement of the personality in specified stages. Nursing intervention involves mainly the use of the therapeutic interpersonal process.

A nurse using Peplau's model might devise a care plan such as the following:

Nursing Diagnosis	Goal	Intervention
Tension of anxiety based on physiologic demands threatening psychologic need for independence and role identification.	Growth through resolution of anxiety	Assign clinical specialist to establish relationship with patient; then help patient explore anxious behavior, needs, and threats, and plan for positive growth from experience of illness.

THE RIEHL INTERACTION MODEL—DATA BASE FOR THE CASE STUDY

In assessing a patient in a symbolic interaction framework, the nurse's main function is to interpret the patient's action. In this case, Dr. Ambrose was obviously continuing to control everyone, including himself, as he had done prior to having an M.I. As a result, a role reversal occurred since he refused to fit into the system and act like a patient. Because he was a physician, and nurses are used to taking orders from physicians, the nursing staff inadvertantly supported his actions and allowed him to be in charge. His actions also indicated that he denied his illness and refused to believe that he had an M.I. He convinced himself that his active participation in sports, his large successful practice, his regular checkups, etc., made it impossible for this to happen to him. His continuing to give orders to his family and to the nurses—to bring him a telephone in order that he might conduct business as usual, to accelerate his activity plan, thus allowing him to regulate his own care—and his incessant loquaciousness all indicate he feared loss of control of himself, either temporarily or permanently by death.

The goals are stated in behavioral terms and are action oriented. This approach is based on the premise that social acts are noted, interpreted, and assessed by actors in the situation confronting them and that since acts are dynamic, with the actors' insight they can cause a change in behavior.

The key factor in intervention is to become the patient's advocate. To do this the nurse must get inside the defining process of the patient-actor in order to understand him. In other words the nurse asks, "What would I do if I were wearing his shoes?" Since the nurse cannot see inside and accurately second guess the patient, the nurse must have the involved parties role-play, each taking the role of the others in turn. With practice, this can be accomplished in a very sophisticated way. Role playing provides the nurse with actions that can be observed and thus with objective data to develop and evaluate the plan of care.

The following is a representative approach. Certainly other possibilities could be considered.

Nursing Diagnoses	Goal	Intervention
1. Role reversal in patient/ nurse relationships, i.e., patient rather than the nurse is in charge of his actions which frustrates the nursing staff	1. a. To enlighten nursing staff about situation. b. To enlighten patient about situation c. To reverse the situation so patient plays patient role which is necessary for recovery.	1. a. Have inservice with nursing staff and have them role-play this patient and themselves. b. Discuss patient, physician, and nurse roles with patient and encourage him to role-play his impression of how a patient acts. c. Encourage patient to continue to play patient role and allow nurse to take care of him.
2. Denial of illness and the sick role	2. To make patient aware that he has had an M.I.	2. Ask patient if he knows his diagnosis. If not, tell him he has had an M.I. Explore with him what this means to him, his life and his family, and his career. Have him and family role-play this.
3. Fear of loss (of control) of self and others	3. To provide as much control to patient as possible within confines of illness	3. Involve patient and family in patient-care plan, delegating tasks (considering physical strength and ability) to everyone, including nurses.

SIMILARITIES AND DIFFERENCES IN CASE STUDY ANALYSES

The case of Dr. Ambrose has been considered from the viewpoint of five nursing models. Each analysis of the data base, diagnoses, goal, and interventions will be examined for similarities and differences in the approaches of the various models.

The first similarity noted in the discussion of the data base is that each case study presentation focuses on patient behavior. The analyses according to Roy, Johnson, Peplau, and Riehl make direct reference to patient behavior or action in their initial discussions. The Orem discussion assumes behavioral data in the discussion of health-deviation self-care demands. We will see, however, that the observation of behavior has a different meaning within each model. For each theorist, behavior is noted as evidence of a different type of deviation. These differences are explored in the discussion of the respective nursing diagnoses.

The descriptions of the data base according to each model begin to show differences when we ask what data is noted in addition to patient behavior.

Roy adds an enumeration of stimuli affecting the maladaptive behaviors, while Johnson's section joins the behavioral data with a sketch of the structural units of the subsystem that are out of balance. The further data according to Orem are the self-care deficits. Peplau directs the reader to note the needs, threats, and tension underlying the behavior. Similarly, Riehl aims to interpret the patient's action.

From their data bases, the five models produce quite different nursing diagnoses. However, some similar general tendencies in these diagnoses may be noted. First, the issues of independence and control, along with role performance, are subsumed in the diagnoses arrived at through use of each of the nursing models. Secondly, it has been noted that both Peplau and Riehl focus on underlying needs and that these needs are implied within the diagnoses. Roy's diagnoses also include an underlying need. Similarly, Johnson's concept of set may reflect a need.

Given these initial similarities, a reading of the first column of each of the plans for nursing care for Dr. Ambrose reveals that each theorist has a unique perspective on the nature of nursing problems. For Roy, the basic description is maladaption caused by conflict of needs with environmental demands; for Johnson, the behavioral instability of dominance and insufficiency is caused by rigid set, limited choices, and lack of goal, set, and choices; for Orem the problem is knowledge and motivational deficits without a specified etiology; for Peplau the problem is anxiety, due to conflict of physical demands and threatening needs; and for Riehl it is limited perception and inappropriate role interaction based on a need.

These differing views of the nursing diagnoses are reflected in the goals set according to each nursing model. Again, however, there is at least one general similarity in the goals. Four out of five of the models expect some temporary dependency behavior on the part of the patient. Only the Peplau model does not specify whether or not the dependent behavior will be increased.

Still, the meaning of this dependent behavior and the means of bringing it about differ with each of the five models. Roy seeks cognitive and affective restructuring, allowing adaptive behavior. Johnson intends behavioral stability through modification of goal, set, and choice. Orem proposes increased self-care theough an unspecified educative process. Peplau's goal is anxiety resolution bringing about growth. And Riehl hopes to bring about perceptual change, which makes for appropriate role interaction.

Though there have been some similarities in the analyses discussed thus far, basically the views of the different theorists lead to quite different nursing diagnoses and goals for Dr. Ambrose. These differences are based on the fundamental differences in how each theorist views nursing, the problems it deals with, and the goals it seeks to accomplish.

What, then, are the implications of these varying viewpoints for the actual nursing care this patient will receive? Surprisingly, the last column of intervention shows more similarities than differences. Four basic approaches to this patient seem to be used. All the statements of proposed interventions allow for the patient's expression of his feelings. Likewise, all would maintain as much independent behavior as possible and would provide new ways for meeting independence needs. Four of the five models—Roy, Johnson, Orem, and Riehl—specifically employ health education of the patient. Lastly, only the Johnson analysis mentions rewarding dependent behavior. However, this could be considered an appropriate intervention according to the other models.

The general means of intervention vary with the different models, as follows: Roy—manipulating stimuli; Johnson—stimulating, protecting, and so forth; Orem—guiding and teaching; Peplau—establishing an interpersonal relation; and Riehl—using role playing. Yet, when it comes to the actual nursing action, the prescriptions are very similar.

This curious result merits some discussion. The simplistic conclusion is that it doesn't matter much which model you use. The language and meaning of what you observe and do are different, but the actual practice of nursing is the same. Another possibility is that the nurses devising the analyses based on each model are bound by what is current nursing practice and devise their interventions accordingly. Perhaps greater research into the intervention modes of each model would reveal additional possible interventions that have not been tried before.

SUMMARY

This case study has served to further clarify the implications of some of the nursing models explored in this book. Certain similarities have been noted. For example, each model includes in its data base a description of patient behavior; most models focus on the same basic issues with a given patient and try to identify an underlying need; and the outcome criteria within the goals, as well as the nursing approaches, display a striking uniformity. However, there are great differences in the language used, and according to the viewpoints of the various models, the meaning behind observations and actions. Only further work on the use of these models can determine whether the differences noted are real or illusory.

Joan P. Riehl

32

Nursing Models in Current Use

Since the nursing literature indicates that conceptual frameworks, or models, are being taught and utilized more and more in nursing, it seemed appropriate to conduct a survey to ascertain some facts on the subject, specifically, which models were being taught in schools of nursing and to what extent they were being used in clinical practice.

METHODOLOGY

As a means of obtaining this information, a questionnaire was sent to the three types of nursing schools in the United States. It was known that nursing models were being taught in many college programs but there was uncertainty about their inclusion in other nursing schools. So, rather than contact only the deans of baccalaureate and higher degree programs, it was decided that all three levels of nursing schools, be included i.e., the former, associate degree, and diploma schools.

The criteria for selection of the schools that would constitute the sample were fourfold: (1) the school must have received NLN accreditation in 1976. (2) Representatives of the three types of undergraduate nursing schools from every state and graduate programs without undergraduate schools were included. (3) The sample was restricted to three baccalaureate degree programs, one associate degree program, and one diploma school per state. Whenever there were no diploma schools in the state, an AD program was substituted for it and vice versa, and when there were less than three baccalaureate schools, substitutions were made with A.D. programs. (4) When more than one school had NLN accreditation in any given state, the ones with the most graduates were used. A total of 265 schools were contacted. Of these, 149 were baccalaureate degree, 55 were A.D., and 48 were diploma schools. Thirteen programs offering a master's degree were also included that did not duplicate the schools already in the study. Of course, some baccalaureate programs had a master's or A.D. program as well. In these cases, the questionnarie was addressed to the person in charge of the given program selected for that state. Since there were 1360 nursing schools in the United States in 1976, the survey was small but representative, nevertheless.

RESULTS AND DISCUSSION

Table 1 presents a summary of the total number of accredited nursing programs by type of school, the number of questionnaires sent and received, and the percent returned by the schools in the study. Only 27 percent of the total accredited programs were included in the study as a result of our selection method for the sample. Of this figure, 43 percent of the questionnaires were returned, so that the results represent 12 percent of the accredited programs in the continental United States in 1976.

In Table 2, the questions, with such forced-choice answers as yes, no, or don't know, are given. The purpose of these questions, was to discover (1) if conceptual models were taught in the classroom and implemented in the clinical area by the students, and (2) if the faculty maintained a clinical practice and what nursing model they employed, if any.

In the graduate programs, models were taught in theory and used in practice in all cases. Fifty percent of this faculty practiced nursing and utilized models. Their clinical endeavors consisted, primarily, of providing consultative services to others.

In the baccalaureate group of 78 schools reporting, 29 of these had graduate programs as well, and 6 of them A.D. programs, which meant that 43 were 'pure' baccalaureate schools. Since the questionnaire was sent to the deans of the four-year program, these answers were considered as emanating

TABLE 1.   The Number and Percent of Questionnaires Returned from the Nursing Schools

NLN Accredited Programs		Questionnaires Sent	Questionnaires Received	Percent Returned
Baccalaureate	254	149	78	52
Associate Degree	268	55	17	31
Diploma	382	48	17	35
Masters	65	13	2	15
Total:	969	265	114	43 (average)

TABLE 2. Percentage of Teaching and Implementation of Models

	Master's		Baccalaureate		Associate Degree		Diploma	
	Yes	No	Yes	No	Yes	No	Yes	No
Models taught in theory	100		91	9	88	12	47	53
Models implemented by students	100		89	11	88	12	41	59
Department heads practicing nursing	50	50	46	54	59	41	35	53
Faculty practicing nursing	50	50	98	2	88	12	82	6
Department heads using models	50	50	62	38	41	6	24	66
Faculty using models	50	50	77	23	41	59	41	12

Note: In some instances, the person completing the questionnaire was uncertain whether or not other faculty (including deans, if the associate completed the form) either practiced nursing or made use of a model in practice. This accounts for the percent discrepancy in the above table on these items.

from that source. The presence of the other programs may have influenced the results, however. Conceptual models were taught in 91 percent of these schools, and in 89 percent of them the models were implemented in the clinical areas. Of the deans, 46 percent maintained some form of clinical practice with 62 percent of this group using a model in their work. On the other hand, as many as 98 percent of the faculty practiced nursing but only 77 percent of them employed a model.

Eighty-eight percent of associate degree programs teach the theory of nursing models to their students and require them to implement this knowledge in their practicum. Fifty-nine percent of the department chairmen have some contact with patients, and 88 percent of this group of educators use a conceptual framework. This faculty is similar to the baccalaureate group in that many of them (88 percent) practice nursing but only some (41 percent) use a model in their work. Perhaps it is phenomenal that even this number can actually implement a model in practice, particularly if they do staff nursing in an acute-care hospital, some of which are still highly regimented.

Diploma-school paradigms are similar to those discussed above. Forty-seven percent of them teach some form of a nursing model in the classroom, and 41 percent of this group implement this framework in the students' clinical area. Similarly, 35 percent of their chairpersons maintain a clinical practice, and 24 percent of the group use a model. Eighty-two percent of this faculty participate in some form of clinical activity while 41 percent of them utilize a model in their work.

The question asked to obtain the information for Table 3 was open-ended which resulted in a wide variation of written answers. For example, some listed the broad classification of systems models while others specifically supplied the name of the systems model they were using, such as the Orem or the adaptation model. This influenced the content of Table 3, but since specific information is more informative, it was decided to include exact answers when given. Table 3 shows which nursing models are being taught and employed in practice across the nation and which models the faculties favor in their clinical endeavors. As shown in the table, multiple theories are taught at the master's degree level while eclectic approaches or student-selected models are employed in practice. The faculty who are involved with clinical work serve primarily as consultants, and their clients, who are usually other nurses, select the models of their choice. The Orem and Levine models are popular with faculty, especially in the Chicago area.

In the baccalaureate, associate degree, and diploma programs, the system models are the most frequently used by the faculty, the most frequently taught, and the most frequently implemented in practice by students under faculty supervision. The developmental models rank second in theory and practice in the baccalaureate and A.D. programs and are used by 18 percent of the baccalaureate faculty. Interaction models are the third most popular in

TABLE 3. Conceptual Models Taught and Implemented in Nursing Practice (by percent)

Model	Master's	Baccalaureate	Associate Degree	Diploma
Multiple theories				
theory	100			
practice	100	17		
faculty	50			
Orem/Levine (System)				
theory		9		
practice		7		
faculty	100	10		
Systems				
theory		51	24	35
practice		46	24	12
faculty		50	18	
Developmental				
theory		39	18	12
practice		39	29	
faculty		18		
Interaction				
theory		30		
practice		37		
faculty		13		
Adaptation (System)				
theory		27	12	17
practice		21	12	17
faculty		20		17
Health-Care				
theory		18		
practice		7		
faculty		3		
Nursing Process				
theory		10	18	
practice		7	12	12
faculty		10		
Stress				
theory		8	12	
practice		12	12	
faculty		12		

the baccalaureate programs in theory and practice, and 13 percent of the faculty prefer them in their clinical work. The adaptation models are the next most frequently taught and practiced in all three types of undergraduate nursing schools; about 18 percent of the baccalaureate and diploma faculty use such models. A health-care model, including health-illness problems, is also taught in 18 percent of the schools responding but it is implemented in only 7 percent of the clinical areas of the baccalaureate schools.

The nursing process was listed as a model being used in theory (10 percent), in practice (7 percent), and by the faculty (10 percent) of baccalaureate programs. It is also taught (18 percent) and practiced (12 percent) in AD programs. Although it was not reported as being taught in the diploma schools, 12 percent of these students use it in their clinical areas. The stress model is the last of this group being taught in several of the baccalaureate and AD programs; it is equally popular (12 percent) in both groups in theory and practice and is used by the baccalaureate faculty as well (12 percent).

Other models and approaches that were mentioned as being taught, practiced by students, and implemented by faculty are as follows: King, Rogers, Schlotfeldt, behavioral, crisis, problem-solving, client-patient, needs, homeostatis, pathophysiology, Orlando-Wiedenbach, Neuman, and Carl Rogers in the baccalaureate schools; needs, Orem, coping-adaptation, wellness-illness, physiologic, total person approach, problem-oriented, nursing problems, and interaction in the A.D. programs; developmental-stress, equilibrium, health-care, and interaction in the diploma schools.

CONCLUSION

It is evident from the foregoing study results that nursing models are fairly well established in the theory and practice curricula of all types of nursing schools in this country. Those who were not currently teaching conceptual frameworks to their students often added a comment that their curriculum was being revised to include such content in the near future. Presently the systems models are the most widely taught and used by faculty and students in all types of nursing programs, and the developmental and adaptation models and the nursing-process approach are also in the curriculum of all three undergraduate schools. Interaction models are popular, and the Orem, stress, and health-care frameworks are used about equally in the baccalaureate schools. The last are also taught in A.D. programs.

In some baccalaureate and in all graduate programs, multiple frameworks are taught and eclectic or student-selected models are employed in practice. This is certainly understandable at this level. If the faculty's choice of model is any indication of future trends, systems models will continue to dominate the field, with the developmental, interaction, adaptation, stress, and Orem models all running about an equally popular second.

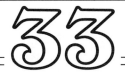

Joan P. Riehl,
Sister Callista Roy

A Unified Model
of Nursing

In the first edition of this text, debate was left open on the question of whether the profession of nursing should adopt a single unified nursing model. The advantages and disadvantages were listed, and the former seemed to outweigh the latter. At this time, we are willing to take a stand on the matter. Although we want to identify the unique perspective a model can give us, we wish to maintain the pluralism of theories that promotes productivity.

The answer seems to lie in the relationship between models and theory that was noted in Chapter 1. A model provides an overview of the person who becomes the nurse's client, and a guide for assessment, diagnosis, goal intervention and evaluation. Specific theories stem from the nature of nursing problems, or diagnoses, and nursing interventions. By virtue of the fact that the client presents himself to the nurse, he displays irregular subjective and objective signs and symptoms. The nurse's primary goal is to resolve these adversities. Since these are givens, it is proposed that nursing move toward the perspective of a single view of the person and of the goal of nursing, and also toward a multiplicity of theoretical approaches to the problems and interventions of nursing. This would allow both model stability and the freedom to grow and learn. In time, diagnoses and interventions that prove to be accurate and effective will likewise become more crystallized.

THE RECIPIENT OF NURSING CARE

Many of the nursing theorists whose models are presented in this book view man similarly. Chrisman, Johnson, Neuman, Preisner, Rogers, and Roy emphasize that man is a system in interaction with his environment. Differences only begin to appear when one looks at what each individual theorist considers to be the component parts of the system of a person. The explication of the subsystems of an individual vary from broad outlines to more precise definitions. Chrisman describes a person as an interlocking biologic, interpersonal, and intrapersonal system. Neuman states that the patient is a dynamic composite of the interrelationship of three variables: physiologic, sociocultural, and developmental, Preisner and Johnson refer to behavioral subsystems. Johnson specifies these as achievement, affiliative, aggressive-protective, dependency, eliminative, restorative, and sexual. According to Roy man has four adaptive modes. The physiologic mode is subdivided into the following need systems: exercise and rest, nutrition, elimination, fluids and electrolytes, oxygen and circulation, and regulation, including temperature, senses, and endocrine system. Other adaptive modes are self-concept, role functioning, and interdependence.

In the selection of a view of the individual's subsystems to be used in a unified nursing model, preference should be given to the design that provides the most complete view of the person, that is, as complete a view as possible with the least number of catagories. Several models meet these criteria. The Johnson and Roy models provide categories that appear all-inclusive of human activity and, therefore, should be considered.

Further validation of the appropriate view of an individual's subsystems might be found in any one of several of the systems models presented in this book. A study could be designed to test each view by the use of assessment tools based on each of the models in diagnosing the problems of the same patients. The approach resulting in the most complete list of nursing diagnoses would be considered the most appropriate view of the subsystems of a person for a unified model of nursing.

An overview of all the concepts of the individual presented by the nursing theorists in this book provides additional insights for a unified model. Neuman points out that, in his interaction with his environment, a person has a flexible line of defense and a normal line of defense as well as an internal set of resistance factors. Johnson, on the other hand, refers to man's regulating and control mechanisms. The concepts of lines of defense and internal regulating mechanisms that serve as resistance factors can well be added to the developing concept.

In addition, Rogers has directed some important work that seems to specify how subsystems act. She identifies the principles of homeodynamics as complementarity, helicy, and resonancy. Initial research has shown these to be significant principles for a viewing of an individual's interaction with his changing environment.

Considering the similarities and differences of nursing models, the general approach of a unified nursing conceptual framework to the recipient of nursing care may be stated as follows: A person is a unified whole composed of subsystems, with a flexible and normal line of defense; his internal regulating mechanisms help him to cope with a changing environment; he functions by the principles of homeodynamics.

THE GOAL OF NURSING CARE

In the earlier discussion of a person as the recipient of nursing care, a systems approach to a model of nursing was assumed. In specifying the goal of nursing care, it is necessary to make this assumption more explicit, and to specify the relationship among the types of nursing models. The goal of nursing will depend on this relationship among the model types.

A systems approach has been discussed as one means of handling the analysis of complex situations. The use made of systems approach by nursing theorists in this book and others (*Nursing Clinics of North America 1971* and *Proceedings Second Theory Conference 1969*) is applicable to the analysis of a person. This person is a system who interacts with his environment by means of reciprocal inputs and outputs. Every system has two types of goals—one of maintaining itself and one of something beyond maintenance as a viable, accurate system. The second is developmental, a goal directed toward an identifiable end. For example, an incentive to be a good employee is to earn a promotion, which encourages one to work toward that objective.

It is at this point that developmental models can be related to systems models. We remind the reader inherent in the developmental model is the concept of change. This is particularly true of the model's postulates, which state that the person passes through stages to reach his maximum potential. This maximum potential may be considered the goal of the system. Thus the two types of models are related in that the system is the working means for achieving the goal specified as the highest stage of development. Interaction models will be related to systems models later.

Some of the nursing models studied emphasize the system maintenance goal, others specify the developmental goal, and others combine the two goals. Preisner mentions the dynamic state of equilibrium, Neuman believes that the system should move toward the highest potential level of stability, and Johnson discusses behavioral balance and the maintenance of stability. However, beyond this Johnson sees the goals of the whole behavioral system as the survival, reproduction, and growth of the human organism. Roy states her goal as the support and promotion of adaptation, which will free energy for overcoming illness or maintaining health. Chrisman's combined goal is stated as positive adaptation to stress, which culminates in active survival with a sense of well-being, and promotes individual growth and strength.

When an interactionist approach is added to the concept of goal, we can state that beyond the maintenance of itself and the attainment of its final goal, the system must provide for harmonious exchange with the external environment. Rogers has stressed this aspect of the nursing goal. She has stated that the goal of nursing is to promote concordant interaction between the individual and the environment, to strengthen the coherence and integrity of the human field, and to direct and redirect the patterning of the human and environmental fields for realization of maximum health potential. In Riehl's model, the goal emphasis is placed on the social acts that are noted, interpreted, and assessed by the actors in the situation confronting them. With interpretation comes insight and changes in the actors' behavior.

In summary, the goal of a unified model of nursing may be stated as the maintenance of a person's systems for the purpose of realizing his maximum potential including health and harmonious interaction with his environment.

THE STRUCTURE OF NURSING DIAGNOSES AND INTERVENTIONS

Acceptance of a view of the individual and a goal as discussed above would provide two common basic structures. To the former could be added as necessary pertinent questions that would supplement the assessment of our client and facilitate an accurate diagnosis. These might vary with a particular specialization, as they now do in medicine. The medical specialist reviews or obtains the history and physical and then adds to it; the cardiologist and the neurologist order differing diagnostic tests and their plans of care vary accordingly. Similarly, depending on the nursing area of specialization, one might consider various nursing diagnostic and interventive approaches. Keeping diagnostic and intervention segments open would allow for the pursuit of knowledge where it is needed most, and at the same time encourage the development of nursing theory. This open-endedness is essential for the furtherance of a science of nursing.

METHODOLOGY

All the proponents of nursing models seem to agree that the nursing process is primarily a problem-solving process. The steps of this process include assessment, diagnosis, intervention, and evaluation. This has been and should continue to be the methodological approach. Assessment data may be grouped, if feasible, according to the Weed (SOAP) method. In this way the subjective and objective symptoms would be clearly identified in the assessment, and the plan of care scientifically based on the data collected and the most current knowledge available. The Weed method is simply a refinement of what is called the nursing process. Some nursing models do not go beyond the broad basic outlines of assessment, diagnosis, intervention, and evaluation. Others do, however, and they specify more clearly the approaches to be taken. The above suggestion concerning the maintenance of open-ended diagnostic and intervention approaches should meet with approval of these theorists.

SUMMARY AND CONCLUSIONS

Any analysis of the nursing models presented in this book indicates that they are more similar than different. Though details within the models may vary, it is not very difficult to sketch the broad outline of a unified nursing model. This unified model views an individual, the recipient of nursing care, as a unified whole consisting of subsystems. In interacting with the environment, this person maintains lines of defense and internal regulating mechanisms which function by the principles of homeodynamics. The goal of nursing is to maintain the system of the person and to help this individual realize his maximum potential, which includes health and harmonious interaction with the environment. Nursing fulfills this goal through a problem-solving process that includes the use of various diagnostic and intervention means in an interactive framework.

A unified nursing model allows for a common structure in the areas of recipient of care and goal of nursing, and for an expanding structure in nursing diagnoses and interventions.

Index

Page numbers in *italics* indicate illustrations; followed by *n* indicate footnotes; followed by *t* indicate tables.

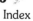

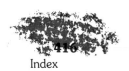